Communicable Disease Control Handbook

Dr Jeremy Hawker *Deputy Director, Local and Regional Services, Health Protection Agency, UK*

Dr Norman Begg *Director of Medical Affairs, GlaxoSmithKline, Uxbridge, UK*

Dr Iain Blair *Consultant in Communicable Disease, Health Protection Agency, Hampshire, UK*

Professor Ralf Reintjes *Professor for Epidemiology and Public Health Surveillance, Hamburg University of Applied Science, Germany*

Professor Julius Weinberg *Pro-Vice Chancellor, City University, London, UK*

Second edition

Blackwell
Publishing

© 2005 Jeremy Hawker, Norman Begg, Iain Blair, Ralf Reintjes and Julius Weinberg
Published by Blackwell Publishing Ltd
Blackwell Publishing, Inc., 350 Main Street, Malden, Massachusetts 02148-5020, USA
Blackwell Publishing Ltd, 9600 Garsington Road, Oxford OX4 2DQ, UK
Blackwell Publishing Asia Pty Ltd, 550 Swanston Street, Carlton, Victoria 3053, Australia

First published 2001
Reprinted 2002 (twice), 2003, 2004
Second edition 2005

4   2008

Library of Congress Cataloging-in-Publication Data

Communicable disease control handbook / Jeremy Hawker ...[et al.].— 2nd ed.
    p. ; cm.
  ISBN 978-1-4051-2424-9
  1. Communicable diseases—Handbooks, manuals, etc.   I. Hawker, Jeremy.
  [DNLM: 1. Communicable Disease Control—Handbooks.
  WA 39 C7333 2005]
  RC112.C626 2005
  616.9—dc22   2005004899

A catalogue record for this title is available from the British Library

Set in 8/11 StoneSerif by TechBooks, New Delhi, India
Printed and bound in Singapore by Utopia Press Pte Ltd

Commissioning Editor: Maria Khan
Development Editor: Claire Bonnett/Fiona Pattison
Production Controller: Kate Charman

For further information on Blackwell Publishing, visit our website:
http://www.blackwellpublishing.com

The publisher's policy is to use permanent paper from mills that operate a sustainable forestry policy, and
which has been manufactured from pulp processed using acid-free and elementary chlorine-free practices.
Furthermore, the publisher ensures that the text paper and cover board used have met acceptable
environmental accreditation standards.

Contents

Section 4: Services and organisations

Section 5: Communicable disease control in Europe

Appendices

Foreword

In the mid 1960s, a belief began to grow that communicable diseases might soon be confined to the history books, as a major health problem of past centuries. Events over the last two decades have shown how misguided such ideas were. Infection continues to present fresh challenges, both here in this country and worldwide.

Events such as the severe acute respiratory syndrome (SARS) outbreak in 2003 demonstrate very clearly that natural threats are ever present. Worldwide, HIV and AIDS continue to cause devastating loss of life, economic ruin and poverty. Collectively, political leaders as well as the international scientific and medical community have yet to find an effective means of prevention and control. Closer to home, tuberculosis and antimicrobial resistance, including the spread of infections such as methicillin-resistant *Staphylococcus aureus* (MRSA), challenge the population's health and the safety of healthcare. The emergence of diseases like West Nile virus in hitherto unaffected parts of the world (the USA and Canada) are a warning of the ever present threat of new and emerging infectious diseases. In 2003, the identification of two incidents associated with European bat lyssa virus (a rabies virus), in England and in Scotland was just another example of how we need to expect the unexpected.

The spread in the last one to two years of avian influenza in Eastern Asia presents a real and present danger to public health worldwide. Those countries that have the responsibility for dealing with potential infection in humans, who have contact with infected poultry, need to be able to respond appropriately. The global community generally must prepare for the possibility of the emergence of a pandemic influenza strain. Influenza pandemics occur in regular cycles over the years and we need to be constantly vigilant, with the help of the World Health Organization (WHO) and its surveillance mechanisms, to ensure early detection of such an event.

Added to these conventional threats, the spectre of bioterrorism now looms large. This brings consequences for identifying and managing previously rare diseases such as anthrax or plague, or an eliminated disease like smallpox. It underlines the need for international co-operation. SARS, although a naturally occurring disease, demonstrated how international medical and scientific networks can respond really effectively to meet the challenges posed by significant global threats. Learning, constantly updating our knowledge and experience are key components of effective disease control. Consequently, I am very pleased to see the emphasis given in this edition of the handbook to international health.

In 2002, in recognition of these various wide ranging and ongoing needs I published my strategy for Infectious Diseases *Getting Ahead of the Curve*. To make sure the UK was well placed to maintain and extend existing arrangements for protecting the public, this recommended the establishment of a new Health Protection Agency. The agency came into force in 2003 and brings expertise in infection (and toxicology and radiology) together with emergency preparedness. It builds on previously strong arrangements provided by the former Public Health Laboratory Service. The agency's aims are to develop and integrate the surveillance of disease, and also co-ordinate the response, linking in to hospitals, communities and other organisations. Veterinary surveillance networks are being aligned with health systems. Consultants in communicable disease control remain at the forefront of delivery of local infection services, together with many others – infectious disease doctors and nurses, microbiologists, community and hospital infection control nurses immunisation co-ordinators.

Today, infection is everyone's business – citizens, political leaders, doctors, scientists and other health professionals alike. It is no longer a quiet backwater of interest only to the specialist. This comprehensive and practical handbook will provide a very accessible source of detailed information for everyone in the field of communicable disease control.

Sir Liam Donaldson
Chief Medical Officer
England

Abbreviations

ACDP	Advisory Committee on Dangerous Pathogens	HUS	Haemolytic uraemic syndrome
AIDS	Acquired immunodeficiency syndrome	ICD	Infection control doctor (hospital)
		ICN	Infection control nurse
BCG	Bacille Calmette–Guérin (vaccine against TB)	ICT	Infection control team (hospital)
		IDU	Intravenous drug user
CCDC	Consultant in Communicable Disease Control (local public health doctor with executive responsibilities for CDC)	IFA	Indirect immunofluorescent antibody test
		IgG	Immunoglobulin class G
		IgM	Immunoglobulin class M
		IPV	Inactivated poliovirus vaccine
CDC	Communicable disease control	LA	Local Authority
CDR	Communicable disease report	MMR	Measles, mumps and rubella vaccine
CDSC	HPA Communicable Disease Surveillance Centre	MRSA	Methicillin-resistant *Staphylococcus aureus*
CICN	Community infection control nurse	NCJDSU	National CJD Surveillance Unit
CJD	Creutzfeldt–Jakob disease	OPV	Oral poliovirus vaccine
CNS	Central nervous system	Pa	Pertussis vaccine (acellular)
CSF	Cerebrospinal fluid	PCR	Polymerase chain reaction
DNA	Deoxyribonucleic acid	PHLS	Public Health Laboratory Service (now part of HPA)
DTP	Diphtheria, tetanus and pertussis		
ECDC	European Centre for Disease Prevention and Control	PT	Phage type
		RCGP	Royal College of General Practitioners
EHO	Environmental health officer		
ELISA	Enzyme-linked immunosorbent assay	RNA	Ribonucleic acid
		RSV	Respiratory syncytial virus
EM	Electron microscopy	SARS	Severe Acute Respiratory Syndrome
EU	European Union	SCIEH	Scottish Centre for Infection and Environmental Health
GI	Gastrointestinal		
GP	General practitioner (primary care physician)	sp.	Species
		STI	Sexually transmitted infection
GUM	Genitourinary medicine	TB	Tuberculosis
HA	Health Authority	TSE	Transmissable spongiform encephalopathy
HAI	Hospital-acquired infection		
HBV	Hepatitis B virus	UK	United Kingdom of Great Britain and Northern Ireland
HCV	Hepatitis C virus		
HCW	Health Care Worker	VHF	Viral haemorrhagic fever
Hib	*Haemophilus influenzae* type b	VRE	Vancomycin resistant *Enterococcus*
HIV	Human immunodeficiency virus	VTEC	Verocytotoxin producing *Escherichia coli*
HNIG	Human normal immunoglobulin		
HP	Health Protection	VZIG	Varicella-zoster immunoglobulin
HPA	Health Protection Agency	WHO	World Health Organization (OMS)

Section 1
Introduction

1.1 How to use this book

This book has been written for those working in the field of communicable disease control. It aims to provide practical advice for specific situations and the important background knowledge that underlies communicable disease control (CDC) activities. As such it should be of interest to public health physicians, epidemiologists, public health nurses, infection control nurses, Environmental Health Officers and microbiologists as well as students in the medical, public health and related fields.

In the four years since the publication of the first edition, there have been many important changes in CDC and health protection. New threats have been identified, such as the increased risk of a deliberate release of a biological, chemical or radioactive hazard after 9/11; the emergence of new diseases such as SARS; and the extension of the range of existing diseases such as West Nile fever. There have been successes, such as the introduction of meningococcal C vaccine and the control of *Salmonella enteritidis* PT4 in many countries, improvements in knowledge (often leading to updating of consensus guidelines) and new laboratory tests, particularly in relation to molecular epidemiology. The combination of these with major administrative changes in the European Union, with the accession of 10 new member states and the creation of a new European Centre for Disease Prevention and Control (ECDC), and in England, where CDC has been merged with specialist services for chemical and radiological hazards (a trend that has already spread to Scotland and Hong Kong) has led to major revisions in the content of the *Communicable Disease Control Handbook*.

The structure of the book follows the following format:

Section 1 contains important background material. Chapter 1.2 runs through the basic principles of transmission and control, which underlie later chapters. Chapter 1.3 is a new chapter aimed primarily at those who undertake on-call duties but do not practice in mainstream CDC or health protection and those undertaking health protection response duties for the first time.

Section 2 addresses topics in the way they often present to CDC staff in the field, i.e. as syndrome-related topics rather than organism-based, such as an outbreak of gastroenteritis of (as yet) undetermined cause, or a needlestick injury. A new chapter in this section addresses common queries from the public and professionals in relation to immunisation. In these chapters, we discuss the differential diagnosis (infectious and non-infectious), including how to decide the most likely cause based on relative incidence, clinical and epidemiological differences and laboratory tests. We also give general advice on prevention and control, including how to respond to a case or cluster when the organism responsible is not yet known. When the organism becomes known, Section 3 should be consulted.

Section 3 addresses CDC in a more traditional way, by disease/organism. We identify, where possible the elements that are most relevant to European countries. We have used England and Wales (or the UK, if appropriate) as an example in each instance, although where important differences in the epidemiology exist in other European we have drawn attention to this. For differences relating to surveillance and control in other countries, the relevant country-specific chapter in Section 5 should be consulted (e.g. those working in Germany should consult Chapter 5.10). British readers will mainly be spared this exercise.

The chapters in Section 3 conform to a standard pattern, which we hope will make instant reference easier. Most chapters are ordered as follows:

1 A short introduction mentioning the syndrome(s), common synonyms and the main public health implications of the organism.

2 A box of *suggested on-call action*. This relates only to what needs to be done if cases are reported outside of normal office hours. Further action may be needed during the next working day, which will be identified in 'response to a case'.

3 *Epidemiology* will give the relevant points on burden of disease. Important differences by age/sex/season/year/risk group in the UK are given, and important differences within Europe are noted.

4 Two sections deal with diagnosis of the infection: *clinical features* and *laboratory confirmation*. Both sections highlight the important points to practising CDC professionals. They are not meant as a substitute for clinical and microbiological textbooks.

5 *Transmission* details the main sources, reservoirs, vehicles and routes of spread of the organism. The main aim of this section is to give the investigator clues as to how a case or outbreak may have arisen, so as to aid identification and control.

6 *Acquisition* deals with the incubation period, infectious period (if communicable), infective dose (if known) and any important factors affecting immunity or susceptibility.

7 The final five sections relate to control of infection. These are mainly based on current practice in the UK (supplemented by our own views) although the principles will be equally relevant to European readers. These sections are as follows:

- Actions likely to be effective in the *prevention* of infection,
- *Surveillance* activities relevant to the organism,
- Suggested public health actions to be taken in *response to a case,*
- Suggested approach to an *investigation of a cluster* of cases of that organism, and suggested actions to help *control of an outbreak,* including a *suggested case-definition* for use in an epidemiological study.

New chapters have been added on SARS and West Nile virus, and for the most likely candidate organisms, a new chapter section on *Response to a deliberate release*. Diseases that are generally less of a public health issue in Europe are summarised in the tables that follow Section 3.

Section 4 refers to the organisation of CDC services and could be titled 'how to run a CDC service'. For the three authors who have worked as Consultants in Communicable Disease Control (CCDC), this is the textbook that we wished we'd had on appointment! It deals with the services that a CDC department is expected to provide, including the non-communicable disease functions that

have been attached to the CCDC/CPHM post in the UK. Some of those chapters are, of necessity, UK focused, although many (e.g. surveillance, outbreak management, hospital infection, clinical governance) will be of equal use to European colleagues. A new chapter on the public health response to a deliberate release has been added to this section.

Section 5 gives a brief overview of structures for infectious disease notification and Public Health action in the 25 EU Member States (including new chapters on each of the 10 new members states), plus Norway and Switzerland. The objective of this section is to allow an orientation on Public Health structures relevant for infectious disease control in various European countries and to offer a starting point for further information on individual countries. Lengthy descriptions have been avoided, but Internet addresses for contact points in the countries and for further information, reports and data have been given. Those readers interested in more detailed or extended information on infectious disease control structures in Europe could consult the report and dataset of the 'EU-Inventory on Communicable Disease Control', which was compiled by the Italian, English and Swedish national surveillance centres and financed by the European Commission.

Finally the two appendices and two lists of useful Websites detail further sources of information and advice for those undertaking communicable disease control functions routinely or on-call.

We are indebted to a number of individuals who have helped us in commenting on parts of the book, including Bob Adak, Nicky Connor, Natasha Crowcroft, Iain Gillespie, Douglas Harding, Marian McEvoy, Fortune Ncube, Pat Saunders, John Simpson and numerous advisors for the country-specific chapters, including Jiri Beran, Antra Bormane, Arnold Bosman, Hedwig Carsauw, Benvon Cotter, Ágnes Csohan, Salvador de Mateo, Manuela de Sousa, Cristina Furtado, Charmaine Gauci, Chrystalla Hadjianastassiou, Christos Hadjichristodoulou, Pierrette Huberty-Krau, Alenka Kraigher, Chintia Lemos, Rasa Liausediene, Eva Maderova, Patrick Mathys, Christine Meffre, Laura Papantoniou, Jurijs

Perevoscikovs, Magdalena Rosinska, Roland Salmon, S Samuelson, Reinhild Strauss, Johanna Takkinen, Alberto Tozzi, Juta Varjas. Linda Parr's administrative skills were essential as was the help of Claire Bonnet at Blackwell Science. Finally, we are grateful to our families and work colleagues for their patience and support whilst we were preoccupied with this project.

1.2 Basic concepts in the epidemiology and control of infectious disease

The epidemiological framework

Identification

Infections can be identified by their clinical features, epidemiology and the use of appropriate laboratory procedures.

Infectious agent

The traditional model of infectious disease causation is the epidemiological triangle. It has three components: an external agent, a susceptible host and environmental factors that bring the host and the agent together.

The agent is the organism (virus, rickettsia, bacterium, fungus, etc.) that produces the infection. Host factors influence an individual's exposure, susceptibility or response to a causative agent. Age, sex, socio-economic status, ethnicity and lifestyle factors such as smoking, sexual behaviour and diet are among the host factors that affect a person's likelihood of exposure, while age, genetic makeup, nutritional and immunological status, other disease states and psychological makeup influence susceptibility and response to an agent. Environmental factors are extrinsic factors that affect the agent and the opportunity for exposure. These include geology, climate, physical surroundings, biological factors, socio-economic factors such as crowding and sanitation and the availability of health services.

Occurrence

The occurrence or amount of an infectious disease will vary with place and time. A persistent low or moderate level of disease is referred to as *endemic* and a higher persistent level is called *hyper-endemic*. An irregular pattern with occasional cases occurring at irregular intervals is called *sporadic*. When the occurrence of an infection exceeds the expected level for a given time period, it is called *epidemic*. The term outbreak or cluster is also used. When an epidemic spreads over several countries or continents it is called *pandemic*. Epidemics vary in size and duration. An *epidemic curve*, a frequency histogram of number of cases against date of onset (see Figs 4.3.1–4.3.3), should be plotted. If exposure to the infectious agent takes place over a relatively brief period, a *point source* outbreak occurs. Intermittent or continuous exposure broadens the peaks of the epidemic curve, and so an irregular pattern is observed. An outbreak that spreads from person to person is called a *propagated* outbreak. In theory the epidemic curve of a propagated outbreak would have a series of peaks at intervals approximating to the incubation period. Usually the epidemic wanes after a few generations because the number of susceptible people falls below a critical level. Some epidemic curves have both common source epidemic and propagated epidemic features because of secondary person-to-person spread. These are called *mixed epidemics*.

Two rates are commonly used to describe the occurrence of infectious diseases:

Incidence =

$$\frac{\text{New cases over a given time period}}{\text{Persons at risk}}$$

Prevalence =

$$\frac{\text{Existing cases at a given point in time}}{\text{Persons at risk}}$$

The chain of infection

Transmission occurs when the agent leaves its *reservoir* or host through *a portal of exit* and is conveyed by a mode of *transmission* and enters through an appropriate *portal of entry* to infect a susceptible host. This is the *chain of infection*.

Reservoir

The reservoir of an infectious agent is any person, animal, arthropod, plant, soil or substance (or combination of these) in which the infectious agent normally lives and multiplies. The reservoir may be different from the *source* or *vehicle* of infection. This is the person, animal, object or substance from which an infectious agent actually passes to a host. Many of the common infectious diseases have human reservoirs, which include clinical cases, those who are incubating the disease and convalescent carriers. *Colonisation* is the presence of a microorganism in or on a host, with growth and multiplication, but without evidence of infection. Shedding of an organism from a colonised host may be intermittent. Infectious diseases that are transmissible from animals to humans are called *zoonoses*. The *portal of exit* is the path by which an agent leaves the source host, which usually corresponds with the site at which the agent is localised, for example respiratory tract, genitourinary system, gastrointestinal system, skin or blood. The *portal of entry* is the route by which an agent enters a susceptible host.

For any given infection, understanding the chain of infection allows appropriate control measure to be recommended.

Mode of transmission

This is the mechanism by which an infectious agent is spread from a source or reservoir to a susceptible person. The mechanisms are detailed in Table 1.2.1.

Natural history of disease

This refers to the progress of a disease process in an individual over time without intervention. Following exposure to an infectious agent there is then a period of subclinical or inapparent pathological changes, which ends with the onset of symptoms. This period is known as the *incubation period*. For a given infectious disease, the incubation period has a range and a mean value. For hepatitis A the range is about 2–6 weeks with a mean of 3 weeks. During the incubation period, pathological changes may be detectable with laboratory or other tests. Most screening programmes attempt to identify the disease process during this early phase of its natural history, since early intervention may be more effective than treatment at a later stage. The onset of symptoms marks the transition from the subclinical to the clinical phase. Most diagnoses are made during this stage. In some people the disease may never progress to a clinically apparent illness. In others the disease process may result in a wide spectrum of clinical illness, ranging from mild to severe or fatal.

Infectious period

This is the time during which an infectious agent may be transferred directly or indirectly from an infected person to another person. Some diseases are more infectious during the incubation period than during the actual illness. In others such as tuberculosis, syphilis and *Salmonella* infection the infectious period may be lengthy and intermittent. The infectious period may be shortened by antibiotic treatment (though in some infections antibiotics may prolong carriage and hence the infectious period).

Susceptibility and resistance

This describes the various biological mechanisms that present barriers to the invasion and multiplication of infectious agents and to damage by their toxic products. There may be inherent resistance in addition to immunity as a result of previous infection or immunisation. The following terms are used to describe the outcomes of exposure to an infectious agent:

Infectivity: the proportion of exposed persons who become infected, also known as the *attack rate*.

Pathogenicity: the proportion of infected persons who develop clinical disease.

Virulence: the proportion of persons with clinical disease who become severely ill or die (case fatality rate).

Table 1.2.1 Modes of transmission of infectious agents

Types of transmission	Examples
Direct transmission Transmission by direct contact such as touching, biting, kissing, sexual intercourse or by droplet spread onto the mucous membranes of the eye, nose or mouth during sneezing, coughing, spitting or talking. Droplet spread is usually limited to a distance of 1 m or less.	*Direct route* Infections of the skin, mouth and eye may be spread by touching an infected area on another person's body or indirectly through a contaminated object. Examples are scabies, head lice, ringworm and impetigo. Sexually transmitted infections are also spread by the direct route. *Respiratory route* Sneezing, coughing, singing and even talking may spread respiratory droplets from an infected person to someone close by. Examples are the common cold, influenza, whooping cough and meningococcal infection. *Faecal–oral route* Gastrointestinal infections can spread when faeces are transferred directly to the mouth of a susceptible host.
Indirect transmission This may be *vehicle-borne* involving inanimate materials or objects (*fomites*), such as toys, soiled clothes, bedding, cooking or eating utensils, surgical instruments or dressings; or water, food, milk or biological products such as blood. The agent may or may not multiply or develop in or on the vehicle before transmission.	*Faecal–oral route* Faeces contaminate food or objects like toys or toilet flush handles. Animal vectors such as cockroaches, flies and other pests may transfer faeces. Environmental surfaces may be contaminated. This is particularly important in viral gastroenteritis when vomiting occurs since the vomit contains large numbers of infectious viral particles. Examples of infections spread in this way are food poisoning and hepatitis A.
It may be *vector-borne*. This in turn may be *mechanical* and includes simple carriage by a crawling or flying insect as a result of soiling of its feet or proboscis or by passage of organisms through its gastrointestinal tract. This does not require multiplication or development of the organism. It may be *biological* when some form of multiplication or development of the organism is required before the arthropod can transmit the infected form of the agent to man when biting.	*The blood-borne route* There is transfer of blood or body fluids from an infected person to another person through a break in the skin such as a bite wound or open cut or through inoculation, injection or transfusion. Blood-borne infections include infection with HIV and hepatitis B and C infections. Spread can also occur during sexual intercourse. *Respiratory route* Droplets from the mouth and nose may also contaminate hands, cups, toys or other items and spread infection to others who may use or touch those items.
Air-borne spread Air-borne spread is the dissemination of a microbial aerosol to a suitable portal of entry, usually the respiratory tract. Microbial aerosols are suspensions of particles that may remain suspended in the air for long periods of time. Particles in the range of 1–5 microns are easily drawn into the alveoli and may be retained there. Droplets and other larger particles that tend to settle out of the air are not considered air-borne. Microbial aerosols are either droplet nuclei or dust.	Examples are infection with *Legionella*, *Coxiella* and in some circumstances tuberculosis.

Table 1.2.2 Standard precautions to prevent the spread of infection

Hand hygiene: handwashing with soap and water or use of an alcohol hand rub or gel. Cover wounds or skin lesions with waterproof dressings.
Use of personal protective equipment: disposable gloves and aprons and eye protection.
Handle and dispose of sharps safely.
Dispose of contaminated waste safely.
Managing blood and body fluids: spillages and collection and transport of specimens.
Decontaminating equipment including cleaning, disinfection and sterilisation.
Maintaining a clean clinical environment.
Prevention of occupational exposure to infection and managing sharps injuries and blood splash incidents.
Manage linen safely.
Place patients with infections in appropriate accommodation.

Hepatitis A in children has low pathogenicity and low virulence. Measles has high pathogenicity but low virulence, whereas rabies is both highly pathogenic and highly virulent. The *infectious dose* is the number of organisms that are necessary to produce infection in the host. The infectious dose varies with the route of transmission and host susceptibility factors. Because of the clinical spectrum of disease, cases actually diagnosed by clinicians or in the laboratory often represent only the tip of the iceberg. Many additional cases may remain asymptomatic. People with subclinical disease are nevertheless infectious and are called carriers.

Preventing spread of infection: standard precautions

It is not always possible to identify people who may spread infection to others, therefore standard precautions to prevent the spread of infection must be followed at all times (see Table 1.2.2). In incidents involving diarrhoea and/or vomiting enteric precautions should be followed (see Table 1.2.3).

The UK National Institute of Clinical Excellence has published guidelines on measures for preventing infections associated with three specific aspects of healthcare: the use of long-term urinary catheters,

Table 1.2.3 Enteric precautions when managing diarrhoea and vomiting

Handwashing	See Table 1.2.2
Disposal of excretions and soiled materials	Patients should normally use a flush toilet
	Attendants should wear disposable plastic gloves
	Wash hands thoroughly
Soiled clothing and bed linen	Flush faecal material into toilet bowl
	Wash in washing machine on 'hot cycle'
	Soaking in disinfectant before washing is not necessary and may bleach coloured fabrics
Disinfection, especially important in schools, nursery schools and residential institutions	Toilet seats, flush handles, wash-hand basin taps and toilet door handles should be cleaned daily and after use with bleach-based household cleaner, diluted according to manufacturer's instructions
	Alcohol-based wipes may be used on seats and other hard surfaces.
	Empty bedpans and urinals into toilet bowl and then wash with disinfectant and rinse
Education	Emphasise personal hygiene and hygienic preparation and serving of food
	Children and adults in jobs likely to spread infection should stay away from school for 48 h after the diarrhoea has stopped

Wet hands, apply soap and use the following procedure

1. Rub palm to palm

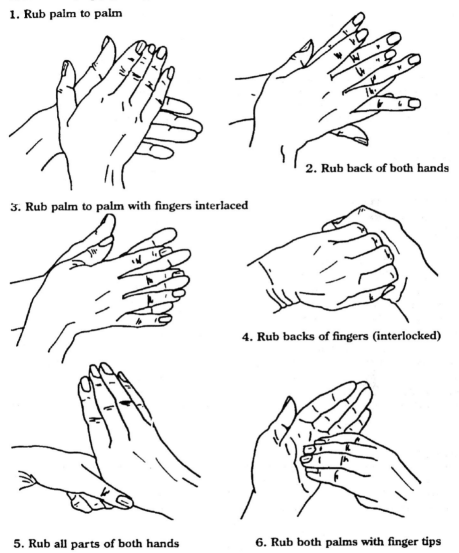

2. Rub back of both hands

3. Rub palm to palm with fingers interlaced

4. Rub backs of fingers (interlocked)

5. Rub all parts of both hands

6. Rub both palms with finger tips

7. Rinse hands under running water and dry thoroughly on a clean towel.

This handwashing technique is based on procedure by G.A.J Ayliffe *et al. J.Clin. Path.* 1978; 31: 923. We would like to gratefully acknowledge ICI Pharmaceuticals UK for providing drawings.

Fig. 1.2.1 How to wash hands correctly and reduce infection.

enteral feeding systems and central venous catheters. Each of these includes education of patients, carers and healthcare personnel (http://www.nice.org.uk/page.aspx?o =71777).

Handwashing

Handwashing is the single most important part of infection control. The technique illustrated in Fig 1.2.1 should be used when washing with soap and water or when using an alcohol gel or rub. Hands should be washed before contact with patients, after any activity that contaminates the hands, after removing protective clothing and gloves, after using the toilet and before handling food. Alcohol hand gels and rubs are a practical alternative to soap and water, but hands that are dirty or contaminated must be washed with soap and water and dried thoroughly before use. Nails should be kept short, rings should not be worn, artificial nails should be avoided and cuts and abrasions should be covered with a waterproof dressing. Adequate handwashing facilities must be available in all patient areas. Liquid soap dispensers, paper hand towels and foot-operated waste bins should be provided.

1.3 Health protection on-call

During office hours health protection activity is usually undertaken by individuals who are expert in their field and have access to a full range of supporting services. Outside of office hours, this is not always the case, e.g. in the UK, health protection on-call at a local level is integrated with general public health rotas and laboratories also offer a much-reduced service.

Requirements for on-call staff

Undertaking health protection on-call should present few problems for those adequately trained in public health, as the skills applied are the same as those used in everyday public health practice, i.e.

- defining the problem,
- collecting the necessary information,
- undertaking a risk assessment,
- identifying good practice,
- implementing the response and
- evaluating the outcome.

A basic element of specialist health protection knowledge and experience is needed and this is broadly equivalent to that defined by the UK Faculty of Public Health 'RITA' competencies, in particular,

- completely understand fully local on-call procedures for the control of infectious diseases.
- understand the role of others in the control of infection, including environmental health, microbiology, genitourinary medicine departments, infection and TB control nurses, hospital control of infection committees.
- appreciate the general principles of outbreak management, and understand the role of (e.g. in England) the local health protection unit, Primary Care Trust, Strategic Health Authority, Local Authority and CDSC.
- deal with the public health consequences of single cases of common communicable disease, e.g. meningitis, meningococcal infection, food poisoning, gastroenteritis, hospital-acquired infection, blood-borne viruses, TB and hepatitis A.
- provide public health management of an outbreak with practical experience of at least two of the following: meningitis, food poisoning, gastroenteritis, hospital-acquired infection, blood-borne viruses, TB and *Legionella*.
- be familiar with the law relating to public health.
- prepare press releases and deal with the media with respect to an incident.

In addition, where the on-call duties include non-infectious environmental hazards

- be familiar with the general principles of emergency planning and managing a major chemical incident and
- contribute effectively to the management of an actual or simulated chemical or other major incident.

These competencies need to be maintained by incorporating them into the continuous professional development plan for each individual. One useful method is attending an on-call updating course every 3 years or so, plus participating in simulations and exercises.

Access to knowledge on-call is important and is available from

• this handbook: on-call actions and underlying theory are given for all the most common pathogens.
• a local on-call pack, detailing local policies, procedures, plans and contact details.
• National guidance documents (see Appendix 2).
• websites, including those of the national CDC or health protection organisation (see inside covers).
• local, regional and national specialist on-call, e.g. the local acute hospital will usually have a consultant medical microbiologist on-call and the national health protection organisation will usually provide access to a communicable disease epidemiologist.

Public health response to a case of infection

The two key questions in dealing with a case of communicable disease are as follows:

• *Where did the case get it from?* This is important because there may be a continuing source that needs to be controlled and because there may be others who have also been exposed and need advice and/or treatment. Others exposed may be known to the case (e.g. household or fellow tourists), but this is not always the case (e.g. a *Legionella* source in the environment).
• *Is the case likely to pass it on?* This may be to close contacts (e.g. household or sexual contacts) that need to be protected by advice to the case and perhaps prophylaxis for the contacts (e.g. hepatitis B), or it may be via the patient's occupation, e.g. a food handler who has a gastrointestinal (GI) infection.

Syndromes and diseases

At the time that health protection issues emerge, the causative agent may not yet be clear, e.g. an outbreak of diarrhoea and vomiting in a hospital or an outbreak of respiratory disease at a nursing home. This may be particularly the case on-call. Section 2 of this book looks at problems from this angle. The important issues to consider are as follows:

• What investigations are needed to identify the agent (e.g. *Salmonella*), the cause of the incident (e.g. poor hygiene practices) and, if relevant, the vehicle of infection (e.g. a particular food served to guests)? Such investigations usually have microbiological, environmental and epidemiological components.
• What generic control measures can be applied to limit morbidity, whilst awaiting confirmation, e.g. enhanced handwashing, environmental cleaning and excluding ill food handlers in outbreaks of GI illness?

Public health action on-call

There are two key questions that define what action is taken on-call:

• Is public health action necessary?
• Does it need to be done now?

The factors in deciding whether public health action is necessary are a combination of the following:

• Is the index case at risk of a poor outcome? A death from meningitis or any case of a viral haemorrhagic fever are examples that lead to public anxiety and media interest.
• Is the index case likely to pass infection on to others? If so, action may be required to limit onward transmission from the index case and any infected contacts.
• Is there likely to be an ongoing source that needs controlling? Some stages in investigating possible sources take considerable time, so the earlier they are started, the sooner the result.
• Do contacts or others exposed to the same source need to be traced? This will be important if their outcome can be improved by an intervention or if it will help limit onward transmission.
• Do the public need information or reassurance? This is often affected by the 'scariness' of the disease, whether particularly vulnerable groups are exposed (e.g. children) and issues of 'blame'.

If public health action is necessary, it does not automatically follow that it should occur out-of-hours. Issues that affect timing include the following:

• The seriousness of the disease. Some infections such as viral haemorrhagic fevers, diphtheria or *Escherichia coli* O157 may require prompt action to prevent even one more additional case in vulnerable groups, whereas others such as norovirus or mumps are less of a threat to most individuals.

• How transmissible is the infection? Not only are some infections more transmissible than others, but some cases of the same infection can transmit more easily than others (e.g. e-antigen positive hepatitis B or smear positive TB).

• How long is the incubation period? Secondary (or co-primary) cases of meningococcal infection may present very quickly, but the incubation period for TB is weeks or months.

• How vulnerable are the people that may have been exposed? Some pathogens are particularly likely to lead to infection or a poor outcome in particular groups, e.g. *E. coli* O157 in young children and the frail elderly or chickenpox in immunosuppressed patients. This will heavily influence speed of response.

• What is the public, media or political reaction? Even if it is not a health protection priority to react on-call (e.g. a HIV positive healthcare worker), action may be required if information becomes public.

• What is 'expected' or good practice?

• When will normal service be resumed? The risk of delaying until normal office hours is obviously proportional to the length of time until a 'normal' response can be activated. Thus, action is more likely on a Saturday morning before a public holiday Monday than on a Sunday night before a normal working Monday.

Collection of baseline data

Collecting information and recording it in a systematic way is important in order to

• aid management of the incident: the information will be useful to you and to others who take over management later in the incident.

• be available for later scrutiny, either for professional purposes (audit, lessons learnt) or legal purposes (public inquiries or civil actions).

A good basic minimum dataset is usually required, preferably by completion of a standard form, covering the following:

• Administrative details for those providing information (name, organisation/position, contact details) and cases and contacts (name, address, phone, GP, hospital).

• Epidemiological information on cases in relation to person (age, sex, occupation), place (residence, travel, institution) and time (onset).

• Diagnosis, consisting of clinical and laboratory information.

• Record of advice given.

Risk assessment

The next stage is usually to undertake a risk assessment, which includes the principles identified above (see section Public Health Action On-Call), but often also includes an assessment of whether contacts have been put at significant risk. The three general questions that are asked in assessing the likelihood of transmission are as follows:

• How infectious is the source (or case)?

• How close is the contact?

• How susceptible are those exposed?

An example of how this is applied for a particular disease is given in Box 3.79.2.

Possible interventions

If it is decided that action is required, possible interventions include

• action to improve outcome for cases by ensuring appropriate care provided. This may include provision of immunoglobulins (rabies), antitoxins (diphtheria), antidotes (chemicals) or different antibiotics to usual (e.g. *Legionella*).

• action to trace others exposed to source or cases in order to provide advice, antibiotics or vaccines (e.g. for contacts of meningococcal disease, all three may be provided).

• action to prevent others being exposed to cases or contacts. For example by rendering them non-infectious by use of antibiotics and/or isolation (e.g. diphtheria or TB); by provision of hygiene advice and/or exclusion from work or school (e.g. GI illness) or by closure of premises associated with incident (e.g. cooling tower or food premises).

• action to identify a possible source so that control measures can be implemented and monitored.

Communications

Communication is vital in public health incidents. Communication needs can be considered from a number of perspectives:

• Who needs to know for public health purposes? Some may need to be contacted on-call (may include the case (or parents), contacts or clinicians) and some can wait until the next working day (e.g. school).

• Who needs to know before the press? This may include officers of local public health organisations (press officer, chief executive, Director of Public Health) and regional or national organisations (e.g. in England, the Regional Director of Public Health, CDSC and the Department of Health may sometimes need to be told).

• Who can offer advice or help in management of the incident? Such individuals may be able to contribute from a microbiological, epidemiological or environmental health aspect.

• Is there any advantage in wider dissemination of information or advice? This may be to primary or secondary healthcare services (e.g. identification and treatment of cases) or the public and press (e.g. to allay anxiety).

Governance issues

Ensuring an appropriate quality of response on-call can be considered as a mixture of preparation and follow up.

Preparation for on-call includes the following:

• Access to an up-to-date on-call pack.

• Access to up-to-date local policies and contingency plans.

• Undertaking appropriate training and updating.

• Exercising contingency plans and multiagency response.

• Ensuring effective authorisation for use of legal powers.

• Ensuring access to required support, including surge capacity.

Follow-up issues include

• debrief to review individual cases with local health protection team as learning exercise,

• systematic audit,

• adverse incident reporting,

• written reports, including any lessons learnt and

• review of policies and plans.

Section 2
Common topics

2.1 Meningitis and meningism

Meningitis is inflammation of the meninges. Meningism is the group of signs and symptoms that accompanies the inflammation. The symptoms of meningism are headache, neck stiffness, nausea or vomiting and photophobia. The classical physical sign of meningism is a positive Kernig's test; however, this may be negative in mild cases. Typical features of meningism are uncommon in infants and young children, who are usually simply floppy and pale with fever and vomiting. A bulging fontanelle may be present in a young infant.

Meningitis is a notifiable disease in many countries. This is however a rather unhelpful term for CDC purposes, as bacterial meningitis (particularly due to *Neisseria meningitidis*), can present as septicaemia without any features of meningitis, and many types of meningitis require no public health action. Meningococcal septicaemia presents with a typical haemorrhagic rash (see Plate 1 *facing p. 20*), which may be accompanied by shock, circulatory collapse, and confusion or coma. Many patients with meningococcal disease will have features of both meningitis and septicaemia (see Chapter 3.48).

Infectious and other causes

Meningitis is the most common cause of meningism; however, meningism can occur in the absence of meningitis (Table 2.1.1). It may accompany upper lobe pneumonia, urinary tract infection and other febrile conditions. Cerebrospinal fluid (CSF) examination is normal in these conditions. Meningism without fever can also occur in non-infectious conditions, the most important of which is subarachnoid haemorrhage; malignancy affecting the meninges can also present as meningism.

Clinical and epidemiological differences

Many infectious agents can cause meningitis. Acute meningitis is nearly always either viral or bacterial; fungal and protozoal infections occasionally occur, mainly in the immunosuppressed patient.

The overall incidence is relatively stable across Europe, except for countries that have implemented mass immunisation against serogroup C meningococcal disease (UK, Spain, Ireland, Belgium, Netherlands), where the incidence has declined in recent years. In 2003, there were 1472 notified cases of acute meningitis in England and Wales, compared to a peak of 2623 cases in 2001 (http://www.hpa.org.up/infections/topics_az/moids/annuallab.htm). Hib meningitis is generally well controlled as all countries in Europe routinely vaccinate in infancy.

Viral meningitis

Viral meningitis is common. However, most cases are mild or inapparent. In 2003 there were 235 notified cases in England and Wales (Table 2.1.2). This represents only a small

Table 2.1.1 Differential diagnosis of meningism

Cause	Distinguishing features
Viral meningitis	Fever, clear CSF with a lymphocytosis and raised protein
Bacterial meningitis	Fever, purulent CSF with a neutrophil pleiocytosis, raised protein and lowered glucose
Other febrile conditions	Fever, normal CSF
Subarachnoid haemorrhage	No fever; abrupt onset, rapid deterioration; bloodstained CSF
Meningeal malignancies	No fever; insidious onset; variable CSF features

Table 2.1.2 Notifications of meningitis by cause in England and Wales in 2003

Meningococcal (excluding septicemia)	646
Pneumococcal	205
Haemophilus influenzae	63
Viral	235
Other specified	115
Unspecified	208
All causes	1472

fraction (approximately 1%) of the true incidence, as only the more severe cases are investigated.

The most common cause is an enterovirus infection (either an echovirus or coxsackie virus) (Table 2.1.3). In enterovirus meningitis there is sometimes a history of a sore throat or diarrhoea for a few days before the onset of headache, fever and nausea or vomiting. The headache is severe; however, there is no alteration of neurological function. Meningism is usually present to a greater or lesser degree. Recovery is usually complete and rapid (within a week). The CSF is clear, with 40–250 cells, all lymphocytes, elevated protein and normal glucose. An enterovirus infection can be confirmed by detection of virus in a faecal sample or by serology. Enterovirus meningitis occurs mainly in later summer. It affects all age groups, although it is commonest in preschool children.

Mumps can cause meningitis, although it is now rare in countries where MMR vaccine is

Table 2.1.3 Causes of viral meningitis

Common
  Echovirus
  Coxsackievirus
Rare
  Poliovirus
  Mumps virus
  Herpes simplex type 2
  Herpes zoster
  Influenza types A or B
  Arbovirus
  Rubella
  Epstein–Barr virus

used. It is easily recognised by the accompanying parotitis. The diagnosis can be confirmed by detection of specific IgM in blood or saliva, or by serology.

In herpes simplex meningitis, the illness is more severe and may persist for weeks. It is associated with primary genital herpes.

Non-paralytic poliomyelitis can present as meningitis, indistinguishable clinically from other causes of enteroviral meningitis. Poliovirus is detectable in faeces or CSF.

Bacterial meningitis

Bacterial meningitis is a medical emergency. The clinical presentation depends on the age of the patient and the infecting organism (see Table 2.1.4 for causes of bacterial meningitis). In the neonate, the presentation is non-specific, with features of bacteraemia. The infant is febrile, listless, floppy and does not take feed. There may also be vomiting, drowsiness, convulsions or an abnormal high-pitched cry. In this age group, the commonest causes are *Escherichia coli* and group B streptococci.

Signs and symptoms in older infants and young children are also non-specific. Meningococcal infection is the commonest cause at this age and is often accompanied by a haemorrhagic rash (see Chapter 3.48).

In older children and adults the symptoms are more specific. Fever, malaise and increasing headache are accompanied by nausea and often vomiting. Photophobia may be extreme. Meningism is usually present. Meningococcal infection is also the commonest cause in this group and the typical rash of meningococcal septicaemia may be present. Patients with rapidly advancing meningococcal disease may, over the course of a few hours, develop hypotension, circulatory collapse, pulmonary oedema, confusion and coma.

Other causes of acute bacterial meningitis in older children and adults are uncommon. *Haemophilus influenzae* meningitis occasionally occurs in unvaccinated children or adults; it has a slower onset than meningococcal meningitis and a rash is rare. Pneumococcal meningitis also has a more insidious

Table 2.1.4 Causes of bacterial meningitis

Neonate	Infant/preschool child	Older child/adult
Common		
E. coli	*N. meningitidis*	*N. meningitidis*
Group B streptococci		*S. pneumoniae*
Uncommon		
Listeria monocytogenes	*H. influenzae*	*L. monocytogenes*
N. meningitidis	*S. pneumoniae*	Staphylococci
Staphylococci		*H. influenzae*
		Myocobacterium tuberculosis

onset and the symptoms are less specific than meningococcal meningitis. It usually occurs in adults with an underlying risk factor such as dura mater defect due to trauma or surgery, chronic intracranial infection, asplenia, terminal complement deficiency or alcoholism. *Listeria* meningitis presents either as a neonatal infection following intrapartum exposure or as a food-borne illness in older children and young adults, often in the immunosuppressed.

Tuberculous meningitis is a manifestation of primary tuberculosis, which occurs mainly in children and young adults. It has an insidious onset; meningism is usually mild and other features (except fever) are often absent.

Laboratory diagnosis

With the exception of tuberculosis, bacterial meningitis causes neutrophil pleiocytosis in the CSF, with raised protein and lowered glucose. A Gram's stain will often demonstrate the typical appearance of the infecting organism, allowing a definitive diagnosis to be made.

Conventional culture of CSF and blood should always be carried out; however, these may be negative, particularly if the patient has been given antibiotics before hospital admission. In addition a CSF specimen may not be available, as clinicians are often reluctant to undertake a lumbar puncture.

A number of non-culture diagnostic techniques are now available. These include poly-

merase chain reaction (PCR) diagnosis for meningococcal disease (see Box 3.48.1 for suggested investigations) and serology. Other useful investigations include throat swab and microscopic examination of a rash aspirate, if present.

General prevention and control measures

• *Hygiene.* Enteroviral meningitis usually spreads as result of environmental contamination, particularly under conditions of crowding and poor hygiene. General hygiene measures such as handwashing will help prevent spread. This is particularly important in hospitals.

• *Pregnancy.* Group B streptococcal meningitis in neonates can be prevented by intrapartum antibiotic treatment of colonised women.

• *Immunisation.* Childhood immunisation schedules in Europe ensure protection against meningitis caused by mumps, polio and *H. influenzae* type b (Hib). In some countries, including the UK, *N. meningitidis* group C and tuberculosis are also in the schedule. Polysaccharide vaccines are available for *N. meningitidis* (serogroups A, C, Y and W135) and *Streptococcus pneumoniae* (23 serogroups) although neither of these vaccines is currently suitable for routine use in infants. A 7-valent conjugate pneumococcal vaccine is licensed in Europe, but has not yet been used in any national mass immunisation programme (unlike in the USA where it has been in routine use for many years).

• *Chemoprophylaxis* is indicated for close contacts of meningococcal and Hib disease (see Chapters 3.48 and 3.35) and investigation for close contacts of TB (Chapter 3.79). It is not necessary for contacts of pneumococcal or viral meningitis.

• *Food safety*. *Listeria* meningitis is preventable by avoiding high-risk foods such as soft cheese, pate and cook-chill foods, particularly for the immunosuppressed and in pregnancy.

• *Optimising case management*. In cases of suspected meningococcal disease, general practitioners and casualty officers should be urged to administer preadmission benzyl penicillin (see Chapter 3.48).

Response to a case or cluster

A case or cluster of meningitis is a highly emotive and newsworthy event. The first priority when a case is notified is to establish the diagnosis. This requires close liaison with clinicians and microbiologists to ensure that appropriate investigations are carried out. If the initial diagnosis is viral meningitis, then no further action is needed at this stage, although it may be necessary to provide information to GPs and parents if the case appears to be linked with others.

If bacterial meningitis is suspected, then further measures will depend on the cause. Again, optimum investigation is essential as the nature of the public health response differs for each organism. Typing of the organism is needed to determine whether cases are linked. Chemoprophylaxis, and sometimes also vaccination, is indicated for cases due to *N. meningitidis* or *H. influenzae* (see Chapters 3.48 and 3.36). With the introduction of Hib vaccine, meningococcal infection is by far the most likely diagnosis in a patient with acute bacterial meningitis and it may sometimes be appropriate to initiate control measures before laboratory confirmation.

In the UK, useful information leaflets on meningitis are available from the National Meningitis Trust and the Meningitis Research Foundation (see Appendix 1).

2.2 Gastrointestinal infection

Every year in the UK, approximately 1 in 30 people attend their general practitioner with an acute gastroenteritis (usually diarrhoea and/or vomiting) and many more suffer such an illness without contacting the health service. Although an infectious cause is not always demonstrated, there is strong epidemiological evidence to suggest that most of these illnesses are caused by infections. A wide variety of bacteria, viruses and parasites may cause gastrointestinal (GI) infection: the most commonly identified ones in the UK are listed in Table 2.2.1. Less common but highly pathogenic infections may be imported from abroad including amoebic or bacillary dysentery, cholera, typhoid and paratyphoid fevers. Other infectious causes of gastroenteritis include other *Escherichia coli*, *Bacillus subtilis*, *Clostridium difficile*, *Giardia lamblia*, *Vibrio parahaemolyticus*, *Yersinia enterocolitica* and viruses such as adenovirus, astrovirus, calicivirus and coronavirus. Non-infectious causes of acute gastroenteritis include toxins from shellfish, vegetables (e.g. red kidney beans) and fungi (such as wild mushrooms), and chemical contamination of food and water.

Laboratory investigation

Identification of the causative organism is dependent upon laboratory investigation, usually of faecal samples. It is important that such samples are taken as soon after the onset of illness as possible, as the likelihood of isolating some pathogens (e.g. viruses) decreases substantially within a few days of onset. Collecting at least 2 mL of faeces and including the liquid part of the stool will increase the chances of a positive result. Delay in transport to the laboratory, particularly in warm weather should be minimised. If delay is likely, samples should be refrigerated or stored in a suitable transport medium. A local policy on sampling and transport should be agreed with

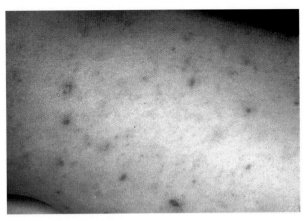

(a)

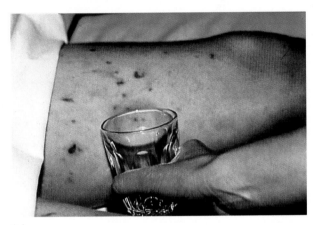

Plate 1 Testing for the non-blanching rash of meningococcal septicaemia with a glass. (a) Early-stage rash; (b) tumbler test.

(b)

the local microbiology laboratory. Samples of vomit may sometimes be helpful. In both cases, the patient should receive instructions on the collection and storage or transport of the specimen. Serum samples may be helpful, particularly if some cases become jaundiced. It is often difficult to distinguish between bacterial and chemical food-borne gastroenteritis on clinical grounds, although some toxins cause an unpleasant taste and/or burning in the mouth or throat. If a chemical cause is suspected, advice on sampling should be obtained from a toxicologist (e.g. public analyst).

A suitable list of organisms to test for in all community outbreaks of gastroenteritis is:
- Salmonellae
- *Campylobacter* species
- *Shigella* species
- *E. coli* O157
- Norovirus
- Protozoa (*Cryptosporidium* and *Giardia*)

Plus, if food poisoning is suspected or if clinical features suggest (see Table 2.2.1):
- *Bacillus* species
- *Clostridium perfringens*
- *Staphylococcus aureus*

Also consider the following if clinical or epidemiological features suggest or if the first list above is negative:
- Rotavirus
- *Vibrio* species
- *Yersinia* species
- *Clostridium difficile*
- Other *E. coli*
- Other viruses
- Toxins or poisons

In hospitals, the most common causes of outbreaks are
- Norovirus,
- *Clostridium difficile*,
- Salmonellae and
- Rotavirus.

Prevention and control

Vaccines are not yet available against the major causes of GI infection and so public health efforts concentrate on reducing exposure to the organisms responsible. Most GI infections are either food-borne or spread person to person. The role of the consumer in demanding safe food via pressure on government and food retailers is under-developed in many countries, including the UK.

At the local level, prevention of GI or food-borne infection is achieved by
- working with food businesses and staff to reduce the likelihood of contamination of food (from the environment, food handlers or cross-contamination), inadequate cooking and storage at inadequate temperatures. The Hazard Analysis Critical Control Point (HACCP) system has proven to be a powerful tool for use by the food industry in identifying and assessing hazards in food, and establishing control measures needed to maintain a cost-effective food safety programme. Important features are that HACCP is predictive, cheap, on-site and involves local staff in the control of risk. In the UK, this approach is reinforced by inspection of premises by the Environmental Health Department of the Local Authority and other enforcement agencies.
- use of statutory powers: UK Local Authorities can exclude cases or carriers of infection from work or school and compensate them for any loss of earnings. Other powers include seizure of food and closure of premises that present an 'imminent risk to Public Health'. Officers of the Environmental Health Department usually exercise these powers. The Meat Hygiene Service (part of the Food Standards Agency) is the enforcing authority for licensed fresh meat/poultry premises in Great Britain.
- advising the public on safe food handling and the reduction of faeco–oral spread. This includes the importance of handwashing immediately after going to the toilet and before handling or eating food. This is of vital importance, as approximately 80% of people with GI infection do not consult the health service when ill.
- adequate infection control policies in all institutions including hospitals, nursing and residential homes, schools and nurseries, including use of enteric precautions (see Chapter 1.2) for cases of diarrhoea or vomiting.
- regular surveillance to detect outbreaks and respond to individual cases. Food poisoning

Table 2.2.1 Differential diagnosis of GI infection

Organism	Laboratory confirmed (annual average, England and Wales*)		Incubation period (Approx.)		Clinical clues in outbreaks		Other features
	Cases (No.)	Outbreaks (No.)	Usual	Range	Symptoms	Severity	
Campylobacter	47,600	9	2–5 days	1–10 days	D† often with blood Abdominal pain ± fever	Usually lasts 2–7 days	Peaks in early summer
Rotavirus	15,800	18	24–72 h	24–72 h	Watery D, fever vomiting ± respiratory symptoms	Usually lasts a few days, but occasionally severe	Usually children, common in winter & spring
Salmonella	15,100	50	12–36 hs	6–72 hours	D often with fever. May be myalgia, abdominal pain, headache	Can be severe Lasts several days to 3 weeks	Peaks in late summer
Cryptosporidium	4,270	8	6–13 days	1–28 days	D, bloating and abdominal pain common	Self-limiting but lasts up to 4 weeks	Severe in immunocompromised Increases in spring and autumn
Giardia lamblia	3,410	1	7–10 days	3–25 days	D, malaise, flatulence smelly stools; cramps, bloating	Often prolonged May be malabsorption and weight loss	Often travel associated Possibility of water-borne outbreak
Norovirus	2,680	322	15–50 h	4–77 hours	Nausea/vomiting common Cramps, mild D may occur	Usually mild lasts 1–2 days	Secondary spread common More common in winter
Hepatitis A	1,100	n/a	Mean = 28 days	15–45 days	Fever, nausea, malaise Jaundice fairly specific but not sensitive	Worse in adults Lasts up to 4 weeks	Children may be asymptomatic

Organism				Symptoms	Duration/severity	Notes
Shigella sonnei	720	2	24–72 h	12–96 h	Often watery D May be mucus	Self-limiting in 3–5 days	Often children or institutions: secondary spread common
E. coli O157	680	14	3–4 days	1–9 days	D, blood not uncommon	Variable, may be very severe, e.g. HUS, TTP	Consider in all cases of bloody diarrhoea
Other shigellae	360	<1	24–72 h	12–96 h	D, mucus, blood, fever and colic common	Lasts average of 7 days Often severe	Often imported, secondary spread common
C. perfringens	360	10	8–18 h	5–24 h	D, abdominal pain common (vomiting and fever are rare)	Usually mild and short-lived lasts ~1 day	Usually failure of temperature control post-cooking
Bacillus cereus	80	<1	1–6 h for syndrome of nausea, vomiting and abdominal pain 6–24 h for syndrome of diarrhoea and abdominal pain			Usually mild and short-lived lasts ~1 day	Often from rice or pasta High attack rate
Staphylococcus aureus	30[‡]	1	2–4 h	0.5–8 h	Vomiting, abdominal pain (diarrhoea rare) Often abrupt onset	May be very acute	Food handler may have skin infection

* Average number of reports p.a. to HPA/CDSC, 2001–2003, (cases) or 1999–2003 (outbreaks).
[†] D = Diarrhoea, which can be defined as three or more loose stools in 24 h.
[‡] 1990–1999.

(proven or suspected and including water-borne infection), dysentery and viral hepatitis are all statutorily notifiable in Great Britain, as are cholera, paratyphoid and typhoid fever in almost all European countries. There are, however, no generally accepted clinical case-definitions for these notifiable infections in the UK and there may often be no laboratory confirmation of the organism responsible. It is, therefore, often necessary to initiate action before the causative organism is known. Arrangements should also be in place for reporting of isolates of GI pathogens from local microbiology laboratories (see Chapter 4.2). However, around 90% of cases seen by general practitioners are not identified by either of these systems: obtaining surveillance data from computerised primary care providers may help address this.

At national level in the UK, the Food Standards Agency has set a target of achieving a 20% reduction in food-borne disease. This is to be achieved by measures to control pathogens in foods, particularly poultry, eggs, red meat and dairy products, and improving food handling and preparation, both in catering and hospitality businesses, and in the home. The target will be monitored using laboratory reports of human infection with *Campylobacter jejuni*, *Salmonella* spp., *C. perfringens*, *E. coli* O157 and *Listeria monocytogenes*.

Response to an individual case

It is not usually possible to identify the organism causing gastroenteritis on clinical grounds in individual cases. The public health priorities in such cases are as follows:

• To limit secondary spread from identified cases by provision of general hygiene advice to all and by specific exclusion from work/school/nursery of those at increased risk of transmitting the infection (see Box 2.2.1). This is usually until 48 hours after their last episode of diarrhoea or vomiting, except when certain organisms such as *E. coli* O157 or typhoid/paratyphoid have been identified (see relevant chapters). Ideally all cases should not attend work, school or other institutional settings, even if not in risk groups, for a similar period.

• To collect a minimum dataset to compare to other cases to detect common exposures or potential outbreaks. It is best to collect such data on standardised forms and a subset should be entered on a computerised database for both weekly and annual analysis. A possible dataset is given in Box 2.2.2.

• Ideally, a faecal sample would be collected from all clinical notifications of food poisoning or dysentery to detect for clusters by organism/type, to detect potentially serious pathogens requiring increased intervention and to monitor trends.

Box 2.2.1 Groups that pose an increased risk of spreading GI infection

1 Food handlers whose work involves touching unwrapped foods to be consumed raw or without further cooking.
2 Staff of healthcare facilities who have direct contact, or contact through serving food, with susceptible patients or persons in whom an intestinal infection would have particularly serious consequences.
3 Children aged less than 5 years who attend nurseries, nursery schools, playgroups or other similar groups.
4 Older children and adults who may find it difficult to implement good standards of personal hygiene, for example, those with learning disabilities or special needs; and in circumstances where hygienic arrangements may be unreliable, for example, temporary camps housing displaced persons. Under exceptional circumstances (e.g. *E. coli* O157 infection) children in infant schools may be considered to fall into this group.
  Source: PHLS Salmonella Committee, 1995 (revision in progress, 2005).

Box 2.2.2 Possible district dataset for investigation of cases of GI infection

Administrative details (name, address, telephone, date of birth, GP, unique number*)

Formally notified?   Yes/No

Descriptive variables (age*, sex*, postcode*)

Date* and time of onset

Symptoms

Diarrhoea	Yes/No
Nausea	Yes/No
Fever	Yes/No
Abdominal pain	Yes/No
Blood in stool	Yes/No
Malaise	Yes/No
Headache	Yes/No
Jaundice	Yes/No

Others (specify):_____

Duration of illness

Stool sample taken? (source, date, laboratory)

Microbiological result (organism details*, laboratory, specimen date)

Food history: functions, restaurants, takeaways

Food consumed in last 5 days (for unknown microbial cause)

Raw water consumed outside the home in previous 14 days

Other cases in household?

Travel abroad?

Animal contact?

Occupation, place of work/school/nursery

Advised not to work?

Formally excluded?

Part of outbreak?*

   Organism specific questions may be added if microbiological investigation reveals an organism of particular public health importance (e.g. *E. coli* O157, *Cryptosporidium*, *Salmonella typhi*, *Salmonella paratyphi*).

Minimum dataset to be recorded in computerised database

A local policy to address these priorities should be agreed with local EHOs, microbiologists and clinicians. The role of the primary care practitioners in public health surveillance and in preventing secondary spread is of particular importance and needs to be emphasised regularly (e.g. via a GP newsletter).

Response to a cluster

The most common setting for a cluster of clinical cases of gastroenteritis is in an already defined cohort, e.g. a nursing home or amongst attendees at a wedding. Such a situation is slightly different to investigate than a laboratory-identified cluster:

• It is important to discover the microbiological agent. Following discussion with the relevant microbiologist (e.g. the local HPA Laboratory in England) stool specimens should be obtained without delay from 6 to 10 of the patients with the most recent onset of illness and submitted to the laboratory for testing for all relevant organisms, (see list given above; the laboratory may not test for all these unless requested). The identity of the agent will dictate the urgency of the investigation (e.g. to prevent further exposure to a source of *E. coli* O157), the control measures to be introduced (e.g. to limit person to person spread of norovirus in institutions) and provide valuable clues as to how the outbreak may have happened (e.g. inadequate temperature control in a *Bacillus cereus* outbreak).

• As microbiological results will not be available for a number of days, clinical details should be collected from all reported cases so that the incubation period, symptom profile, severity and duration of illness can be used to predict which organism(s) are most likely to be the cause (Table 2.2.1). The likelihood of different microbiological causes also varies by season (Figs 2.2.1 and 2.2.2). There may also be clues as to whether the illness is likely to be food-borne or spread person to person (Box 2.2.3). In many such outbreaks a formal hypothesis-generating study is not necessary, and it is often possible to progress to an analytical study to investigate possible food vehicles early in the investigation (see Chapter 4.3).

• The environmental component of the investigation is often illuminating as to why the outbreak happened, i.e. how did an infectious dose of the organism occur in the identified food vehicle. This investigation will look at the following:

(i) Food sources, storage, food preparation, cooking procedures, temperature control after cooking and reheating.

(ii) Symptoms of GI or skin disease, or testing for faecal carriage in food handlers.

(iii) General state of knowledge of the staff and condition of the premises.

(iv) Examination of records of key controls, such as temperature and pest controls.

(v) Whether samples of food are available for examination/analysis and whether environmental swabbing or water sampling is appropriate.

• General control measures to prevent spread from those affected can be instituted early, as can addressing important problems identified in the environmental investigation. This

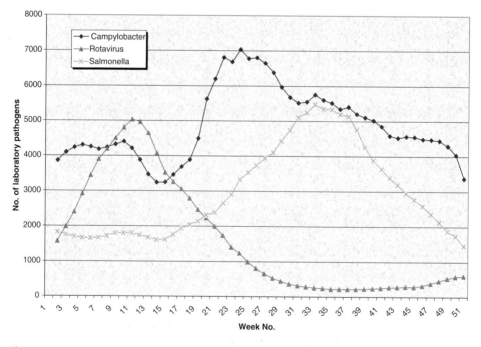

Fig. 2.2.1 Seasonal distribution of GI pathogens, 1999–2003, England and Wales (3-week rolling averages).

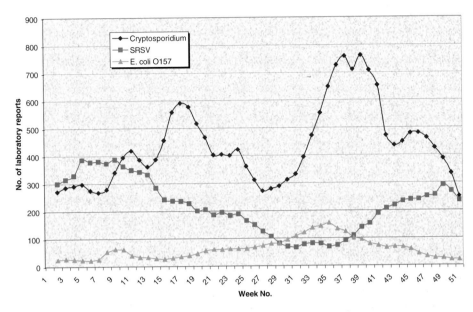

Fig. 2.2.2 Seasonal distribution of GI pathogens, 1999–2003, England and Wales (3-week rolling averages).

Box 2.2.3 Clues as to whether an outbreak of gastroenteritis could be food-borne or spread person to person

May suggest food-borne	May suggest person to person
Dates of onset (epidemic curve) clustered indicating a point source outbreak.	Dates and times of onset do not cluster but occur in waves coinciding with the incubation period of the responsible pathogen.
All wards, classes, buildings or units supplied by the kitchens or food supplier are affected.	Patients and staff in a single ward, class, building or unit are affected.
Food handlers and catering staff are affected.	People in the households of staff-members or pupils are also affected.
Clinical features and laboratory tests indicate an organism predominantly spread via food and water rather than person to person, e.g. *C. perfringens, B. cereus*.	Clinical features and laboratory tests suggest organism predominantly spread person to person, e.g. rotavirus, *Shigella*.
Environmental investigation reveals poor food handling practices or premises.	Environmental investigation reveals poor infection control practice or hygiene facilities.

Warnings

These are not invariable rules, assess each outbreak on its own merits, e.g.
- some food-borne outbreaks may be prolonged by person-to-person spread.
- food-borne outbreaks may be due to a continuing source.
- some outbreaks may be augmented by environmental contamination.

includes the exclusion from work of infected foodhandlers and measures to avoid secondary spread from cases. More specific measures can be instituted when the organism and vehicle are identified (see organism-specific chapter in Section 3).

• In institutions, such as hospitals and nursing homes, institute measures to reduce risk of person-to-person spread (see Chapter 3.53 for details).

2.3 Community-acquired pneumonia

Respiratory tract infections are the most common infectious diseases in developed countries and pneumonia remains one of the most common causes of death. Community (as opposed to hospital) acquired pneumonia (CAP) affects all ages, although its incidence increases dramatically beyond 50 years of age. Other risk factors include chronic respiratory disease, smoking, immunosuppression (including HIV/AIDS) and residence in an institution. Approximately 20% of cases require hospitalisation, of which 5–10% die.

In general, the symptoms of CAP are fever, cough, sputum production, chest pain and shortness of breath, with accompanying chest X-ray changes. The most common causes of CAP are listed in Table 2.3.1. Although the clinical picture cannot be used to diagnose individual cases, clues may be obtained to help identify the causes of outbreaks.

Rare causes of pneumonia for which there may be an environmental cause (most likely abroad, but perhaps due to deliberate aerosol release) include anthrax, brucellosis, hantavirus, histoplasmosis, leptospirosis and plague. Respiratory infection may also be caused by rare or emerging organisms such as SARS-coronavirus, avian influenza, metapneumovirus and *Moraxella catarrhalis* or in immunosuppressed individuals, opportunistic pathogens such as *Pneumocystis carinii*. Similar symptoms may also be seen in exacerbations of chronic respiratory disease and non-infective respiratory conditions, e.g. pulmonary oedema, pulmonary infarction, alveolitis (may follow exposure to inorganic particles) and eosinophilic pneumonias (may be associated with drugs or parasites).

Laboratory investigation

Microscopy and culture of sputum remains the mainstay of diagnosis. However, about a third of pneumonia cases do not produce sputum, culture is only moderately sensitive and contamination with oropharyngeal flora is not an uncommon event. Blood culture is highly specific but relatively insensitive.

Serology has been the mainstay of diagnosis for viral and 'atypical' causes, but this is often not diagnostic until 2–6 weeks into the illness. Mycoplasma specific IgM may be apparent rather earlier. Influenza and RSV may be cultured from nasopharyngeal swabs or aspirates, and viral antigen or DNA may also be detected from these specimens (as may *Chlamydia pneumoniae* DNA). *Legionella* antigen may be detected in urine and pneumococcal antigen in sputum, serum or urine, even if antibiotics have already been given.

A proportion of cases may be infected with more than one pathogen.

Prevention and control

• Immunisation of elderly and those with chronic disease and immunocompromised with influenza and pneumococcal vaccines.
• Immunisation of children against *Haemophilus influenzae* type b. Pneumococcal vaccination of children is also under consideration in many European countries.
• Reduction of smoking.
• Promotion of breastfeeding.
• Avoiding overcrowding, especially in institutions.
• Good infection control in institutions.
• Environmental measures to reduce *Legionella* exposure.
• Surveillance of CAP, especially for influenza, *Mycoplasma*, *Legionella*, *Coxiella* and *Chlamydia*

psittaci. Surveillance of antibiotic-resistant pneumococci.
• Reporting of outbreaks in institutions to public health authorities.

Response to a case

• If resident or attender at institution, or if severely ill, investigate to obtain microbiological cause.
• Follow up individual cases of legionellosis, psittacosis and Q fever for source of organism.
• Advise personal hygiene, particularly handwashing, coughing and disposal of secretions.
• Limit contact with infants, frail elderly and immunocompromised.

Response to a cluster

• Discuss investigation with microbiological colleagues. A suitable set of investigations could be as follows:
  (i) Take nasopharyngeal aspirates or nose and throat swabs from most recently infected cases for virus culture, PCR and antigen testing.
  (ii) Take serum samples from recovered cases or those with date of onset 10 days or more ago.
  (iii) Send sputum samples for microbiological culture and possibly pneumococcal antigen.
  (iv) Send blood cultures from febrile cases.
  (v) Send urine for *Legionella* and pneumococcal antigen.
• If an institutional cluster, isolate or cohort cases until cause known. Stop new admissions. Avoid discharges to institutions containing elderly, frail or immunocompromised individuals. Measures should aim to limit transmission by large droplets, droplet nuclei, respiratory secretions and direct contact. In RSV season, also consider transmission via inanimate objects.
• Collect data on immunisation history (influenza, pneumococcus), travel, exposure to water and aerosols, animals, birds and other potential sources of *Legionella*, *Coxiella* and *Chlamydia psittaci*.

• Advise community cases on hygiene measures (handwashing, coughing, discharges, etc.) and to avoid individuals susceptible to severe disease (e.g. elderly, chronically ill).
• Specific interventions as appropriate to identified organism (see organism specific chapter).
• During influenza season give anti-influenza prophylaxis to contacts in residential care institutions for elderly, whilst awaiting diagnosis (see Chapter 3.38).
• A cluster of CAP could arise as a result of a deliberate release of an aerosol of a serious or rare infection such as anthrax or plague (see Chapter 4.14).

2.4 Rash in pregnancy

Infectious and other causes

There are many possible causes of a rash in a pregnant woman. Most causes are non-infectious and include drug reactions and allergies. The important differentiating feature from an infectious cause is the absence of fever. Infectious causes are relatively uncommon, but important because of the potential harm to the developing fetus. Rubella, parvovirus B19, varicella and syphilis can all cause severe congenital disease or intrauterine death.

Clinical and epidemiological differences

Viral infections in pregnancy are often mild or inapparent with variable or absent fever. The exceptions are varicella, which presents with a characteristic rash, and measles. Bacterial infections are more severe and are usually accompanied by a high fever (with the exception of syphilis). The clinical presentation of each of the infections in Table 2.4.1 is described in more detail in the relevant chapters.

The most common infections in pregnancy are parvovirus B19 (1 in 400 pregnancies), varicella (1 in 500 pregnancies) and the enteroviruses. Rubella and measles are now both

Table 2.4.1 Differential diagnosis of community-acquired pneumonia

Organism	Percent of cases*	Incubation period	Clinical clues†	Epidemiological clues
Streptococcus pneumoniae	29	1–3 days (exogenous)	Acute. Rusty sputum, fever, chest pain. Prominent physical signs.	More common in infants, elderly, unvaccinated and in winter.
Mycoplasma pneumoniae	9	6–32 days (median = 14 days)	Gradual onset, scanty sputum, headache, malaise, sore throat.	Epidemics every 4 years. Often affects younger patients or military
Influenza A	8	1–5 days (median = 2 days)	Headache, myalgia, coryza, fever, sore throat.	May be seasonal community epidemic. Affects the unvaccinated.
Chlamydia pneumoniae	6	Unclear: 10–30 days?	Hoarseness, sore throat, prolonged cough, scanty sputum, sinus tenderness. Insidious onset.	Often affects young adults. No obvious seasonality.
Gram negative bacteria	6	Variable	Severe. Acute onset. Redcurrent jelly sputum.	Particularly common in nursing homes. More likely if chronic respiratory disease, diabetes, alcohol.
Haemophilus influenzae	5	Unclear: 2–4 days?	Purulent sputum. Onset may be insidious.	Often associated with chronic lung disease and elderly.
Legionella pneumophila	4	2–10 days (median = 5.5 days)	Anorexia, malaise, myalgia, headache, fever. Some with diarrhoea, confusion and high fever. Upper respiratory symptoms rare. Often severe.	May be associated with aerosol source. More common in summer and autumn. Mostly over 30; male excess.

Organism		Incubation period	Clinical features	Notes
Staphylococcus aureus	4	1–4 days (exogenous)	Often serious. May be ring shadows on X-ray.	May complicate influenza infection. More common in nursing homes.
Parainfluenza	2	3–6 days	Croup, wheezing or hoarseness. Ear or upper respiratory infection.	Mostly affects children and immunocompromised. Para 1 and 2 more common in autumn or early winter (but para 3 endemic)
Chlamydia psittaci	2	4–28 days (median = 10 days)	Fever, headache, unproductive cough, myalgia. May be rash. Often severe.	Possible link to birds. May be severe. Mostly adults, more often males.
Influenza B	1	1–5 days (median = 2 days)	Headache, myalgia, coryza fever, sore throat.	May be seasonal community epidemic. Affects the unvaccinated.
Coxiella burnetii	1	14–39 days (median = 20 days)	Fever, fatigue, chills, headache, myalgia, sweats. May be weight loss, neurological symptoms or hepatitis.	Possible link to sheep, other animals or animal products. May increase in April–June. Male excess, rare in children.
RSV	1	2–8 days (median = 5 days)	Wheezing, rhinitis, fever.	Peaks every December and January. Causes outbreaks in nursing homes.
Adenovirus	0.7	4–5 days average	Fever, sore throat, runny nose.	Usually children or young adults (e.g. military recruits). Highest in January–April.

* Average from a number of prospective studies of patients admitted to hospital (Farr and Mandell, 1988). Will vary according to epidemic cycles.
† Clinical picture is not a reliable indicator of organism in individual cases.

Table 2.4.2 Infections that may present with a rash in pregnancy

Viral
  Rubella
  Parvovirus B19
  Varicella-zoster
  Measles
  Enterovirus
  Infectious mononucleosis
Bacterial
  Streptococcal
  Meningococcal
  Syphilis

rare, due to successful immunisation programmes. Bacterial causes of rash in pregnancy are very uncommon.

Laboratory investigation

The laboratory investigation of suspected meningococcal and streptococcal disease and syphilis is described in Chapters 3.48, 3.73 and 3.26, respectively.

Where a viral infection is suspected, it is important to exclude varicella, parvovirus B19 and rubella. Varicella can usually be diagnosed on the basis of the typical vesicular rash, but where there is doubt, serology should be performed. Rubella and parvovirus B19 can both be diagnosed by detection of IgM in saliva or serum.

The investigation of a pregnant woman who has been in contact with someone with a rash illness is more complex. The aim of investigation is to determine whether the contact case has varicella, rubella or parvovirus B19, and whether the pregnant patient is susceptible to these three infections. The three algorithms in Figs 2.4.1–2.4.3 describe the laboratory investigation recommended in the UK.

Prevention and control

Rubella infection in pregnancy can be prevented both directly, by vaccination of susceptible women of childbearing age, and indirectly, by universal childhood immunisation (which reduces circulation of wild virus and

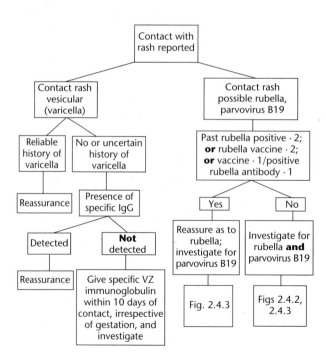

Fig. 2.4.1 Investigation of a pregnant patient in contact with a rash illness.

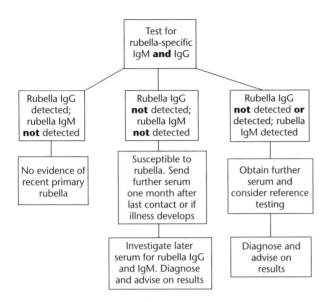

Fig. 2.4.2 Investigation for rubella of a pregnant woman exposed to a rash illness.

thus prevents exposure). All pregnant women should be screened for rubella in each pregnancy and vaccinated postpartum. Rubella vaccine (now given as MMR) is a live vaccine and should not be given during pregnancy, although the risk to the fetus is theoretical and immunisation in pregnancy is no longer an indication for termination of pregnancy.

Varicella vaccine is licensed in most countries in Europe, including the UK, and can be used for both direct prevention of varicella in pregnancy (by vaccination of susceptible women) and indirect prevention (universal childhood immunisation). A specific varicella zoster immunoglobulin (VZIG) is also available for post-exposure prophylaxis of

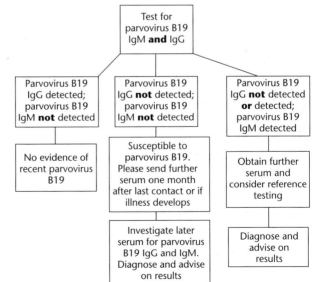

Fig. 2.4.3 Investigation for parvovirus B19 of a pregnant woman exposed to a rash illness.

susceptible women exposed in pregnancy (see Chapter 3.7).

No specific measures are available for prevention of parvovirus B19 in pregnancy, although pregnant women may wish to avoid outbreak situations, and healthcare workers who have been in contact with B19 infection should avoid contact with pregnant women for 15 days from the last contact or until a rash appears (see Chapter 3.56).

Response to a case

Laboratory investigations should be undertaken as described above. Pregnant women with varicella, rubella or parvovirus B19 should be counselled regarding the risks to the fetus and managed accordingly by the obstetrician. The public health management of the close contacts is the same as for non-pregnant cases (see Chapters 3.7, 3.56 and 3.66).

Response to a cluster

As for response to a case, but consider community-wide vaccination programme for clusters of rubella or measles.

2.5 Rash and fever in children

Rashes in children are common (Table 2.5.1). Where fever is present, this usually means the cause is infectious. In the absence of a fever, a non-infectious cause (e.g. allergy or drug reaction) is the most likely cause, although in some infections, e.g. enterovirus infections, the fever may be mild or absent.

Clinical and epidemiological differences

In addition to fever, other features that suggest an infectious cause are the presence of swollen lymph nodes, general malaise, and a history of

Table 2.5.1 Causes of rash in children

Common
Infection
Drug reaction
Allergy
Rare
Inherited bleeding disorder
Leukaemia
Purpura

recent contact with another case. A full vaccination history should always be obtained from a child with a rash.

There are four main types of rash: vesicular, maculopapular, punctate and haemorrhagic. Vesicular rashes have a blister-like appearance and sometimes contain fluid. Maculopapular rashes are flat or slightly raised and there is sometimes joining together of areas of the rash. Punctate rashes have small, discrete pinpoint lesions. Haemorrhagic rashes look like bruising. The main causes of each type are shown in Table 2.5.2.

Laboratory investigations

General investigations that are useful in differentiating infectious from non-infectious causes are a full blood count, erythrocyte sedimentation rate, blood culture, specimens for viral culture and an acute serum sample for serology. Other investigations will depend on the possible differential diagnoses. A saliva test should be obtained if measles or rubella is suspected.

Prevention and control

General hygiene measures such as handwashing may help limit the spread of some infectious causes of rashes. Transmission of measles, rubella, meningococcal disease (serogroup C) and chickenpox are all preventable by vaccination (see Chapters 3.47, 3.66, 3.48 and 3.7, respectively).

Table 2.5.2 Types of rash

	Prodrome	Fever	General malaise	Distribution of rash	Pruritus	Special features
Vesicular rashes						
Chickenpox	None or short coryzal	Mild to moderate	Mild	Mostly truncal	Yes	Contact with sufferers is common; crops
Dermatitis herpetiformis	Nil	Nil	Nil	Trunk	Yes	Sporadic cases eventually leave depigmentation
Eczema herpeticum	Nil	Moderate to high	Moderate	In areas of eczema	Yes	May be seriously ill
Hand, foot and mouth disease	Nil	Minimal	Minimal	Palms, soles and inside mouth	No	Often occurs as minor epidemics
Herpes simplex gingivostomatis	Nil	Moderate to high	Moderate (may be dehydrated)	Mouth and lips	Yes (at onset)	Frequent history of contact with cold sores
Impetigo	Nil	Nil	Nil	Face and hands	Yes	Vesicles often replaced by yellow crusting
Insect bites	Nil	Nil	Rare	Variable	Yes	Usually isolated lesions
Molluscum contagiosum	Nil	Nil	Nil	Variable	Yes	Characteristic pearly vesicles with central dimples
Maculopapular and punctate rashes						
Enteroviral infections	Short	Mild	Mild	General	No	Rash often pleomorphic
Fifth disease	Uncommon; mild fever and respiratory symptoms	Mild, if any	Minimal	Face ('slapped cheeks') trunk and limbs	No	Rash may come and go; heat brings it out; can have a reticular pattern
Glandular fever	Malaise, mild fever and sore throat	Moderate	Common	General	No	Exudate in throat especially marked; swollen glands and spleen
Kawasaki disease	Mild fever, malaise and sore throat	Moderate to high and persistent	Mild to moderate	General	No	Palms and soles, lips and conjunctivae affected

Continued on p. 36

Table 2.5.2 *Continued*

Measles	Rising fever, cough and conjunctivitis	Moderate to high	Substantial	Around ears, then face, then trunk. Confluent	No	Koplik's spots in mouth before rash on 4th day of illness
Meningococcal disease	None or short with coryza or fever	Variable	Profound	Variable	No	Petechial rash may be preceded by maculopapular rash
Pityriasis rosea	Nil	Nil	Nil	Trunk	Initially	Usually in older children; herald patch at onset
Roseola infantum	High fever and irritability	Moderate	Moderate	Trunk then face	No	Dramatic improvement in child when rash appears on 4th or 5th day
Rubella	Short, mild fever and malaise	Mild	Mild or absent	Face then trunk and limbs	No	Posterior occipital lymphadenopathy
Scarlet fever	Fever and sore throat	Moderate to high	Moderate	Face, then rapidly generalized	No	Rash blanches on pressure; strawberry tongue and perioral pallor
Haemorrhagic rashes						
Acute lymphoblastic leukaemia	Mild, non-specific	Absent or mild/moderate	Moderate	Anywhere, including mucous membranes	Nil	Pallor, lymphadenopathy and hepatosplenomegaly may be present
Henoch-Schönlein purpura	Mild, sometimes symptoms of upper respiratory tract infection	Mild or moderate	Moderate	Mainly limbs, especially legs and buttocks	No	Rash is urticarial initially. Arthralgia, joint swelling and abdominal pain often present
Idiopathic thrombocytopenic purpura	Nil to mild	Nil	Nil	Anywhere, including mucous membranes	Nil	Child is usually well, apart from effects of bleeding
Inherited bleeding disorder	Nil	Nil	Nil	Anywhere, including mucous membranes	Nil	Spontaneous bruises. Family history may be present
Meningococcal disease	None or short with coryza or fever	Variable	Severe	Variable	No	Petechial rash may be preceded by maculopapular rash

Source: From E.G. Davies *et al.*, *Manual of Childhood Infections*, British Paediatric Association, 1996, with permission.

Response to a case

• Obtain clinical details, especially whether fever present.
• Check vaccination status.
• Obtain history of contact with other case(s).
• Most childhood rashes are mild and do not warrant any specific public health action.
• Exclusion from school is indicated for the vaccine-preventable diseases (see above) and for scarlet fever (see Chapter 3.73).
• Chemoprophylaxis (and sometimes vaccination) should be given where meningococcal infection is suspected (see Chapter 3.48).

Response to a cluster

As per a case, although it will often be important to give out information to parents and GPs to allay anxiety and to increase disease awareness.

2.6 Illness in returning travellers

The possibility of imported infection should always be considered in the investigations of infectious disease. Imported infections may well present where they are unfamiliar, failure to consider them can have disastrous consequences (see also Chapter 4.10).

Fever in the returned traveller

Fever in the returned traveller may result from a tropical infection or an illness common to non-travellers, such as pneumonia or urinary tract infection, or be due to a non-infectious cause of fever, such as neoplasia.

Infectious causes of fever

The organisms that should be considered depend upon the location(s) visited, the season and the activities undertaken. Careful travel histories are important; it may be necessary to consult an expert who knows the local epidemiology of disease.
• Where has the person been (country)?
• Which districts (urban, rural)?
• Staying where (luxury hotels, camping)?
• Doing what (healthcare, animals)?
• Exactly when (incubation periods)?
• Precautions taken (vaccines, prophylaxis, lifestyle)?

The possibility of a highly infectious exotic infection, such as a viral haemorrhagic fever (VHF) should be considered and advice sought as necessary. VHF is more likely if an individual has been staying in rural areas, or has been in contact with other possible cases. As the geographical range of these diseases is not known they should be considered whenever the clinical picture warrants, although confirmed cases are rare. Caution should be exercised when the patient has been involved in caring for others who were ill, or in healthcare worker (see Chapter 3.84).

The common imported causes of fever include malaria, enteric fevers, pneumonias (including Legionnaires' disease), hepatitis, tuberculosis, rickettsiae and schistosomiasis. Falciparum malaria is a medical emergency. Malaria has a variety of clinical presentations (see Chapter 3.46) and usually presents within 3 months of return, but may occasionally take 1 year.

Other illnesses in travellers

Travellers' diarrhoea usually occurs during travel or soon after return. The most frequently identified pathogen causing traveller's diarrhoea is toxigenic *Escherichia coli*. In some parts of the world (North Africa and South-east Asia), *Campylobacter* predominates. Other common causative organisms include *Salmonella*, *Shigella*, rotavirus, and the Norwalk agent. The longer the history, the more likely the cause is to be parasitic, e.g. *Giardia*, *Entamoeba histolytica* or *Cyclospora*, rather than bacterial or viral.

Pharyngitis may be due to diphtheria, and in a febrile patient who has visited rural West Africa, Lassa fever. Diphtheria and leishmaniasis may both present with cutaneous lesions. Hepatitis A, B, C and E viruses may all be contracted abroad.

Response to a case of illness in a traveller

For febrile illnesses
• determine likely exposure;
• malaria should be excluded if there is any possible exposure in a patient who is unwell;
• enteric precautions for cases with diarrhoea;
• exclusion and contact tracing as appropriate for cholera, diphtheria, hepatitis A or B, paratyphoid and typhoid fevers (see specific chapters in Section 3);
• if haemorrhagic fever or other highly contagious imported infections such as SARS is seriously considered, the nearest unit with special expertise should be contacted urgently;
• inform national surveillance unit of incidents of potential significance, e.g. VHF, SARS, Legionnaires' disease, outbreak of food poisoning and imported infections that should be reported to WHO under the International Health Regulations (yellow fever, cholera, plague).

Acute travellers' diarrhoea is usually self-limiting and does not require antibiotic therapy. Chronic bowel problems that persist after returning home may be postinfectious sequelae, such as lactose intolerance or irritable bowel syndrome or an initial presentation of inflammatory bowel disease. Rare infectious causes of chronic bowel symptoms include *Giardia intestinalis* (see Chapter 3.25), *Cyclospora cayetanensis* (see Chapter 3.17), *Cryptosporidium* species (Chapter 3.16) and *Entamoeba histolytica* (Chapter 3.1).

Investigation of a cluster

The absence in Western Europe of essential vectors in the life cycle of an organism and better sanitary conditions mean that the conditions for onward transmission do not exist for many imported infections. Secondary cases are unusual. For those that can occur in UK, determine if cluster is a result of primary exposure abroad (tell national centre), or secondary transmission in UK (investigate mechanism).

Surveillance

Surveillance of travel-related infection is largely unsystematic and there are few good estimates of the risks of acquiring an infection when visiting a particular location. This makes basing advice on good evidence difficult.

Travel-associated infections and clusters of travel-associated infection should be reported to the public health authorities so that an improved picture of communicable disease risk can be developed.

2.7 Sexually transmitted infections

Sexually transmitted infections (STI) are infections that are spread by direct sexual contact. Table 2.7.1 lists the common infectious agents that cause STIs, their clinical features and common sequelae. Diagnosis depends on clinical features and the results of laboratory investigations including culture, serology, ELISA and PCR (see Table 2.7.1).

STIs are an important cause of ill health and may lead to long-term complications such as infertility, ectopic pregnancy and genital cancers. These complications specifically affect young women. The costs of NHS services for diagnosing and treating STIs and their complications are considerable. STIs such as gonorrhoea in men can be an indicator of sexual behaviour, which may carry a risk of transmission of HIV infection. STIs, which result in genital ulceration, may enhance HIV transmission. Interventions that reduce STI incidence have great potential for health gain.

Surveillance in England and Wales

As with any infectious disease, control of STIs depends on good surveillance. The main UK sources of surveillance data are shown in Table 2.7.2.

Table 2.7.1 Clinical features and laboratory confirmation of acute STIs

Infection and infectious agent	Clinical features and sequelae	Diagnosis
Genital chlamydial infection *Chlamydia trachomatis*	Many cases asymptomatic. In women may be cervicitis and urethritis. May be complicated by pelvic inflammatory disease, tubal damage, infertility and ectopic pregnancy. In men, urethritis and possibly epididymitis. Incubation period 7–14 days but many cases are asymptomatic.	Infection may be confirmed by enzyme immunoassay, direct fluorescent antibody test, ligase chain reaction (may be used on urine), polymerase chain reaction or culture of cervical or urethral samples.
Bacterial vaginosis *Gardnerella vaginalis*, anaerobic coccobacillus, other anaerobes including *Bacteroides*	Vaginal discharge and itching. There is debate about the importance of sexual transmission.	Wet mount of the discharge reveals vaginal epithelial cells studded with so-called clue cells.
Chancroid *Haemophilus ducreyi*	A painful ulcerating genital papule appears 4–10 days after exposure. If untreated, suppurating lymphadenopathy follows.	Diagnosis is confirmed by a Gram-stained smear or culture on special media.
Genital candidiasis *Candida albicans*	Vaginitis with irritation and discharge. *C. albicans* is a vaginal commensal and infection is often endogenous although sexual spread may occur. In males, infection is often asymptomatic but irritation and a rash on the glans penis may occur.	The organism can be identified in a Gram stain or wet mount or by culture.
Genital herpes Herpes simplex virus (HSV). Usually HSV-2 but HSV-1 causes 20% of cases	Primary infection produces painful vesicles or ulcers on the penis, labia, cervix and adjacent genital areas. There may be fever and malaise. Incubation period is 2–10 days. Healing occurs within 17 days. In the majority of cases, recurrent secondary episodes, usually less severe, occur as often as once a month due to HSV latency in local nerve ganglia. Precipitating factors include menstruation, sexual intercourse and stress. Subclinical attacks are common and are important in transmission. Serious HSV infection of the neonate may be acquired during delivery	Genital herpes has a typical appearance and can be confirmed by viral isolation.
Genital warts Human papillomaviruses (HPV)	Sessile warts are 1–2 mm in diameter and affect dry areas of skin. Condylomata acuminata are large fleshy soft growths and occur particularly when cellular immunity is depressed. Genital warts are often multiple and may occur anywhere on the external genitalia and within the vagina. Subclinical HPV infections of the genitalia are common. Certain HPV types are associated with genital tract neoplasia Possible sequelae are carcinoma of anus, cervix, penis and vulva. Incubation period is from 1 month to several months.	HPV cannot be cultured. Diagnosis may be made histologically on examining cervical cytology specimens. Polymerase chain reaction-based assays are now available that are capable of distinguishing more than 25 different HPV types.

Continued on p. 40

Table 2.7.1 (*Continued*)

Infection and infectious agent	Clinical features and sequelae	Diagnosis
Gonorrhoea *Neisseria gonorrhoeae*	Cervicitis in females and urethritis in males, with purulent discharge. Anorectal and oropharyngeal infection can occur. Incubation period is 2–5 days. Subclinical infection is common and an important source of transmission. Salpingitis is a complication in 10–15% of females but local complications in males are uncommon. Possible sequelae are neonatal infection, pelvic inflammatory disease, ectopic pregnancy, infertility, epididymitis, urethral stricture, septic arthritis.	Urethral or cervical swabs should be requested. Gram-negative diplococci may be seen on microscopy. *N. gonorrhoea* may be cultured.
Non-chlamydial non-gonococcal urethritis	*Ureaplasma urealyticum* and *Mycoplasma hominis* are causes of urethritis and pelvic inflammatory disease. Possible sequelae are infertility and ectopic pregnancy.	Specific diagnostic tests for these organisms are not usually clinically indicated.
Granuloma inguinale *Calymmatobacterium granulomatis*, a Gram-negative coccobacillus	Destructive ulcerating genital papules appear 1–12 weeks after exposure. Possible sequelae are genital lymphoedema, urethral stricture.	Biopsy of the edge of the ulcer shows Donovan bodies on appropriate staining.
Human T-cell lymphotropic virus	Leukaemia, lymphoma, tropical spastic paraparesis.	Tests for HTLV specific antibodies are available.
Lymphogranuloma venereum Types L-1, L-2 and L-3 of *Chlamydia trachomatis* distinct from those that cause trachoma and oculogenital infection	Starts with a painless penile vesicle 1–4 weeks after exposure. This heals but is followed 1–2 weeks later by fever and regional lymphadenopathy, which leads to suppuration and fibrosis that become chronic.	Diagnosis is made by serology, culture of aspirates or direct fluorescence of smears.
Syphilis *Treponema pallidum*	The clinical manifestations of syphilis are varied. The primary and secondary stages are characterised by mucocutaneous lesions. The primary chancre occurs on average 21 days after exposure. A variable secondary rash follows after 6–8 weeks, often with fever and malaise. Gummata (tertiary lesions) appear after several years. Almost any organ of the body can be affected. Transplacental spread of *T. pallidum* may result in fetal death, prematurity or congenital syphilis. Possible sequelae are fetal and neonatal infection, neurological and cardiovascular disease.	The diagnosis of syphilis is based upon clinical examination and demonstration of *T. pallidum* in early infectious lesions by dark ground microscopy. Serological tests aid the diagnosis of secondary, latent and tertiary syphilis.
Trichomoniasis *Trichomonas vaginalis*, a flagellated protozoan	Vaginitis with offensive discharge. Asymptomatic urethral infection or colonization common in males. Incubation period is 5–21 days.	Motile organisms may be seen on unstained wet preparation.

Table 2.7.2 The main UK sources of surveillance data

Surveillance type	UK example	Comment
Routine clinical	KC60 Returns	Aggregate data reported by GUM clinics, episodes of diagnosed STIs by diagnosis, sex, age group and homosexual acquisition for selected infections in males. Since clinics do not serve defined catchment populations KC60 aggregate data is of limited use below regional or national level. However the individual patient data that is aggregated to produce the KC60 returns is available from each clinic including area of residence and ethnic group. Surveillance systems based on these data are now being established.
Routine laboratory	Laboratory reporting of STIs	Laboratory reports of acute STIs from all healthcare settings by sex and age group.
Sentinel	The Gonococcal Resistance to Antimicrobials Surveillance Programme (GRASP)	Sentinel surveillance of gonococcal isolates by selected GUM clinics and laboratories, age group, sex, ethnic group, sexual orientation, previous infection, sexual lifestyle, antimicrobial susceptibility.
Enhanced	Enhanced syphilis surveillance	GUM clinics in E&W, reports of infectious syphilis, age group, sex, ethnic group, sexual behaviour and network, where infection acquired.

Outputs from these surveillance sources are published regularly by the Health Protection Agency on its website http://www.hpa.org.uk/infections/topics_az/hiv_and_sti/default.htm.

In the UK, STIs declined in the 1980s and early 1990s but have increased substantially since 1995. New attendances at GUM clinics in England, Wales and Northern Ireland doubled between 1991 and 2001. Increases in STI diagnoses slowed in 2003 but clinic workload has continued to increase.

The burden of STIs falls disproportionately on young men and women, homosexual and bisexual men and those of black ethnic origin. London has the greatest burden of STIs and the epidemiology of most STIs in London is influenced more by homosexually acquired infections than in other areas.

Increase in high risk sexual behaviour accounts for these increases in STIs and increases in condom use have been offset by even greater increases in unsafe sex.

There are major variations in the epidemiology of individual STIs with respect to the scale of the increase, the gender, age group, sexual preferences and ethnic origin of those predominantly affected and the reporting area (see Chapter 3.25).

The decreases in certain STI diagnoses seen recently in some areas and within some population subgroups may be due to sexual health promotion campaigns and other interventions, although STI surveillance data is susceptible to changes in consulting patterns, clinical practice and ascertainment factors.

Increases in STI diagnoses has put pressure on GUM clinic services especially in disadvantaged urban areas, which have the highest infection rates. This is producing marked health inequalities.

The recent epidemiology of the main STIs is summarised in Table 3.26.1.

Prevention and control of STIs

The source of STIs is controlled by early diagnosis of cases of infection and prompt effective treatment. Contacts are actively followed up and offered diagnostic testing and prophylactic antibiotics, if appropriate.

All pregnant women are screened for syphilis by serology and increasingly there is opportunistic screening for genital chlamydia infection in women at increased risk.

GUM clinics are open access clinics that offer free, confidential services and treatment for all STIs including HIV infection. A national network of GUM clinics was created as a result of the Venereal Disease Regulations 1916.

Transmission of STIs is controlled by promoting safer sexual behaviour, including condom use through education and information.

Vaccines are not available for the major STIs, but susceptible individuals and populations may be offered hepatitis A and hepatitis B immunisation.

2.8 Jaundice

Differential diagnosis

The differential diagnosis of jaundice includes many infectious and non-infectious causes (see Tables 2.8.1 and 2.8.2). In a previously well patient with acute onset of jaundice, the most likely cause is viral hepatitis.

Viral hepatitis can be clinically distinguished from other causes of jaundice by the presence of a prodrome of fever, anorexia, nausea and abdominal discomfort. The liver is often enlarged and tender. There may be a history of travel to endemic areas, contact with a case

Table 2.8.1 Non-infectious causes of jaundice

Drug reaction (paracetamol, phenothiazines, alcohol)
Recent anaesthetic
Haemolysis (e.g. due to G6PD deficiency, sickle cell disease)
Physiological (in the neonate)
Toxin causing liver damage
Primary biliary cirrhosis
Gallstones
Biliary or pancreatic cancer
Genetic disorders

Table 2.8.2 Infectious causes of jaundice

Common
  Viral hepatitis
  Malaria
Uncommon
  Acute infections of the biliary system
    (cholecystitis, cholangitis, pancreatitis)
  Leptospirosis
  Epstein–Barr virus infection
  Cytomegalovirus
  Yellow fever

or high-risk behaviour. Bilirubin is present in the urine, and serum transaminase levels (ALT, AST) are markedly elevated.

In viral hepatitis, the fever usually subsides once jaundice has developed. If the fever persists, other liver infections should be considered, such as Epstein–Barr virus or leptospirosis.

Laboratory investigations to distinguish between the different types of viral hepatitis and other liver infections are covered in the relevant chapters.

Prevention and control

General measures for the prevention of gastrointestinal infection (Chapter 2.2) and blood-borne virus infection (Chapter 2.10) will help prevent jaundice due to viral hepatitis. Malaria prophylaxis is covered in Chapter 3.46. Vaccines are available for hepatitis A (Chapter 3.30), hepatitis B (Chapter 3.31) and yellow fever (Chapter 3.88).

Response to a case

Determine whether infectious or non-infectious cause. No specific public health measures are needed for non-infectious causes. For infectious causes, specific measures will usually be indicated, depending upon the causal agent. Assume blood, body fluids and (until 1 week after start of jaundice) stools are infectious until cause known.

Investigation of a cluster and response to an outbreak

Investigate to determine whether infectious or non-infectious cases. For non-infectious cases, consider common toxic exposure. For infectious cases, the response will depend upon the causal agent.

2.9 Infection in the immunocompromised

It has become increasingly common for patients to have impaired immunity due to, e.g., ageing, treatments or underlying disease. Infection should always be considered when an immunocompromised person becomes unwell; the risk of infection by both common and unusual pathogens is increased and infection may present in unusual ways in unusual sites.

Particular opportunistic infections may be associated with specific immune defects (e.g. invasive aspergillosis with neutropenia and intracellular organisms with T-cell defects), therefore knowledge of the immune defect may guide preventative measures, investigation and therapy. Treating infection in the immunocompromised is highly specialised; this chapter concentrates upon issues that might be of concern to a public health specialist.

Epidemiology

Organism and syndrome(s)

Infections with common organisms usually respond to routine treatment. Of major concern is infection with antibiotic-resistant or unusual organisms that may not be recognised. Immunocompromised patients are often exposed to healthcare facilities, and to courses of antimicrobials, and are therefore at increased risk of infection with resistant organisms.

The major public health role is in identifying and ensuring systems are in place to minimise the risk of infection in the immunocompromised. Activities can be considered by cause of compromise or by preventative action.

Causes of immunosuppression

• Physiological: extremes of age.
• Impaired anatomical barriers, e.g. burns, catheters, intubation.
• Impaired cellular or host defence: genetic or acquired, underlying malignancy, chronic infection, immunosuppressive drugs.

Specific causes of immunosuppression and public health issues

Underlying conditions

HIV

Associated infections: *Pneumocystis*, TB, *Cryptosporidium*, CMV.

HIV-positive patients are particularly at risk when they associate with other immunocompromised patients in healthcare surroundings. Services should be organised to minimise transmission of likely pathogens, in particular TB. Outbreaks of resistant TB associated with healthcare have occurred.

Post-splenectomy

Associated infections: capsulate bacteria, malaria.

Post-splenectomy or as a consequence of hyposplenism, patients are at risk of infection from capsulate bacteria, particularly *Streptococcus pneumoniae*, *Neisseria meningitidis*, *Haemophilus influenzae*. Asplenic children under 5 years, especially those with sickle cell anaemia or splenectomized for trauma, have an infection rate of over 10%. Most infections occur in the first 2 years following splenectomy; however, the increased risk of dying of serious infection is almost certainly lifelong.

Splenectomized patients and those with functional hyposplenism should receive (asplenia is not a contraindication to routine immunisation) the following:

• Pneumococcal immunisation.
• *H. influenzae* type b vaccine (if not already immune).
• Conjugate meningococcal group C immunisation.
• Influenza immunisation.
• Prophylactic antibiotics, probably lifelong (oral phenoxy-methylpenicillin or an alternative).

Asplenic patients are at risk of severe malaria, so the importance of preventive measures should be stressed for travellers.

Patients should carry a card to alert health professionals to their risk of overwhelming infection. Splenectomized patients developing infection despite measures must be given a systemic antibiotic and urgently admitted to hospital.

Prevention of infection in the immunocompromised

Prevention through immunisation

• Pneumococcal infection
• *H. influenzae*
• Influenza
• Meningococcal C
• Varicella vaccine for close nonimmune contacts of immunocompromised where continuing contact is unavoidable (e.g. sibling of a child with leukaemia)

Note: Live vaccines are contraindicated in many immunocompromised patients.

Avoid giving live vaccines (except MMR and BCG) to siblings of immunocompromised patients. Immunoconpromised children should avoid close physical contact with children vaccinated with OPV for 4–6 weeks following administration (this does not require school withdrawal).

Prevention through prophylaxis

• Pneumocystis (oral trimethoprim/sulphamethoxazole)
• Malaria chemoprophylaxis
• Penicillin in hyposplenism

Prevention through managing the environment

Boiling water: the Bouchier Report of 1998 on *Cryptosporidium* in water supplies clarifies which groups are at particular risk of *Cryptosporidium* infection. Patients with T-cell deficiency are advised to boil their drinking water. This group includes
• HIV-positive patients with a low T-cell count,
• children with severe combined immunodeficiency (SCID) and
• others with specific T-cell deficiencies.

Fungal infection and building work

Outbreaks of fungal infection have been associated with building work occurring close to healthcare areas that immunocompromised patients have frequented. Consideration to relocating services should be made if major building work is undertaken.

Reducing exposure

Treatment of TB and HIV-positive: examining the geographical layout of services so that infected and at-risk patients do not come into contact.

Avoid healthcare staff who are zoster susceptibles working with immunocompromised individuals, or vaccinate nonimmune healthcare workers.

Travel advice

Immunocompromised patients are at increased risk of travel-related infection. Asplenic patients are at risk of severe malaria, and patients with AIDS are at risk from GI parasites. Advising such patients requires detailed knowledge of the epidemiology of disease in the area they are planning to visit and the underlying cause of immunosuppression.

Laboratory diagnosis

A search for infection, including blood and urine cultures and a chest X-ray, will be necessary as soon as an immunocompromised patient spikes a fever. Opportunistic organisms that do not cause disease in the immunocompetent must be sought, but it should be remembered that immunocompromised patients are most often infected by common pathogens.

Surveillance

All units treating significant numbers of immunocompromised patients should have ongoing surveillance of infection in place, and be aware of the risk of outbreaks in the patient population.

Investigation of a cluster

Clusters of infection in the immunocompromised should be investigated with urgency. A cluster suggests a group of vulnerable people exposed to a common source, e.g. fungal spores following building work near a ward containing immunocompromised patients, or exposure on a unit for HIV-positive individuals to a case of open TB.

Control of an outbreak

- Rapid removal of any source.
- If necessary closure of a ward if environmental contamination is feared.

2.10 Blood-borne viral infections

Human immunodeficiency virus, hepatitis B and hepatitis C are the main blood-borne viruses of public health importance. These are covered in detail in individual chapters.

Preventing exposure in the health and social care workplace

Health and social care workers should work safely to prevent occupational exposure to blood-borne viruses. The precautions shown in Table 2.10.1 are recommended:

Table 2.10.1 Preventing occupational exposure to blood-borne viruses in the health and social care workplace

Handle and dispose of sharps safely	Avoid using needles and sharp instruments if possible. Handle sharps safely, and do not re-sheath needles. Dispose of sharps in a container that conforms to UN Standard 3291 and British Standard 7320. Do not overfill the container. Where available use innovative products that reduce the risk of sharps injuries.
Managing blood and body fluids: spillages	Clean up spillages of blood immediately, and follow written workplace policy. Open wounds must be covered with a waterproof dressing. Wear gloves and apron. Use scoop for broken glass. Cover spillage with chlorine-releasing granules to soak up the spillage or use paper towels and sodium hypochlorite (10,000 ppm available chlorine). Use *spillage kit* if available.
Collection and transport of specimens	Follow written policy. Use personal protective equipment (PPE) as appropriate. Only staff who have been trained should collect and handle specimens. Ensure specimens are transported in accordance with *Safe Transport of Dangerous Goods Act 1999*.
Prevention of exposure to infection and use of personal protective equipment (PPE)	Avoid puncture wounds, cuts and abrasions in the presence of blood. Protect eyes, mouth and nose from blood splashes. Use PPE including gloves, plastic aprons, impermeable gowns, protective eyewear and masks.

Continued on p. 46

Table 2.10.1 (*Continued*)

Dispose of waste safely	Health and social care staff should have a written policy on waste and should be instructed in the safe handling and disposal of waste. Clinical waste is defined in the Controlled Waste Regulations 1992 as waste that arises from the treatment of humans or animals and is capable of causing infection or other harm. It includes human and animal tissue, blood, surgical dressings, syringes, surgical implements, microbiological cultures, bodily waste and some pharmaceutical products and chemical waste. Clinical waste has been further classified into five categories (Health Services Advisory Committee, *Safe Disposal of Clinical Waste,* HSE Books, 1999, ISBN 0 7176 2492 7). Healthcare workers who produce waste are bound by a duty of care imposed by Section 34 of the Environmental Protection Act 1990 and the Environmental Protection (Duty of Care) Regulations 1991 in the UK. Producers of waste should conduct a local risk assessment to determine the most appropriate storage, collection, transport and disposal arrangements for the waste. Guidelines (Environment Agency, *Technical Guidance On Clinical Waste Management Facilities*, July 2003) should be followed.
Decontaminating equipment including cleaning, disinfection and sterilisation	Best practice advice on decontamination of medical equipment is available on the Medicines and Healthcare Products Regulatory Agency (MHRA) website http://www.mhra.gov.uk and the decontamination section of the NHS Estates Authority website http://www.decontamination.nhsestates.gov.uk. Wherever possible single-use disposable devices should be used. Re-usable medical devices should be decontaminated in a sterile services department (SSD). An automated process should be used whenever possible. If devices have to be cleaned manually this should be done away from clinical areas. Staff must be properly trained and supervised and should wear PPE. Dedicated equipment and receptacles should be used. The instructions of the device manufacturer should be followed including choice, use and compatibility of decontaminants and dismantling and re-assembly of instruments. Ensure that water used is of a suitable quality, at the correct temperature and avoid producing aerosols. Sterilisers should be correctly sited and maintained and used according to manufacturer's specification. Household bleach is usually supplied at a strength of 100,000 ppm free chlorine. Adding one part bleach to nine parts cold water gives a solution for disinfecting blood and body fluids (10,000 ppm). For general use, such as disinfecting work surfaces, a 1000 ppm solution of bleach is adequate (i.e. 1 in 100 dilution of household bleach). Undiluted Milton is equivalent to a strength of 10,000 ppm. All dilutions become ineffective with time and should be freshly made up every day.
Manage linen safely	Blood-stained linen should not be sorted but should be placed in a water-soluble primary bag. This in turn should be placed within a secondary bag for storage and transport. The washing programme should include a disinfection cycle. Guidelines are available (HSG (95)18: Hospital laundry arrangements for used and infected linen, Department of Health 1995.

Management of blood exposure incidents

Following a needlestick or other sharps injury (from an infected patient) the risk of HIV infection is 0.3%. The risk of HCV is 3% and the risk of HBV is 30%. The risk of acquiring HIV infection from a mucous membrane exposure is less than 0.1%.

Action following a sharps injury, a blood splash or other exposure incident

There should be a written policy detailing the local arrangements for risk assessment, advice, the provision of post-exposure prophylaxis and follow-up. The policy should designate one or more doctors to whom exposed persons may be referred urgently for advice and should ensure that adequate 24-hour cover is available. Primary responsibility usually rests with the occupational health service, with out-of-hours cover provided by accident and emergency departments. These arrangements should be included in the programme of mandatory staff training.

The action to be taken is summarised as follows:
• Follow recognised first-aid procedures. The injured area should be encouraged to bleed and washed with soap and water.
• Wounds should be cleaned, sutured and dressed as appropriate. Tetanus toxoid should be administered if indicated.
• A risk assessment should be carried out based on the type of body fluid involved, the route and severity of the exposure and the likelihood that the source patient has a blood-borne viral infection.
• The source patient should be asked to consent to testing for HIV, HBV and HCV.
• If appropriate the exposed person should be offered post-exposure prophylaxis (PEP) for HBV and/or HIV. There is currently no PEP for HCV.
• A baseline blood sample should be taken from the exposed person for storage. A follow-up blood sample should be taken for testing at 6 months.
• Healthcare providers should follow local policies on reporting occupational exposures.

Some types of occupational exposure are required to be reported under the Reporting of Injuries, Diseases and Dangerous Occurrences (RIDDOR) legislation.
• Use of these post-exposure procedures should be considered in the event of a bleed-back incident from a healthcare worker to a patient. Use of these procedures following exposures outside the healthcare setting is controversial.

Employment policies

In the UK, guidelines for healthcare workers with blood-borne viral infections who carry out *exposure-prone procedures* have been published.

Exposure-prone procedures are those in which there is a risk that injury to the healthcare worker could result in exposure of the patient's open tissues to the blood of the healthcare worker. Such procedures occur mainly in surgery, obstetrics and gynaecology, dentistry and midwifery.

HIV infected healthcare workers are not permitted to carry out exposure prone procedures.

Hepatitis B infected healthcare workers who are e-antigen positive and those that are e-antigen negative but have HBV DNA levels above 10^3 genome equivalents/mL are routinely restricted from performing exposure-prone procedures.

Healthcare workers who have antibodies to hepatitis C virus should be tested for hepatitis C virus RNA. Those found to be positive should not perform exposure-prone procedures.

Draft guidelines (Department of Health. Health Clearance for Serious Communicable Diseases: New Health Care Workers. Draft guidance for consultation, January 2003) propose that all new healthcare workers who will perform exposure-prone procedures should have health clearance for HIV, HCV and HBV in addition to TB.

All staff undertaking exposure-prone procedures should be immunised against HBV and have their immune status confirmed. All other staff at risk of blood-borne infections should ensure that they are fully immunised against HBV.

Advice for people living with blood-borne viral infections

All persons found to be infected with a blood-borne virus should be considered potentially infectious and should be counselled concerning infectivity. The following advice should be given:
• Keep cuts or grazes covered with a waterproof plaster until the skin has healed.
• Avoid sharing your razor or toothbrush (or anything which might cut the skin or damage the gums and cause bleeding). Use your own towel and face cloth.
• If you cut yourself, wipe up any blood with paper tissues and flush these down the toilet. Wipe any surfaces where blood has been spilt with household bleach diluted in cold water (1 part bleach to 10 parts water). Do not use this on your skin or on any fabrics. In these circumstances wash thoroughly with soap and water.
• Tell any helpers that you are a carrier of a blood-borne virus and that blood precautions should be taken. If available they should wear plastic gloves. Otherwise they can use a towel or cloth to prevent them from getting blood on to their skin.
• If your clothing is soiled with blood or other body fluids, wash them using a pre-wash and hot washing machine cycle.
• Dispose of used tampons straight away by flushing down the toilet. Dispose of sanitary towels in your rubbish after first sealing inside a plastic bag.
• If you go for medical or dental treatment, tell your doctor or dentist you have a blood-borne viral infection.
• Do not donate blood or carry an organ donor card.
• Do not have acupuncture, tattooing, ear piercing or electrolysis.
• If you are an injecting drug user do not share your works and dispose of used needles and syringes safely by putting then in a rigid container with a lid. If possible use a local needle exchange scheme. Return used works to the scheme in the special plastic sharps bin.
• Sexual intercourse, pregnancy and birth: See table 2.10.2.

Table 2.10.2 Advice on sexual intercourse, pregnancy and birth, for people infected with a blood-borne virus

	HCV	HBV	HIV
Sexual intercourse	If you are in a stable relationship with one partner you may not feel the need to start using condoms; however, it is advisable to avoid sexual intercourse during a menstrual period. Otherwise condom use should be encouraged and safe sex should continue to be promoted for the prevention of HIV and other sexually transmitted infections.	Condom use recommended until sexual partners are immunised against HBV and have had immunity confirmed.	Condom use recommended.
Pregnancy and birth	The risk of transmission from mother to child appears to be very low. At the present time there is no need to advise against pregnancy based on HCV status alone. Mothers who are viraemic should not breastfeed.	All babies of HBsAg positive mothers should receive hepatitis B vaccine. Those whose mothers are e-antigen positive, HBsAg positive without e-markers (or where e-marker status has not been determined) or had acute hepatitis during pregnancy also require HBIG.	The risk of transmission from mother to child can be reduced by anti-viral treatment in pregnancy, caesarean section and by avoiding breastfeeding.

If you have HCV infection you should limit weekly alcohol consumption to less than 21 units for women and 28 units for men.

Blood-borne viral infections are not infectious under normal school or work conditions. There is no need to stay away from school or work.

2.11 Vaccine queries

Vaccine queries are very common; answering them can generate significant work for the public health practitioner. Those who administer vaccines often receive little or no training on the subject and may rely heavily on the local public health team for support. The questions in this chapter are a selection of those commonly encountered in public health practice. The following websites may be helpful:

- http://www.immunisation.org.uk/faqs.php
- http://www.mmrthefacts.nhs.uk
- http://www.bccdc.org/content.php? item=19

Schedule

One of my patients had the first two doses of the primary schedule as a baby and has now turned up 3 years later for the third dose – do I need to restart the course?

An interrupted immunisation course should be treated as normal – there is no need to restart the course.

A baby in my practice was born at 27 weeks gestation – should I delay his/her immunisations?

It has been shown in several studies that even very premature babies mount an adequate immune response when they are vaccinated starting at 2 months. There is no need to delay.

I've got a 14-year-old patient who has never had any immunisations – is it too late to start now?

It is never too late. Your patient needs a full course of immunisation against all antigens in the national schedule (except for pertussis, which can be omitted in older children). No one should be unprotected.

I've given the first dose of DTPa-IPV-Hib vaccine to a 7-week-old baby by mistake – what should I do?

Although the response may not be optimal, DTP-containing vaccines provide adequate protection from 6 weeks of age. Complete the course at the recommended ages, no extra dose is needed.

A 6-month-old baby was born in Italy and had two injections there – what should I do to complete the course?

The immunisation schedule is different in every country. In Italy, hepatitis B is given but not Men C; other vaccines are the same as in the UK (although the timings are different). The baby will need Men C (three doses) and one more dose of DTPa-IPV-Hib (this could be given as DTPa-IPV-Hib-Hep B, available from the manufacturer, which would complete the hepatitis B course). The WHO publishes immunisation schedules for different countries; see http://www .who.int/vaccines-surveillance/intro.html.

Contraindications

A patient has had a severe reaction to a tetanus booster – does this mean he/she can't have any more?

A further booster would only be indicated if the patient has a tetanus-prone wound more than 10 years later. In this situation it would be OK to give the booster provided there are facilities to deal with a severe reaction.

I've got a patient who is highly allergic to eggs – are there any vaccines he/she can't have?

Non-anaphylactic allergic reactions are not a contraindication to any vaccine. Yellow fever and influenza vaccines should not be given to people with egg anaphylaxis. There is now evidence that MMR can be given to children with severe egg allergy, including anaphylaxis.

MMR

Is there any harm in giving the MMR vaccine as separate injections?

None of the separate components are licensed in the UK, so the vaccine quality or transportation conditions cannot be guaranteed. Separating the vaccines just delays completing the course.

One of my patients is worried about his child having the MMR vaccine and would like a blood test to see if it's needed – can he/she have this?

There is no point in having a blood test, because even if he/she is immune now it does not mean immunity will be lifelong. Having a test will only cause delay.

I've heard the MMR vaccines contain pork – what should I tell my Muslim patients? *Porcine material is used in the manufacturing process of some MMR vaccines, but is undetectable in the final product. Muslim leaders are aware of this and support the use of MMR vaccine.*

One of my patients developed a rash and a temperature after the first dose of MMR vaccine. Is it safe to give the second dose?

Yes – a mild version of measles is a common side effect of MMR and usually resolves spontaneously. Reactions are less common after the second dose as most children will have developed antibodies that neutralise the vaccine virus.

Travel

One of my patients is off to India tomorrow – is it too late to give any vaccines?

Most vaccines will provide reasonable protection within 2 weeks even after a single dose. Give vaccines as appropriate, but advise that protection will not be optimal.

I've got an HIV positive patient who is going on a trip to Africa and Asia – are there any vaccines he can't have?

Yellow fever and BCG vaccines should not be given; a letter of exemption from yellow fever may be required. Give IPV instead of OPV. All other vaccines can be given.

Occupational

I've given two complete courses of hepatitis B vaccine to a nurse but she still hasn't got any antibodies – what should I do?

Some adults are non-responders. Check for HBsAg carriage (if positive, may need to exclude from undertaking exposure-prone procedures). Consider giving a higher dose vaccine (specifically licensed for haemodialysis patients). May need HBIG if a needlestick injury is sustained.

A student nurse had a chickenpox vaccine last week, and now has a vesicular rash – does she need to be off work?

If the rash is localised and a vaccine reaction suspected, the rash should be covered and the nurse can continue to work, unless in contact with high-risk patients (risk assessment needed). If the rash is generalised the nurse should avoid patient contact until all the lesions have crusted.

Storage and administration errors

I came into the surgery this morning and found the cleaner had unplugged the fridge – are the vaccines still OK?

Vaccines are able to survive temperatures outside normal fridge limits for a limited period of time (up to 1 week). The manufacturer should be able to provide more advice on a specific vaccine. If in doubt it is better to discard the vaccines and order more.

Someone turned the fridge up and the vaccines are now frozen – are they still OK?

No – freezing causes irreversible deterioration of the vaccine. Discard and order more.

I've given an adult dose of hepatitis A vaccine to a child – what should I do?

The risk of a vaccine reaction is normally not dose-related, so continue the vaccine course as normal and reassure. In the UK, the incident should be reported to the Committee on Safety of Medicines via a yellow card.

I've given a vaccine that is out of date – do I need to repeat the dose?

There is usually some margin of error (up to a month) for out-of-date vaccine administration – consult the manufacturer. If in doubt repeat the dose.

Other

Which vaccines contain thiomersal?

Some influenza and hepatitis B vaccines contain traces of thiomersal used in the manufacturing process. None of the childhood vaccines in the UK schedule contain thiomersal.

I've got a family of asylum seekers in my practice and they have no medical records. What vaccinations do they need?

Assume they are unimmunised and give a full course of immunisations according to the national schedule. Consider also hepatitis B.

I've heard that babies in America get a pneumococcal vaccine – why don't they get it here?

Can I get the vaccine even though it's not recommended?

The Department of Health is still considering whether routine immunisation is justified in the UK (selective immunisation is already recommended). The manufacturer may be able to supply the vaccine, please contact them directly.

Useful guidance on immunisation of immunocompromised children can be found at: http://www.rcpch.ac.uk/publications/recent_publications/Immunocomp.pdf.

Section 3
Diseases

3.1 Amoebic dysentery

Infection by the protozoan parasite *Entamoeba histolytica* usually presents as an intestinal infection, which may include dysentery.

Suggested on-call action

- Exclude cases in high-risk groups for transmission of gastrointestinal infections (Box 2.2.1).
- If other non-travel related cases known to you or reporting laboratory/clinician, consult local outbreak plan.

Epidemiology

Although much more common in tropical countries, amoebiasis does occur in Europe: approximately 200 cases a year are reported in the UK. Infection is most common in young adults but is unusual in pre-school children, especially infants. Increased risk is reported in institutions for the mentally handicapped, amongst gay men and in travellers to developing countries.

Clinical features

Intestinal infection may be asymptomatic; an intermittent diarrhoea with abdominal pain; amoebic colitis presenting as bloody diarrhoea; and a fulminant colitis with significant mortality in the malnourished, pregnant, immunosuppressed or very young. Extraintestinal disease includes liver, lung and brain abscesses.

Laboratory confirmation

The diagnosis is confirmed by demonstrating either the trophozoites or cysts of *E. histolytica* on microscopy of very fresh stool samples. Three specimens are required to exclude amoebiasis. Many cysts are non-pathogenic (often called *Entamoeba dispar*) but morphologically indistinguishable from *E. histolytica*: immunological and isoenzyme ('zymodeme') differences can be used by reference laboratories to identify these organisms. Invasive disease may be diagnosed by serology.

Transmission

E. histolytica is predominantly spread by environmentally resistant cysts excreted in human faeces. Transmission may occur via contaminated water or food, or direct faeco–oral contact. Cysts resist standard water chlorination. Acute cases pose only limited risk.

Acquisition

The incubation period is usually 2–4 weeks, but a range of a few days to years has been reported. The infectious period depends upon the excretion of cysts in the stool and may last several years. In acute dysentery only trophozoites are passed in the stool; these die within minutes in the environment. Recovered patients appear to be immune to re-infection in almost all cases.

Prevention

- Avoidance of faecal contamination of water supplies, combined with adequate water treatment (e.g. filtration).
- Good personal, toilet and food hygiene.
- Care with food and water for travellers in developing countries.
- Sterilisation of reusable colonic or rectal equipment (e.g. colonic irrigation or medical investigation).

Surveillance

- Cases should be reported to the local public health department: notify as 'dysentery' in UK.
- Laboratory isolates should also be reported to national surveillance systems.

Response to a case

• Exclude cases in groups at increased risk of spreading infection (see Box 2.2.1) until 48 hours after first normal stool. Risk groups 1 and 2 should have one negative faecal sample taken one week after end of treatment before return to work
• If no history of travel abroad, then obtain detailed food history for the period of 2–4 weeks before onset, including drinking water.
• Enteric precautions. Hygiene advice to case and household.
• Screen household or institutional contacts. Discuss with microbiologist for further investigation of positives. Consider treatment for those with prolonged excretion of pathogenic cysts, especially if in risk group for spreading infection.

Investigation of a cluster

• Check to ensure that infection is not due to travelling abroad: inform relevant national centre if associated with particular country.
• Organise further testing to ensure that reported cases have infection with pathogenic *E. histolytica*.
• For symptomatic cases, obtain detailed food and water consumption history for the period of 2–4 weeks before onset of symptoms. Check home/work/travel against water supply areas.
• Look for links with institutions with potential for faeco–oral spread, e.g. young adults with learning difficulties or camps with poor hygiene facilities.
• Consider transmission between gay men.

Control of an outbreak

• Rarely a problem in developed countries. Response will depend upon source identified.
• Enteric precautions for cases and carriers. Exclusion of those in risk groups (Box 2.2.1). Consider treatment if confirmed as *E. histolytica*. Ensure that treatment includes an agent that eliminates cysts (e.g. diloxanide).

• Sanitary disposal of faeces, handwashing, food hygiene and regular cleaning of toilet and kitchen areas.

Suggested case definition for an outbreak

Demonstration of trophozoites or diarrhoea and demonstration of cysts.

3.2 Anthrax

Anthrax is a potentially serious infection caused by *Bacillus anthracis*, an organism that forms spores that may survive for many years. There are concerns that it is a potential bioterrorism agent.

Suggested on-call action

• Ensure that the case is admitted and treated.
• Identify likely source of exposure and other individuals who may have been exposed.
• Ensure exposed individuals are clinically assessed.

Epidemiology

Anthrax is a zoonosis, acquired from contact with infected herbivores or their products, which has been eliminated from the UK and most of northern Europe. There are rare sporadic cases in the UK, usually resulting from occupational exposure, in particular to animal carcasses, hides, hair and wool. There is occasional concern about renovating old buildings where animal hair may have been used in the construction, although these have not been associated with cases.

Anthrax is endemic in many parts of the world, such as the Middle East, Africa and the former Soviet Union. In these areas it is usually a disease of rural herdsmen. Imported infection is rare. Inhalational and intestinal diseases are rare.

Clinical features

The clinical manifestations are dependent upon the route of infection:

Cutaneous anthrax (over 90% of cases): infection is through the skin. Over a few days a sore, which begins as a pimple, grows, ulcerates and forms a black scab, around which are purplish vesicles. There may be associated oedema. Systemic symptoms include rigors, headache and vomiting. The sore is usually diagnostic; 20% of cases are fatal.

Inhalation/pulmonary anthrax: spores are inhaled, with subsequent invasion of mediastinal lymph nodes. An abrupt onset of flu-like illness, rigors, dyspnoea and cyanosis is followed by shock and usually death over the next 2–6 days.

Intestinal anthrax occurs following ingestion of spores, with severe gut disease, nausea, vomiting, anorexia, fever and then septicaemia.

Pulmonary and intestinal disease are usually recognised late and have worse outcomes.

Laboratory confirmation

Swabs from cutaneous lesions, nasal swabs (in inhalational anthrax suspected), blood cultures, lymph node or spleen aspirates, or CSF (if meningitic) show characteristic bacilli on staining with polychrome methylene blue. Colonies may be grown overnight. The definitive test for *B. anthracis* is polymerase chain reaction (PCR).

Transmission

Transmission is usually from contact with contaminated material, such as animal carcasses, hair, wool, hides or bone meal. Spores can remain viable in the soil for many years. Transmission may be by direct contact, inhalation or ingestion (e.g., of spores in meat). There is no recorded person-to-person spread via the inhalational route.

Acquisition

The incubation period varies with disease type: inhalation anthrax 1–7 days, usually within 48 hours; cutaneous anthrax 1–7 days, rarely up to 7 weeks; ingestion 1–7 days.

Secretions from cutaneous lesions may be infectious. Environmental spores may be infectious for decades.

Prevention

• Pretreatment of animal products, and good occupational health cover are the mainstays of control.
• Animals believed to have died of anthrax should be disposed of under supervision. Mass vaccination of animals may reduce disease spread.
• Noncellular vaccines for human use are available for individuals at risk from occupational exposure, such as veterinarians working in endemic areas, zoos, etc. Workers handling potentially infectious raw material should be aware of the risks. In the event of a deliberate release, individual risk would be assessed on a case-by-case basis. Post-exposure prophylaxis with antibiotics can be very effective in preventing disease, if given early enough.

Surveillance

In most countries, including the UK, anthrax is a notifiable disease. Cases should be reported on clinical suspicion as a matter of urgency.

A suspected case includes any previously healthy person with:
• rapid onset of severe, unexplained febrile illness or febrile death,
• rapid onset of severe sepsis not due to a predisposing illness, or respiratory failure with a widened mediastinum and
• severe sepsis with Gram-positive rods or *Bacillus* species identified in the blood or CSF and assessed not to be a contaminant.

Anthrax should be immediately reported to the local Public Health Authorities. Also report to national authorities.

Response to a case

- Set up incident team.
- Remove potentially contaminated clothes to reduce possibility of secondary cutaneous cases. Instruct exposed persons to shower thoroughly. Use standard universal precautions for care.
- Investigate source: search for history of potentially infected animals or animal products (e.g. hide, wool, hair, bones) and trace to place of origin. May need to liaise with veterinary officers. Particularly enquire as to travel and occupational exposure – include exposure to mail.
- Consider bioterrorism if
  (i) single confirmed case of inhalational anthrax;
  (ii) single confirmed case of cutaneous anthrax in individual with no contact with animals or animal hides;
  (iii) two or more suspected cases linked in time and place.
- Initial therapy of inhalational anthrax should be with Ciprofloxacin 400 mg i.v. every 12 hours or Doxycycline 100 mg every 12 hours plus additional antibiotics (rifampicin, vancomycin, chloramphenicol, penicillin, amoxicillin, imipenem, clindamycin, clarithromycin). Benzyl penicillin or amoxicillin should not be used alone.
- Other possible contacts of the source should be identified and placed under clinical surveillance for 7 days since last exposure.
- Contacts of cases are not at risk.

Investigation of a cluster

Check for history of exposure in endemic countries. If none
- undertake full hypothesis-generating study, using semi-structured interviews of all cases and re-interviewing as potential sources identified by other cases. Include full occupational history;

- institute case-finding, both locally and nationally;
- consider bioterrorism.

Control of an outbreak

- Trace exposure as a matter of urgency.
- Remove source.

Response to a deliberate release

- Report to local and national public health authorities.
- Define exposed zone and identify individuals exposed within it (some may have left scene).
- Cordon off exposed zone.
- Decontaminate those exposed: remove clothing and possessions, then shower with soap and water.
- Chemoprophylaxis (currently ciprofloxacin) as soon as possible for those exposed.
- Record contact details for all those exposed.
- Some health and emergency workers may also need prophylaxis.
- Police may take environmental samples.

More general information is given in Chapter 4.14 and specific information on HPA website.

Suggested case definition

Suspected
- Rapid onset of severe, unexplained febrile illness or febrile death.
- Rapid onset of severe sepsis not due to a predisposing illness, or respiratory failure with a widened mediastinum.
- Severe sepsis with Gram-positive rods or *Bacillus* species identified in the blood or CSF and assessed not to be a contaminant.
Confirmed case
A case that clinically fits the criteria for suspected anthrax, and in addition, definitive positive results are obtained on one or more pathological specimens by the reference laboratory.

3.3 *Bacillus cereus*

Bacillus cereus is a rare cause of food poisoning that manifests as one of two mild gastrointestinal syndromes. It is not spread from person to person.

Suggested on-call action
If you or reporting clinician/microbiologist know of associated cases, consult Outbreak Control Plan.

Epidemiology

B. cereus food poisoning occurs worldwide but is rare in the UK, accounting for up to 100 reported cases each year and around 0.2% of sporadic gastroenteritis cases presenting to general practitioners. A much higher incidence has been reported from Hungary, Netherlands and Finland. Reported outbreaks are usually linked to institutions, including restaurants, schools and hospitals.

Clinical features

Two clinical syndromes may occur, caused by different toxins:

(i) A short incubation illness consisting of vomiting accompanied by nausea, abdominal pain and, occasionally, diarrhoea later. This is usually a mild illness, which lasts less than 12 hours and is difficult to distinguish from staphylococcal food poisoning.

(ii) A short-medium incubation illness consisting of diarrhoea usually accompanied by abdominal pain and perhaps tenesmus, nausea or vomiting. Diarrhoea may be profuse and watery and lasts around 24 hours. It is difficult to distinguish clinically from *Clostridium perfringens* food poisoning.

Laboratory confirmation

B. cereus may be cultured from stool or vomit samples but is also found in a small number of healthy controls. It may be cultured from suspect foods; however, large numbers (e.g. $>10^5$/g) are necessary to prove that food was the source of infection. Serotyping is available to compare strains from different cases or with food isolates; however, more than one strain can be associated with an individual outbreak. Phage typing may also be available. Reference laboratories can test the potential of the isolate for toxin production.

Transmission

B. cereus is ubiquitous in the environment and is found at low levels in many raw, dried or processed foods. Contamination of food may easily occur prior to cooking and spores can survive normal cooking. Cell growth occurs between 10 and 50°C (optimum 28–35°C) and so storage of food at ambient temperature after cooking allows multiplication of the organism. *B. cereus* produces two toxins: a heat-stable emetic toxin associated with the short incubation vomiting illness and a heat-labile enterotoxin associated with the longer incubation diarrhoeal illness. Both toxins occur preformed in food, but the latter may also be produced in the gut after ingestion.

Many outbreaks of *B. cereus* vomiting have been linked to the method of making fried rice employed in Chinese restaurants. The rice is boiled, allowed to drain at room temperature (to avoid clumping), stored and then flash-fried at insufficient temperature to destroy preformed heat-stable toxin. Attack rates of near 100% have been reported from such outbreaks.

Other reported food vehicles include pasta dishes, vanilla sauce, cream, meatballs, boiled beef, barbecue chicken and turkey loaf. Attack rates of 50–75% are reported for these outbreaks.

Nosocomial infection and cases in intravenous drug users have also been reported.

Acquistion

The incubation period is approximately 2–3 hours (range 1–6 hours) for the vomiting illness and 8–12 hours (range 6–24 hours) for the diarrhoeal syndrome. *B. cereus* is not considered communicable from person to person because of the high infectious dose required, which is about 10^5/g. People at increased risk of severe infection include those with sickle-cell disease, patients with intravascular catheters, intravenous drug users and those with immunosuppressive or debilitating medical conditions.

Prevention

• Store cooked foods at above 60°C or below 10°C before re-heating or consumption.
• Limit storage time and re-heat thoroughly.

Surveillance

• Infection by *B. cereus* should be reported to local public health departments (in the UK, notify as 'food poisoning') and to national surveillance systems.
• Ensure laboratories test for *B. cereus* when an increase in cases of vomiting or diarrhoea with abdominal pain is noted.

Response to a case

• Collect data on food consumption in 24 hours before onset of symptoms. Ask particularly about meals out of the house.
• Although secondary spread of *B. cereus* does not occur, it is prudent to exclude risk groups with diarrhoea or vomiting until 48 hours after recovery. Microbiological clearance is not necessary before return.
• No need to screen contacts unless as part of an outbreak investigation.

Response to a cluster

• Discuss further investigation, e.g. serotyping and toxin production, with microbiologist.
• Undertake hypothesis-generating study covering food histories particularly restaurants, social functions and other mass catering arrangements.

Control of an outbreak

Identify and rectify faults with temperature control in food preparation processes.

> **Suggested case definition for an outbreak**
>
> *Clinical:* Either
> • vomiting occurring 1–6 hours *or*
> • diarrhoea occurring 6–24 hours
> after exposure to potential source.
>
> *Confirmed*: As above plus *B. cereus* of correct serotype cultured from stool or vomit.

3.4 Botulism

Botulism is caused by a neurotoxin produced by *Clostridium botulinum*. In Europe its main significance is as a rare cause of food-borne infection with a potentially high mortality: one suspected case warrants immediate investigation. It is also a potential bioterrorism agent and a cause of severe illness in intravenous drug users.

> **Suggested on-call action**
>
> A suspected case of botulism should be viewed as an emergency for investigation:
> • Ensure that the case is admitted to hospital
> • Obtain food history as a matter of urgency
> • Obtain suspect foods
> • Identify others at risk
> • Inform appropriate local and national authorities
> More details are given later in section Response to a Case.
>   If deliberate release suspected: see section Response to Deliberate Release at end of this chapter.

Box 3.4.1 *Bacillus subtilis –licheniformis* **group**

Recently recognised food-borne pathogens transmitted via inadequate post-cooking temperature control of foods such as meat or vegetable pastry products, cooked meat or poultry products, bakery products, sandwiches and ethnic meat/seafood dishes.

    B. subtilis causes a predominantly emetic illness with an incubation of 10 minutes to 14 hours (median = 2.5 hours) and *B. licheniformis* a predominantly diarrhoeal illness with incubation period of 2–14 hours (median 8 hours). *B. amyloliquifacians* and *B pumilis* are rarely reported.

    Investigation and control measures are similar to *B. cereus*.

Epidemiology

Only two cases of food-borne botulism were notified in England and Wales during 1994–2003, although an outbreak affecting 26 people occurred in 1989. Reported cases of botulism are more common in Italy (40 cases per annum), Germany (15) and Spain (10). The age–sex and ethnic distribution of cases will usually reflect the consumption patterns of the implicated foods.

In recent years, cases of wound botulism have been reported in intravenous drug users in Europe. This is now the most common type of botulism in the UK and Ireland, with 47 cases reported during 2000–2003.

Infant botulism is very rare in Europe, although cases are reported from Italy and the UK.

Clinical features

The neurotoxin classically causes acute bilateral cranial neuropathies manifesting as a dry mouth, difficulty in swallowing, double vision, slurred speech and blurred vision. Symmetrical descending muscle weakness may follow, affecting upper and then lower limbs and causing shortness of breath with risk of respiratory failure. There may be initial vomiting or diarrhoea followed by constipation. There is usually no fever or sensory loss. Mortality of up to 10% is reported. Other syndromes have been confused with botulism (Table 3.4.1): deep tendon reflexes (may be present initially but diminish or disappear in ensuing days in botulism), brain scan, CSF examination, nerve conduction tests and Tensilon test for myasthenia gravis may help eliminate these other diseases.

Table 3.4.1 Differential diagnosis of botulism

Disease	Distinguishing features
Guillain–Barré and Miller–Fisher syndromes	Anteceding febrile illness, parasthesia, paralysis may be ascending, early loss of reflexes, increased CSF protein, EMG findings
Myasthenia gravis	Recurrent paralysis, sustained response to anticholinesterases, EMG findings
Stroke	Usually asymmetric paralysis, abnormal CNS image
Intoxication (carbon monoxide, organophosphates, mushrooms)	Drug detected in body fluid
Tick paralysis	Parathesias, ascending paralysis, tick bite (or tick in-situ)
Poliomyelitis	Anteceding febrile illness, asymmetric paralysis, CSF changes
Viral syndrome	No bulbar palsies or flaccid paralysis
Psychiatric illness	EMG findings
Paralytic shellfish poisoning	Food history (onset <1 h), parasthesia

C. botulinum may also cause infant (intestinal) botulism and wound botulism, both of which also produce a similar picture of descending flaccid paralysis.

Laboratory confirmation

Urgent confirmation of the diagnosis is important. The toxin may be detected in serum, faeces, vomit, gastric fluid or food. The organism may also be cultured from faeces, gastric fluid and food. The aid of the relevant reference laboratory should be enlisted and suspect foods (or drugs) and clinical specimens sent immediately by courier. As *C. botulinum* is ubiquitous in the environment, any isolate in food should be shown to be of the same 'cultural group' or produce the same toxin type as the cases (there are seven toxin types, designated by letters A–G). Toxin types A, B, E and F are associated with human disease, with type B being the most common in Europe. It may take up to 5 days for reliable negative results to be available.

For wound botulism, pus (or wound swab) and tissue biopsy (from surgical debridement) should also be sent for anaerobic culture. Infant botulism may occasionally be caused by *C. baratii* or *C. butyricum*.

Transmission

Illness results from the ingestion (or injection) of preformed toxin. Although boiling inactivates the toxin, spores may resist 100°C for many hours. These may multiply (producing toxin) when conditions are favourable, i.e. anaerobic, above pH 4.6 and at room temperature (usually 10–50°C, but in some cases as low as 3°C). These conditions occur in underprocessed foods such as home-cured hams or sausages, home-preserved fish or vegetables and foods contaminated after canning and bottling, e.g. bottled vegetables in Italy and canned salmon in the UK. The contaminated food may be consumed directly or used as an ingredient for another product. *C. botulinum* spores are ubiquitous in the environment and can be found in dust, soil, untreated water and

the digestive tracts of animals and fish. Toxin type E is particularly associated with fish products. Inhalation of toxin may also cause disease, but this is extremely rare under natural conditions.

Disease may also result directly from ingestion of spores rather than toxin (intestinal botulism) or the introduction of spores into a wound where they can reproduce in anaerobic conditions, as seen recently in intravenous drug users using contaminated drugs.

Acquisition

The incubation period for food-borne illness is usually 12–72 hours but extremes of 2 hours to 10 days are reported. In general the shorter the incubation period, the higher the ingested dose and the more severe the disease. The incubation for wound botulism may be longer (4–21 days following trauma) and for inhalational botulism may be shorter (<1–72 hours).

Although demonstrable in the faeces of cases, botulism is not communicable from person to person. The dose of toxin needed to cause symptoms is very low with illness resulting from nanogram quantities of ingested toxin. Type F toxin is about 60 times more toxic than type B (order: F > C > A > D > B). Estimated lethal doses of type A toxin are 0.1 μg given intravenously or intramuscularly, 0.8 μg inhaled and 70 μg ingested. Therapeutic botulinum toxin preparations contain only about 2% of the lethal intravenous dose. There appears to be no acquisition of immunity to botulinum toxin, even after severe disease. Repeated illness is well recognised.

Prevention

• Care with commercial or home canning processes and with home preservation of fish to ensure spores are destroyed before storage.
• Avoid consumption from food containers that appear to bulge (possible gas from anaerobic organisms) or containers that are damaged. Avoid tasting potentially spoilt food.

- Refrigeration of incompletely processed foods. Boiling for 10 minutes before consumption would inactivate toxin in home-canned foods.
- High index of clinical suspicion and urgent investigation and response to cases.
- Prevention work with intravenous drug users.

Surveillance

- Botulism is statutorily notifiable in most EU countries (including Belgium, Denmark, France, Germany, Italy, Netherlands, Norway, Spain and Sweden). In the UK, notify cases as 'suspected food poisoning'.
- Clinicians should report suspect cases to local public health authorities for urgent investigation.
- Laboratories should report positive toxin or culture results from patients to the relevant local and national centres as a matter of urgency.

Response to a case

- Clinicians or laboratories should report suspected cases immediately to the relevant public health officer for urgent investigation.
- Take urgent food history from case or, if not possible, other reliable informant (e.g. spouse). Take details of all foods consumed in 5 days before illness. Ask specifically about any canned foods or preserved foods.
- Obtain any leftovers of any foods eaten in last 5 days, including remains from uncollected domestic waste and unopened containers from the same batch. This prevents further consumption and allows storage under refrigeration by the laboratory in case later testing appropriate.
- Organise testing of foods at highest suspicion (e.g. canned food eaten 12–72 hours before onset) with reference laboratory.
- Inform appropriate national public health authority and, if commercial food product suspected, the national food safety agency.
- Case finding: any other suspected cases in local hospitals or laboratories or known to national centre? If so, compare food histories.

- Ensure that the case is admitted to hospital for investigation and treatment, and that others exposed to suspect food are informed and assessed. Arrange for supply of botulinum antitoxin to clinician in charge of case (need not await microbiological confirmation if strong clinical evidence). Appropriate antibiotics and surgical debridement also indicated for wound botulism.
- Person-to-person spread unlikely, but universal precautions sensible for carers, laboratory staff and post-mortems.
- No exclusions required for cases or contacts if well enough to work.
- If no obvious food source, consider intravenous drug use via contaminated illegal drugs; intestinal botulism, especially if child under 2 years of age; mis-injection of pharmaceutical preparation or a deliberate bioterrorism incident.

Investigation of a cluster

- Treat individual cases as indicative of a significant public health risk and investigate as above.
- Instigate case finding with local clinicians and laboratories, and national centre.
- Compare food histories, and specifically ask *each* case about *each* food reported by all other cases.
- Organise laboratory testing of *any* food reported by more than one case.
- Check preparation details of any food reported by more than one case to see if anaerobic conditions could have been created for any component and/or it was stored at room temperature after cooking.
- Remember, as well as canned, bottled or preserved produce, unexpected food vehicles have been reported from recent incidents, including sautéed onions (kept under butter), hazelnut yogurt (canned puree used in preparation), baked potatoes (kept in foil) and honey.
- Consider possibility that cases may be intravenous drug users exposed to contaminated illegal drugs (cases may not just be young males or homeless people).

Box 3.4.2 Severe systemic infection in intravenous drug users

In summer 2000, severe infection with a high case-fatality rate due to toxin-producing *Clostridium novyi* type A was reported in injecting drug users who had injected heroin intramuscularly or intravenously in the UK and Ireland. One hundred and eight cases and 43 deaths were reported between April and August 2000. The most likely cause of the infection was a contaminated batch of heroin.

Drug users are also at risk of other clostridial diseases from contaminated drugs, including wound botulism, tetanus and severe necrosis at injection sites due to *C. histolyticum*. Injecting sites may also become infected with MRSA or group A *Streptococcus*, leading to septicaemia.

Diagnosis:

The illness is characterised by local inflammation at an injection site, which is followed by hypotension and circulatory collapse. There is a very high white blood cell count. Cases usually have a temperature of less than 40°C and may look and feel quite well before deteriorating dramatically over a period of a few hours.

Appropriate microbiological investigations include blood culture, pus sample (or wound swab), tissue sample (from surgical debridement) serum and any available environmental samples (e.g. heroin).

Transmission:

C. novyi type A is found in soil and animal faeces. Spores may contaminate batches of illicit heroin and can survive preparation for injection including mixing with citric acid and heating. When injected into tissues or muscle rather than intravenously, the anaerobic conditions allow multiplication and the production of a toxin that enters the circulation causing damage to vital organs. The infection is not spread from person to person.

Prevention:

Injecting drug users should be advised to
- smoke heroin instead of injecting;
- if injecting, inject into a vein and not into muscle or under skin;
- not share needles, syringes with other drug users;
- use as little citric acid as possible to dissolve the heroin;
- not mix heroin for injection with cocaine;
- seek prompt medical attention if swelling, redness or pain develops at an injection site.

Public health action:

- Drug injectors who develop swelling, pain and redness at an injection site should seek immediate medical attention. Surgical debridement and early treatment with antibiotics active against anaerobes (e.g. penicillin and metronidazole) may be life saving.
- Sudden death is not uncommon in drug users. All possible cases should be compared to the case definition (see below). Cases of infection should be investigated in the usual way. Staff of community drug services may be able to assist. Enquiries should be made about sources of heroin, method of injecting, use of citric acid and other users who may be affected.

Public Health and drug services staff should alert injectors that contaminated heroin is circulating and advise on steps that can be taken to prevent infection.

Case definition:

An IDU admitted to hospital or found dead with soft tissue inflammation (abscess, cellulitis, fasciitis or myositis) at an injection site *and either*
- severe systemic toxicity (total peripheral white blood cell count $>30 \times 10^9$/L and sustained systolic pressure <90 mmHg despite fluid resuscitation), *or*
- evidence at necropsy of a diffuse toxic or infectious process including pleural effusion and soft tissue oedema or necrosis at an injection site.

• Consider possibility of bioterrorism: this could be via air-borne release or contamination of foodstuffs. Consider if cases have similar geographic exposure but no common food exposure; multiple simultaneous outbreaks with no obvious common source; unusual toxin type (C, D, F or G, or E without exposure to aquatic food); or similar cases in animals (liaise with veterinary agencies).

Control of an outbreak

• Identify and remove any implicated food.
• If commercially produced food, organise recall of product.
• If food vehicle identified, organise medical assessment of others that have consumed it.
• If linked to intravenous drug use, liaise with local community drug workers to get public health messages on safer drug use (see Box 3.4.2) out to users and to promote early diagnosis and treatment of cases.

Response to deliberate release

• Activate local and national plans and procedures.
• Decontamination of exposed people, clothing and fomites if air-borne release.
• Identify and monitor exposed individuals, including those who may have left the scene.
• No prophylaxis indicated for those exposed if remain asymptomatic.
• Ensure access to antitoxin and supportive therapy for those who develop symptoms.
• Full biological protective equipment for those entering 'exposed zone'.
• Contaminated area to be made out-of-bounds for few days after release (toxin loses activity during this period).
• Household bleach solution or 0.5% solution of hypochlorite (5000 ppm) are adequate decontamination.
• More general information is given in Chapter 4.14 and more specific information is available on HPA website.

> **Suggested case definition for use in outbreak**
>
> *Confirmed:* Clinically compatible case with demonstration of botulinum toxin in blood, faeces, vomit or gastric aspirate.
> *Clinical*: Acute bilateral cranial neuropathy with symmetrical descending weakness, no sensory loss and afebrile.
> *Provisional*: Any three from dysphagia, dry mouth, diplopia, dysarthria, limb weakness, blurred vision or dyspnoea, in an alert, non-febrile patient with no sensory deficit. Review when clinical investigations complete.
> If exposure known (e.g. food vehicle), then this can be added to the case definition.

3.5 Brucellosis

Bacteria of the genus *Brucella*, usually *B. abortus, B. melitensis, B. ovis, B. suis*, and rarely *B. canis*, cause brucellosis (undulant fever, Malta fever, Mediterranean fever), which may present as an acute febrile disease or a chronic illness.

Epidemiology

About 500,000 cases of human brucellosis are reported worldwide annually. Up to a third of infections may be unrecognised. Fewer than 20 cases have been reported in England and Wales in each of the recent years. Brucellosis has been eradicated in much of Northern Europe and most cases are acquired abroad. Within the Mediterranean area and Southern Europe it is still endemic and outbreaks occur. *B. melitensis* in sheep and goats remains the most important source. Farmers, veterinarians, abattoir workers and consumers of unpasteurised milk products are at particular risk of acquiring disease.

Clinical features

About half the recognised cases present with an acute, often severe, systemic febrile illness, sometimes associated with cough, arthralgia or testicular pain. Others present with localised suppuration, often involving bones or joints, particularly the spine. Splenomegaly and lymphadenopathy occur in about 15% of cases. Chronic disease may last for years, with non-specific features of fatigue, malaise and little or no fever. Neuro-psychiatric features may predominate.

Laboratory confirmation

Routine: definitive diagnosis is provided by culture of *Brucella* from blood, bone marrow or pus. However, the yield is often poor. The laboratory should be prepared to prolong culture, which may take 10 days or longer. Bone marrow culture produces the highest yield and may remain positive for some days after antimicrobial chemotherapy starts.

Reference: serology using agglutination tests remains the mainstay of diagnosis. The 2-mercaptoethanol agglutination, Coombs test and ELISA are in use. Interpretation of results is difficult. Sensitivity in chronic infection is poor. Serologic tests have to be interpreted in the light of clinical data and the local prevalence.

Transmission

Brucellosis is a zoonotic disease. *B. melitensis* and *B. ovis* are associated with goats and sheep, *B. abortus* with cattle, *B. suis* with pigs (occasionally acquired from dogs, deer and elk) and *B. canis* with dogs. Transmission is either by direct contact with infected animals or tissues (blood, urine, aborted foetus, placenta), or following consumption of contaminated milk or milk products. Air-borne infection in stables, laboratories and abattoirs has also been described. A new species of *Brucella* has been identified in seals, whales, dolphins, porpoises, and an otter.

Acquisition

The incubation period is 5–60 days. Presentation of the chronic form or bone or joint disease may take very much longer.

There is no person-to-person spread.

The duration of acquired immunity is uncertain.

Prevention

• The prevention of human disease is dependent on the control of brucellosis in the animal population.
• Mass testing, with slaughter of infected herds, has virtually eliminated endemic brucellosis in N. Europe, USA, Israel and Japan.
• A vaccine is available for cattle but is unsuitable for human use.
• Pasteurisation of milk will diminish the risk to populations in endemic areas.
• Those working with seals or small cetaceans should take suitable precautions.

Surveillance

• Brucellosis is a notifiable disease in many countries. In England and Wales it is statutorily notifiable if occupationally acquired.
• Cases should be reported to public health authorities on suspicion, so that steps can be taken to identify the source.

Response to a case

• Individual cases should be investigated to determine the source of infection.
• The authorities in the country in which the infection is believed to have been acquired should be informed.

- If the case has not been abroad, possible animal exposure should be sought.
- Others who may have been exposed should be offered serological investigation.

Investigation of a cluster

- As cases seen in N. Europe are imported, a cluster usually results from a common exposure at a single point.
- Occasionally the source may be difficult to identify if it is sold widely in an endemic area, through markets or small traders. Outbreaks associated with unpasteurised dairy products (e.g. goats' cheese) have occurred in recent years in S. Europe.

Control of an outbreak

The mainstay of control is the identification and eradication of infected livestock.

Suggested case definition for an outbreak
Clinical: an acute illness characterised by fever, night sweats, undue fatigue, anorexia, weight loss, headache and arthralgia.
Confirmed: clinical case with isolation of *Brucella* spp. from a clinical specimen, or demonstration by immunofluorescence of *Brucella* spp. in a clinical specimen, or fourfold or greater rise in *Brucella* agglutination titre between acute and convalescent serum specimens obtained at least 2 weeks apart.

3.6 *Campylobacter*

Campylobacter species cause diarrhoeal and systemic illnesses in humans and animals, and are the most common bacterial cause of infectious intestinal disease in developed countries. Although food-borne outbreaks are rarely identified, occasional large outbreaks due to contaminated milk or water may occur.

Suggested on-call action:
• Exclude symptomatic cases in high risk groups (Box 2.2.1) • If you or reporting clinician/microbiologist aware of potentially linked cases, consult Outbreak Control Plan.

Epidemiology

About 50,000 laboratory confirmed cases are reported annually in the UK although true community incidence is much higher at an estimated 8.7 per 1000 population. Deaths are rare, with an estimated annual mortality of about 25 in the UK. Infection occurs at all ages. Laboratory reported cases are highest in children under five and show a secondary peak in young adults. Amongst hospitalised patients, a third peak occurs in those aged 60–80. Positivity rates (number of confirmed *Campylobacter* infections per faecal specimen routinely submitted) are highest in 15- to 24-year-olds. There is a slight male excess in cases, particularly in young adults.

Campylobacter infections occur all year round, but there is a sharp peak in late spring and early summer in the UK, slightly earlier than that seen for *Salmonella* (Figure 2.2.1), which then declines in late summer. In Scandinavian countries, the peak is later, probably related to travel abroad. Outbreak associated cases occur regularly in the spring and autumn in the United States. Outbreaks are rarely identified in the UK.

Certain groups are at increased risk of *Campylobacter* infection due to increased exposure, including those with occupational contact with farm animals or meat, travellers abroad (e.g. to Turkey, Portugal, Spain or to developing countries), gay men (including infection with other *Campylobacter* species) and family contacts of cases. *Campylobacter* infection is the most commonly identified cause of travellers' diarrhoea in Scandinavia and the second most common (after enteropathogenic *Escherichia coli*) in the UK. *Campylobacter* infection is hyperendemic in developing countries.

Clinical features

Campylobacter infection may vary from asymptomatic (estimated 25–50% of cases) to a severe disease mimicking ulcerative colitis or acute appendicitis. Most diagnosed cases present as acute enteritis with symptoms of diarrhoea, abdominal pain, fever, malaise and nausea. There may be a prodromal period of fever, headache, myalgia and malaise for approximately 12–24 hours before onset of intestinal symptoms. Diarrhoea varies from loose stools to massive watery stools, with an average of 10 stools per day on the worst day. A third to a half of diarrhoeal cases also have blood in the stool, usually appearing on the second or third day. Abdominal pain may be prominent, is often described as constant or cramping rather than colicky and may be relieved by defaecation.

Most cases settle after 2–3 days of diarrhoea and 80–90% within one week. Complications include reactive arthritis, Guillain-Barré syndrome and haemolytic uraemic syndrome.

Although difficult to distinguish from other causes of intestinal infection in individual cases, *Campylobacter* might be suspected as the cause of an outbreak due to the combination of abdominal pain and fever, and/or the presence of bloody diarrhoea or faecal leukocytes. However, *E. coli* O157 may cause a similar picture.

C. jejuni is responsible for most campylobacteriosis and *C. coli*, which may be less severe, for most of the rest. Other species such as *C. fetus* and *C. lari* are uncommon causes of diarrhoea in immunocompetent individuals, but can cause severe systemic illness in debilitated or immunosuppressed patients.

Laboratory confirmation

The mainstay of diagnosis is culture of the organism from faecal samples. Sensitivity is increased if samples are delivered to the laboratory on the day of collection. If this is not possible, samples should be either refrigerated or stored in a suitable transport medium. Culture of *Campylobacter* requires different conditions than for other enteric pathogens. Provisional results may be available after overnight incubation. Confirmation that the colonies are *Campylobacter* requires simple microscopy, but identification of the species depends upon latex agglutination (quick but costly) or biochemical tests (takes 1–2 days). Typing (e.g. serotype, phage type and/or genotype) of *C. jejuni* or *C. coli* may be available from reference laboratories if required for epidemiological purposes.

Microscopic examination of fresh diarrhoeal stool specimens may permit a rapid presumptive diagnosis, although sensitivity is only 60% compared to culture. *Campylobacter* is sometimes isolated from blood cultures in acute illness. Serological testing may be useful for retrospective diagnosis in countries, like those of north-west Europe, with a low background rate of asymptomatic illness, although it does not differentiate between species and cross-reactions occur. Antibiotic resistance is high in strains from some holiday destinations. *Campylobacter* may be isolated from food or environmental specimens after enrichment culture.

Transmission

Campylobacteriosis is a zoonosis. It is found worldwide in the gastrointestinal tract of birds and mammals. Many animals develop a life-long carrier state. Humans are not an important reservoir. Transmission from animals to man occurs predominantly via ingestion of faecally contaminated food or water. Campylobacters are sensitive to drying, acid, high salt concentrations, chlorine and temperatures over 48°C. The main routes of infection are as follows.

Water-borne

Campylobacter excretion by wild birds causes contamination of open waters, and the organisms can survive for several months in water below 15°C. Large outbreaks have occurred from the use of untreated surface water in community water supplies. There may also be failures in 'treated' water supplies. Smaller outbreaks have occurred from the storage of water in open-topped tanks, which risk contamination by bird or rodent faeces. Deliberate or accidental ingestion of raw water can cause infection in those undertaking outdoor activities, e.g. trekkers, canoeists, etc.

Milk-borne

Campylobacters are commonly found in bulked raw milk samples. Infected animals may contaminate milk with faeces or excrete the organism via infected udders. Campylobacters can survive in refrigerated milk for 3 weeks and, when ingested, milk protects the organisms from the effect of gastric acid. Properly conducted pasteurisation destroys the organism. Consumption of raw or inadequately pasteurised milk has caused large outbreaks of campylobacteriosis, and contributes to endemic infection.

Contamination of milk after pasteurisation may also occur. In the UK, home delivery of milk in foil-topped bottles left on the doorstep is a temptation for birds such as magpies and jackdaws. The birds peck through these tops and contaminate the milk with *Campylobacter*. This may contribute to the early summer peak in infection in certain areas of the UK.

Poultry and other foods

In the majority of sporadic cases in developed countries, *Campylobacter* probably entered the kitchen on contaminated meat. Chicken carcasses are the most commonly contaminated, but pork, lamb and beef (including meat products such as sausages) may also be affected. Contamination of these meats is usually with *C. jejuni*, with the exception of pork for which almost all are *C. coli*. The contamination can lead to illness in one of three ways: contamination of hands leading to accidental ingestion; inadequate cooking, especially of chicken and a particular risk for barbecues; and

cross-contamination of foods, which will not be cooked, either via hands or via utensils such as knives and chopping boards. Fortunately *Campylobacter* does not multiply on food, which reduces the risk of large food-borne outbreaks. Normal cooking kills *Campylobacter*, and viable organisms are reduced 10-fold by freezing, although freezing cannot be assumed to have made contaminated poultry safe.

Other food vehicles that have been reported include shellfish contaminated by sewage and mushrooms contaminated by soil.

Consumption of contaminated food and water is the likely cause of most cases of travel-associated campylobacteriosis.

Direct transmission from animals

Approximately 5% of cases in the UK are thought to occur through contact with infected pets. The most likely source is a puppy with diarrhoea or, less often, a sick kitten and the most likely victim a young child. Transmission from asymptomatic pets has also been reported. Children may also be exposed to excreting animals on farm visits.

Occupational exposure to excreting animals or contaminated carcasses is also well recognised.

Person-to-person spread

Although the transmissibility of *Campylobacter* is low, person-to-person spread does occur. The index case is usually a small child who is not toilet trained. The victim may be the person responsible for dealing with soiled nappies. Vertical transmission has also been documented as has spread by blood transfusion.

Secondary spread has not been documented from asymptomatic food handlers or hospital staff.

Acquisition

The incubation period is inversely related to the dose ingested. Most cases occur within 2–5 days of exposure with an average of 3 days, but a range of 1–10 days incubation is reported.

The infectious period lasts throughout the period of infection, although once the acute illness is over the risk is very low. The average duration of excretion is 2–7 weeks, falling exponentially after the end of symptoms. Treatment with erythromycin usually terminates excretion but it is rarely necessary to attempt to do this. The infective dose is usually 10^4 organisms or above, but food vehicles which protect the organism against gastric acid (e.g. fatty foods, milk, water) can result in an infectious dose of as little as 500 organisms. Immunity develops in response to infection, with antibodies that protect against symptomatic infection against the same strain and cross-reacting strains. Patients with immune deficiencies or chronic illnesses may develop severe disease.

Prevention

• Chlorination of drinking water supplies.
• Pasteurisation of milk for retail sale.
• Reducing infection in poultry and animal farms, particularly from water supplies and other ways of introducing infection into poultry sheds.
• If unable to prevent contaminated meat leaving the slaughterhouse, gamma-irradiation of carcasses is effective, although not popular with the public.
• Adequate hygiene in commercial and domestic kitchens, particularly the avoidance of cross-contamination.
• Adequate cooking of meat, especially poultry.
• Protecting doorstep milk against birds.
• Handwashing after contact with faeces, nappies, meat or animals, including on farm visits.
• Conventional disinfectants are active against *Campylobacter*.
• Advice to travellers abroad.

Surveillance

• *Campylobacter* infection is notifiable in many European countries: in the UK it is notifiable as suspected 'Food Poisoning', of which it is the most commonly reported cause.
• Laboratory isolates of *Campylobacter* species should be reported to local public health departments and the national surveillance system.
• Surveillance schemes may also incorporate typing data, as in the HPA sentinel scheme.

Response to a case

• Enteric precautions for case (see Chapter 1.2).
• Exclude from work/nursery if in risk group (see Box 2.2.1) until 48 hours after first normal stool. No microbiological clearance necessary.
• Antibiotic treatment unnecessary unless severe or prolonged illness.
• Obtain history of food consumption (particularly chicken, unpasteurised milk or untreated water), travel and contact with animals.
• Investigate illness in family or other contacts.

Investigation of a cluster

• Discuss further microbiological investigations of epidemiological relevance with reference laboratory, e.g. typing of strains to see if similar. Ensure that local laboratories retain isolates for further investigation.
• Obtain details from cases on
    (i) source of water supply (failure of treatment?);
    (ii) source of milk supply (failure of pasteurisation?);
    (iii) functions attended (food-borne outbreak?);
    (iv) foods consumed, particularly consumption of undercooked chicken or, if *C. coli*, pork;
    (v) bird-pecked milk;
    (vi) farm visits (age-distribution of cases may support this);
    (vii) occupation/school/nursery;
    (viii) travel abroad or in UK.

Control of an outbreak

• Exclude symptomatic cases if in risk groups and ensure enteric precautions are followed.
• Re-enforce food hygiene and handwashing.

- Transmission is usually thought to be foodborne or, occasionally, water-borne, therefore check for ways in which food or water could have become contaminated.
- Prevent use of unpasteurised milk, untreated water or undercooked poultry.

Suggested case definition for outbreak

Clinical: diarrhoea or any two symptoms from abdominal pain, fever, nausea, with onset 2–5 days after exposure in person with link to confirmed case.

Microbiological: isolate of outbreak strain from faeces or blood. As carriage of any type of *C. jejuni* in asymptomatic controls in the UK is only about 1% but 25–50% of cases of *Campylobacter* infection are asymptomatic, clinical component of case definition could be waived if appropriate typing results are available.

3.7 Chickenpox and shingles (varicella-zoster infections)

Chickenpox is a systemic viral infection with a characteristic rash caused by varicella-zoster virus (VZV), a herpes virus. Its public health importance lies in the risk of complications in immunosuppressed and pregnant patients, and the potential for prevention by vaccination. Herpes zoster (shingles) is caused by reactivation of latent VZV whose genomes persist in sensory root ganglia of the brain stem and spinal cord.

Suggested on-call action

Assess clinical status of close contacts and arrange for VZIG, if appropriate (see Box 3.7.1).

Epidemiology

Chickenpox occurs mainly in children, although the incidence in older children and adults is rising in the UK and some other Western countries. There are epidemics every 1–2 years, usually in winter/spring. More than 90% of adults have natural immunity. Herpes zoster occurs mainly in middle or older age. Mortality is low, although it increases with age. There is an average of 26 deaths from chickenpox in England and Wales annually.

Clinical features

There is sometimes a prodromal illness of fever headache and myalgia. The diagnostic feature is the vesicular rash, which usually appears first on the trunk. They start as small papules, develop into clear vesicles, which become pustules and then dry to crusts (see Plate 2 *facing p. 212* in smallpox chapter). There are successive crops of vesicles over several days. The hands and feet are relatively spared.

A more fulminant illness including pneumonia, hepatitis or disseminated intravascular coagulation may affect the immunocompromised, neonates and occasionally healthy adults, particularly smokers. Congenital varicella syndrome occurs following infections in the first 5 months of pregnancy, although most risk appears to be in weeks 13–20.

Herpes zoster begins with pain in the dermatome supplied by the affected sensory root ganglion. The trunk is a common site. The rash appears in the affected area and is vesicular and rapidly coalesces. It is very painful and persists for several days and even weeks in elderly people.

Laboratory confirmation

This is rarely required as the clinical features are so specific. If necessary, VZV is readily demonstrable from vesicular fluid in both chickenpox and shingles; serology is also available and can be used to demonstrate immunity.

Transmission

Man is the only reservoir. Carriage does not occur. Chickenpox is highly infectious; herpes zoster very much less so. Transmission is by direct person-to-person contact, by air-borne spread of vesicular fluid or respiratory secretions and by contact with articles recently contaminated by discharges from vesicles and mucous membranes. The risk of transmission is high; the attack rate in susceptible exposed children is 87%.

Acquisition

The incubation period for chickenpox is 11–21 days, usually about 15–18 days.

Cases are infectious for up to 5 days before the onset of the rash (usually 1–2 days) until 5 days after the first crop of vesicles. Infectivity may be longer in immunosuppressed patients. Most transmission occurs early in the disease.

Patients with herpes zoster are usually infectious only if the lesions are exposed or disseminated. Infectivity is increased in immunosuppressed patients.

Prevention

• Live attenuated vaccines are available in many European countries, and in the US.
• Selective vaccination policy has been adopted in most of Europe (including the UK), unlike the US where universal vaccination is recommended.
• Aim of selective vaccination is to prevent varicella among those in close contact with individuals who are most at risk from complications of the disease, e.g. nonimmune healthcare workers and household contacts of the immunosuppressed.
• The schedule is one dose in children and two doses a month apart in adults.

Surveillance

• Notifiable in many EU countries (Estonia, Italy, Malta, Spain, Greece, Latvia, Slovakia, Hungary, Lithuania, Slovenia). In the UK, it is only notifiable in Scotland.
• Laboratory diagnosis rare, so local surveillance depends on informal sources such as schools. The public health practitioner may also be contacted with a request for specific immunoglobulin in an immunosuppressed or pregnant contact. Trend data can be obtained from sentinel general practices.

Response to a case

• Exclude children with chickenpox from school until 5 days from the onset of rash. Healthcare workers with chickenpox should stay off work for the same period.
• No exclusion criteria need to be applied to individuals with herpes zoster in the community. Healthcare workers with shingles should inform their Infection Control Team.
• In most circumstances, no further action is required. There are, however, some situations in which post-exposure prophylaxis with human varicella-zoster immunoglobulin (VZIG) is indicated. VZIG is indicated for nonimmune individuals with a clinical condition which increases the risk of severe varicella and who have significant exposure to chickenpox or herpes zoster (Box 3.7.1).
• VZIG is available from public health laboratories in the UK, CDSC and (in Scotland) regional transfusion centres. It should be given within 10 days of exposure.
• The dose (i.m. injection) is
    (i)   0–5 years: 250 mg (1 vial)
    (ii) 6–10 years: 500 mg (2 vials)
    (iii) 11–14 years: 750 mg (3 vials)
    (iv) 15 years and over: 1000 mg (4 vials)

Investigation of a cluster

Look for links to institutions with high levels of susceptible individuals.

Response to an outbreak

• In most outbreaks there will be no specific action in addition to the exclusion criteria and issue of VZIG described above.

Box 3.7.1 How to determine whether VZIG is required post-exposure

1 Is the contact at risk of severe disease? Include
- immunosuppressed patients;
- infants whose mothers develop chickenpox (but not zoster) in the period 7 days before to 7 days after delivery;
- nonimmune infants exposed to chickenpox or zoster (other than via mother) in the first 7 days of life, or while still in intensive/special care;
- pregnant women exposed at any time in pregnancy (N.B. when supplies are short VZIG may be restricted to exposures during the first 20 weeks of pregnancy or within 21 days of the estimated day of delivery).

2 Is the exposure significant? Consider
- type of infection in index case. VZIG is only indicated for exposure to chickenpox or to the following: disseminated herpes zoster, exposed herpes zoster lesions or immunosuppressed patients with herpes zoster.
- timing of exposure. VZIG is only indicated for exposures between 2 days before onset of rash to crusting of lesions.
- closeness and duration of contact. The following are significant: contact in the same room for 15 minutes or more; face to face contact; contact in the same hospital ward.

3 Is the contact already immune?
- Individuals with a history of chickenpox are immune and do not require VZIG. Those without a history should be tested for VZ antibody, as many will be immune.

- Hospital outbreaks pose special problems because of the risk of transmission to immunosuppressed and pregnant patients. All staff in contact with these high-risk groups should be screened for VZ antibody. Nonimmune staff could then either be vaccinated, or where there is significant exposure to VZ virus (see above), excluded from contact with high-risk patients for 8–21 days after exposure.

Suggested case definition for an outbreak

Physician diagnosis of chickenpox or herpes zoster.

3.8 *Chlamydia pneumoniae*

Chlamydia (or Chlamydophila) pneumoniae, also known as TWAR, is a recently recognised pathogen and is a relatively common cause of atypical pneumonia and other respiratory infections.

Suggested on-call action

None required unless outbreak suspected.

Epidemiology

Infection probably occurs worldwide and has been demonstrated in many European countries. Data from the United States shows annual incidence rates of 6–9% in 5- to 14-year-olds falling to 1.5% for adults, leading to an overall seroprevalence of 50% by about 30 years of age. Incidence is low in the under 5 year-olds, but infection/re-infection may occur at any age. No seasonal pattern has been demonstrated but there is evidence of 2–3 year cycles of high and low endemicity.

Clinical features

The most commonly identified manifestations of *C. pneumoniae* infection are pneumonia and bronchitis, which are usually mild but often slow to resolve. Approximately 7–10% of community-acquired pneumonia is caused by this organism. Pharyngitis and sinusitis may occur in isolation or together with chest infection and these together with a usually insidious onset and prolonged cough may help to distinguish an outbreak from other causes of atypical pneumonia. Asymptomatic infection is common.

Laboratory confirmation

Diagnosis is usually confirmed by serology or direct antigen detection. Serology is based on demonstration of a fourfold rise to genus-specific IgG on complement fixation testing, which therefore cross-reacts with *C. psittaci* and *C. trachomatis*. Micro-immunofluorescence detection of *C. pneumoniae* specific antibody, including an IgM test for diagnosis of acute infection, is required for confirmation. IgM rises can be detected after about 3 weeks and IgG, 6–8 weeks after onset. Re-infection provides an IgG response in 1–2 weeks without an IgM response. Direct antigen testing and PCR tests have been developed for pharyngeal swabs, bronchoalveolar lavage and sputum. *C. pneumoniae* is difficult to culture, but throat swabs may be positive on special cultures. Co-infection with other respiratory pathogens is relatively common.

Transmission

No zoonotic or environmental reservoir has been discovered. Spread is likely to be person to person, presumably via respiratory tract secretions. Transmission appears to be slow but outbreaks, particularly in institutions such as nursing homes, schools and the military, do occur.

Acquisition

The incubation period is unclear: estimates range from 10 to 30 days. The infectious period is also unclear but appears to be prolonged. It

is possible that asymptomatic cases may also play a part in transmission. Although strong antibody responses occur, re-infection (even within the same outbreak) is reported. Most severe cases or deaths occur in those with underlying disease.

Prevention

General measures for respiratory infection including the following ones:
- Stay away from work or school when ill.
- Cover mouth when coughing or sneezing.
- Sanitary disposal of respiratory secretions.
- Handwashing.
- Avoid overcrowding.

Surveillance

- Sporadic infection with *C. pneumoniae* is not statutorily notifiable in most countries, including England and Wales.
- However, possible outbreaks or clusters should be reported to local Public Health departments.
- Laboratories should report all clinically significant infections to national surveillance systems.

Response to a case

- Hygiene advice to cases and advice to stay at home whilst coughing/sneezing.
- Check for links to other cases.

Investigation of a cluster

- Seek microbiological advice to confirm as *C. pneumoniae* infection.
- Look for direct contact between cases or attendance at same functions or institutions.

Control of an outbreak

Likely to be difficult due to asymptomatic infectious cases, re-infection, prolonged infectivity and long incubation period. Could include hygiene measures, case finding and treatment, but effectiveness not known.

3.9 *Chlamydia psittaci*

Psittacosis (or ornithosis) is a potentially fatal systemic disease caused by *Chlamydia* (or *Chlamydophila*) *psittaci*. It is a zoonotic infection particularly associated with birds.

Suggested on-call action

• If linked cases suspected, institute outbreak plan.
• If not, ensure case investigated promptly on next working day.

Epidemiology

Much of the reported epidemiology of psittacosis is based on a combination of respiratory symptoms and demonstration of *Chlamydia* group antigen on serology. It therefore requires re-examination in the light of the discovery of the more common *C. pneumoniae* (see Chapter 3.8), which also causes disease fitting such a case definition.

Around 100 cases of psittacosis are reported a year in England and Wales. Cases occur worldwide and are more common in those exposed to birds occupationally or as pet owners. Cases occur mostly in adults and more often in males. There is no distinct seasonal pattern.

Clinical features

Onset may be insidious or non-specific with fever and malaise, followed by an atypical pneumonia with unproductive cough, fever and headache, with 20% mortality if untreated. Other syndromes resemble infectious mononucleosis and typhoid. Asymptomatic infection may occur. Most cases report fever and most (eventually) develop a cough. Headache, myalgia and chills are each reported in about half of cases. Relapses may occur. Ovine strains may cause serious infection in pregnant women, resulting in late abortion, neonatal death and disseminated intravascular coagulation in the mother.

Laboratory confirmation

Culture is rarely used because of the risk of laboratory-acquired illness and diagnosis is usually based on serology. As routine Complement Fixation Tests (CFTs) cross-react with *C. pneumoniae*, further testing may be necessary to confirm which species is responsible. Acute and convalescent samples of serum are usually collected about 3 weeks apart. Microimmunofluorescence (MIF) tests are now available and are specific for *C. psittaci*. Antigen or genome detection may also be possible in some laboratories if rapid results are required.

Transmission

C. psittaci is a zoonotic disease. Animal reservoirs include psittacine birds such as cockatiels, parakeets, parrots, macaws and lovebirds; other birds, particularly ducks, turkeys and pigeons; and less commonly mammals, especially sheep. Infection is transmitted to humans by inhalation of infected aerosols contaminated by droppings, nasal discharges or products of conception (e.g. sheep abortions) in which it may survive for months at ambient temperatures. Birds may be asymptomatic carriers of the organism. *C. psittaci* is destroyed by routine disinfectants such as bleach (1:100), quaternary ammonium (1:1000) and 70% isopropyl alcohol.

Groups at increased risk of disease include those in the pet trade, bird fanciers, poultry workers, abattoir workers, veterinarians and laboratory workers. Owners of pet birds are also at risk: the increase in psittacosis in the UK and Sweden has been linked to importation of exotic birds for pets.

If human-to-human spread of *C. psittaci* occurs at all (earlier reports may actually have been *C. pneumoniae*) then it is rare.

Acquisition

The incubation period has been reported as anything from 4 days to 4 weeks. Most cases probably occur 5–15 days after exposure. Infection may result from only brief, passing exposure to infectious birds. The infectious period in birds may last for months. Human cases are not considered infectious for practical purposes. Protective immunity to re-infection is short lived. Those at risk of severe infection include pregnant women (especially to ovine chlamydial infection) and the elderly.

Prevention

• Quarantine and other controls on imported birds.
• Masks, good ventilation and measures to avoid contamination in poultry plants and other areas where workers might be exposed.
• Pregnant women to avoid exposure to sheep, especially during lambing.

Surveillance

• Although not statutorily notifiable in most of the UK (local exceptions exist), all cases of psittacosis should be reported promptly to local public health authorities. Psittacosis is notifiable in many European countries, including Germany, Sweden, Denmark and Norway.
• Laboratories should report all clinically significant infections to national surveillance systems.

Response to a case

• All cases should be reported promptly by the clinician or microbiologist for investigation by local public health officers.
• Look for exposure to psittacines, poultry, other birds and mammals. Trace source back to petshop, aviary, farm, etc. Involve veterinary

and microbiological colleagues to test animals for infection. Infected birds should be treated or destroyed and the environment thoroughly cleaned and disinfected.
• Ensure other potential cases are tested.
• No need for isolation. Cough into paper towel for safe disposal.

Investigation of a cluster

• Discuss further investigation with microbiologist to confirm *C. psittaci* as cause, and to see if typing is possible.
• Conduct hypothesis-generating study to include pet birds (possibly illegal); pet mammals; hobbies (e.g. pigeon racing); visits to petshops, farms, bird centres, etc.; and occupational exposure to animals. Document less defined exposures, e.g. walking through fields (potentially contaminated pasture?), roofing (exposure to pigeons?), etc. Check if any institution or home visited had a pet bird.

Control of an outbreak

Work with veterinary colleagues:
• Look for infected birds or mammals.
• Treat or destroy infected birds.
• Thoroughly clean and disinfect environment.
• Case finding to ensure those infected receive prompt treatment.
• Action to prevent recurrence.

Suggested case definition for outbreak

Confirmed: Compatible clinical illness, plus
    (a) culture of *C. psittaci*,
    (b) fourfold increase in specific IgG by MIF,
    (c) demonstration of specific IgM by MIF (titre ≥ 16) and
    (d) PCR positive.
Suspected: Compatible clinical illness plus
    (a) epidemiological link to confirmed case, or

Continued

Continued

> (b) fourfold increase by CFT antibody testing, or
> (c) single high IgG title by MIF.
>
> In an epidemiological investigation, may wish to include asymptomatic individuals with clear microbiological evidence of recent infection (see criteria for confirmed cases) to help identify exposure.

3.10 *Chlamydia trachomatis* (genital)

Chlamydia trachomatis is one of three species of the genus *Chlamydia*. One group of serovars cause genital infection, neonatal ophthalmia, pneumonia and adult ocular infection. Different serovars cause lymphogranuloma venereum (L1, L2 and L3) and endemic trachoma.

Genital *Chlamydia* infection is the most commonly diagnosed sexually transmitted infection in the UK.

Suggested public health on-call action
Not usually applicable.

Epidemiology

In 2003 there were 89,818 diagnoses at genitourinary medicine (GUM) clinics in England, Wales and Northern Ireland – a 9% increase compared with 2002. The highest rates of infection were in males aged 20–24 years and females aged 16–24 years. Amongst females aged 16–19 years, diagnostic rates exceed 1% in all English regions. These increases are due in part to increased prevalence but also to increased availability of diagnostic testing, new screening initiatives and increased awareness. Surveys among sexually active women in the UK have found prevalences of 4–12%. Similar results have been reported in European and North American studies. Risk factors for infection include age 25 years or less, recent change of sexual partner, use of oral contraceptives and low socio-economic status.

LGV is common in Africa, Asia and South America, but until recently has been rare in Western Europe. Since 2003 a series of outbreaks due to L2 serovar have been reported from European cities among men who have sex with men (MSM).

Clinical features

Many cases of infection in men and women are asymptomatic. In women there may be a cervicitis and urethritis, which may be complicated by pelvic inflammatory disease, tubal damage, infertility and ectopic pregnancy. In men there is urethritis, which may be complicated by epididymitis.

LGV is a chronic disease that starts with a painless sore that develops into swollen lymph glands and hemorrhagic proctitis.

Laboratory confirmation

A range of tests are available for the laboratory diagnosis of *C. trachomatis*, including culture and nucleic acid amplification tests (NAATs) on urine or swab samples. Less sensitive enzyme immunoassay tests should no longer be used.

Transmission

Transmission is by direct usually sexual contact. Adult eye infection can be spread indirectly by fingers contaminated with infected genital discharges.

Acquisition

The incubation period is 7–14 days and the case will remain infectious until treated. Only limited short-term immunity occurs and reinfection rates are high.

Prevention

• Programmes of opportunistic selective screening, case finding and partner notification are cost-effective.

• Use of condoms during sexual intercourse will reduce individual risk.
• In the UK, diagnostic testing is recommended for men and women with symptoms and women undergoing gynaecological surgery.
• Universal population screening is not recommended but after successful trials, a national programme of selective screening for genital *Chlamydia* is being introduced in England. Screening is offered to all women under 25 years of age who are sexually active and other categories of men and women under 25 years in various clinic settings, including GUM and contraceptive clinics.

Surveillance

• It is not necessary to report individual cases to local health protection teams, but anonymised or aggregated data should be reported to national surveillance systems.
• Cases who attend GUM clinics are reported through the KC60 returns in England and Wales. However, many cases are treated in general practice.
• Laboratories should report positive results through laboratory reporting systems.

Response to a case

• Treatment is with a 7-day course of doxycycline or erythromycin or a single dose of azithromycin.
• During treatment, cases should avoid sexual intercourse.
• Sexual contacts should be traced and treated. Referral of cases to a GUM clinic for management is recommended.

Investigation of a cluster and control of outbreaks

This is not generally applicable but contact tracing, mapping sexual networks, treatment and education may be appropriate.

Suggested case definition
Cases are defined by the results of appropriate laboratory tests.

3.11 Cholera

Cholera is a life-threatening secretory diarrhoea resulting from infection with toxin-producing *Vibrio cholerae* O1 or O139.

Suggested on-call action
• Cases should normally be admitted to an infectious diseases unit and enteric precautions instituted.
• Confirm diagnosis and the toxin production status of the isolate.
• Exclude cases in risk groups 1 to 4 (see Box 2.2.1) for 48 hours after the first normal stool.
• Identify household contacts and those with common exposure, place under surveillance for 5 days from last contact and exclude from food handling.

Epidemiology

Cholera is rare in Europe. The UK has seen about 80 imported cases of cholera between 1990 and 2000. Other European countries such as Germany and Norway see 2–6 imported cases each year. Worldwide, cholera has become more widespread as the virulent El Tor biotype has spread, encouraged by international migration and the breakdown of public health measures, especially associated with war, famine and other disasters. European visitors are unlikely to visit areas where cholera is common. *V. cholerae* O139 has recently been identified as causing epidemic cholera.

Clinical features

Cholera is characterised by a sudden onset of copious, watery diarrhoea and sometimes vomiting. Stool volumes of up to 30 L a day lead to rapid dehydration. There may be severe muscle pain as a result of hypokalaemia. This dramatic presentation is distinctive, but mild or subclinical infections are more common. The outcome depends on the amount of fluid and electrolyte loss and replacement; severe untreated cases have 50% case-fatality, but with correct treatment, less than 1% die.

Laboratory confirmation

Vibrios are small, comma-shaped, motile, Gram-negative bacilli, which may be seen on direct microscopy of stools or cultured from stool or a rectal swab. Various media have been described for culture; colonies can be recognised by fermentation reactions or by using antisera or fluorescent antibody tests. *V. cholerae* O1 is divided into two biotypes: classical and El Tor. Determination of toxin production is important, nontoxin producing organisms are not of public health significance (most *V. cholerae* isolated in the UK are not toxin producers). More recently the polymerase chain reaction (PCR) and other nucleic acid-based rapid techniques have been described.

Transmission

Infection is faeco–oral, commonly through contaminated water; undercooked seafood can also act as a vehicle. Cholera vibrios are sensitive to acidity; most die in the stomach, but achlorhydria increases susceptibility to infection. Following colonisation of the small bowel, an enterotoxin that interferes with intestinal epithelial cell metabolism is produced, causing secretion of electrolytes and water into the intestinal lumen.

Person-to-person spread should not occur where sanitary conditions are acceptable.

Acquisition

The incubation period is 6–48 hours.

Cases are infectious during the period of diarrhoea and up to 7 days after.

Prevention

Control by sanitation is effective, but may not be feasible in endemic areas.
• A parenteral vaccine of whole killed bacteria has been used widely, but is relatively ineffective and is not generally recommended.
• Antibiotic prophylaxis is feasible for small groups over short periods in high-risk situations.
• Breastfeeding in endemic areas protects infants from disease.

Surveillance

• Cholera is a notifiable disease, and the public health authorities should be informed of any case.
• WHO should be informed by the national agency.
• Illnesses caused by strains of *V. cholerae* other than toxigenic *V. cholerae* O1 or O139 should not be reported as cases of cholera.

Response to a case

• See on-call box above.
• Individual cases should be investigated to determine the source.
• Microbiological clearance: when indicated, two consecutive negative stools taken at intervals of at least 24 hours are required.
• Hygiene advice to the case and contacts.

Investigation of a cluster

• Clusters should be investigated in case there is secondary transmission within the household or community. This is rare in Europe.
• If secondary transmission likely, can consider chemoprophylaxis with tetracycline, doxycycline or erythromycin.
• Obtain history of foreign travel.

Control of an outbreak

Outbreaks are rare in developed countries and are controlled through the provision of safe drinking water supplies.

Suggested case definition for an outbreak
Clinical: an illness characterised by diarrhoea and/or vomiting in a contact of a case. *Confirmed*: clinical case with isolation of toxigenic *Vibrio cholerae* O1 or O139 from stool or vomitus.

3.12 CJD (Creutzfeldt–Jakob disease) and other human transmissible spongiform encephalopathies

Human transmissible spongiform encephalopathies (TSEs) are a group of conditions characterised by progressive fatal encephalopathy with typical spongiform pathological appearances in the brain. They include classical Creutzfeldt–Jakob disease (CJD), variant Creutzfeldt–Jakob disease (vCJD) and kuru. The causal agent of vCJD is PrP, a prion protein.

Suggested on-call action
• Undertake risk assessment. • May need to prepare for media interest.

Epidemiology

CJD in its classical form is the commonest of the human TSEs but is still rare, with an annual incidence worldwide of 0.5–1.0 cases per million population. In the UK there are about 35 cases per year, with an average age of onset of 55–75 years.

The first case of vCJD was first identified in 1996. At the time of going to press, 155 definite and probable cases had been reported in the UK, 6 in France and 1 case each in Ireland, Italy, USA and Canada. The future course of the epidemic is unknown: the best estimate of the number of people currently incubating the disease in the UK is 3800 with an upper limit of about 11,000. The age distribution of vCJD is younger than in classical CJD (median age 29 years, range 14–74 years) and cases have a different symptom profile and a different appearance of brain tissue on post-mortem. There may be genetic differences in susceptibility: all cases of vCJD tested to date are homologous for methionine at codon 129 of the prion protein gene, this is similar to cattle, where codon 129 codes for methionine—about 38% of the UK population are of this genotype. No relationship with occupation is apparent.

Kuru is a disease that occurs exclusively in Papua New Guinea; it has now almost disappeared.

Clinical features

The onset of vCJD is with variable psychiatric symptoms. This is typically followed by abnormal sensation at 2 months, ataxia at 5 months, myoclonus at 8 months, akinetic mutism at 11 months, with death at 12–24 months.

Laboratory confirmation

The diagnosis of vCJD is made on the basis of typical clinical features (see case definition) and post-mortem findings of spongiform change and extensive PrP deposition with florid plaques throughout the cerebrum and cerebellum.

Transmission

Most cases of classical CJD are sporadic, about 15% are inherited and around 1% are iatrogenic, transmitted from human pituitary derived growth hormone injections, corneal transplants and brain surgery involving contaminated instruments. Classical CJD is not thought to be transmissible via blood transfusion.

The most likely source of vCJD in humans is cattle infected with bovine spongiform encephalopathy (BSE). The PrP causing vCJD and BSE are indistinguishable from each other, but are different to those causing classical CJD or scrapie. The route of spread is unknown although consumption of infected bovine neural tissue is thought to be the most likely. Such exposure is likely to have been at its greatest before the introduction of effective control measures in 1990. In addition to the CNS tissues (including eye and pituitary) that are infectious in all types of TSE, vCJD also involves the lymphoreticular system and so tissues such as tonsils, appendix, thymus, lymph nodes, spleen, Peyer's patches and possibly bone marrow could all be infectious. Two cases possibly associated with blood transfusion have been reported; iatrogenic transmission from contaminated surgical instruments is also theoretically possible, with CNS and back of eye operations likely to pose the highest risk. Although scrapie, the main TSE of sheep, is not thought to be transmissible to man, it is possible that sheep infected with BSE could have entered the food chain.

Kuru is transmitted by cannibalistic consumption of infected human brain tissue.

Acquisition

The incubation period for vCJD is unknown, but is probably several years; for iatrogenic CJD and kuru the mean incubation is 12 years. The infective dose is unknown, but is likely to be affected by route of exposure. Cattle under 30 months of age are thought to be significantly less likely to be infectious.

Prevention

• Prevent BSE in cattle and transmission of infected tissues to man. This includes banning consumption of potentially infected feed to cattle, avoiding human consumption of nervous and lymphoreticular tissues, safe preparation of carcasses and slaughter of affected herds.

• Effective decontamination of surgical instruments according to best practice. Single-use disposable instruments should be used where possible.
• Incinerate surgical instruments used on definite or probable CJD cases and high-risk groups.
• Quarantine of surgical instruments used on possible cases.
• Use of leucodepleted blood for transfusions.
• Use of non-UK-sourced plasma and blood products.
• Avoid transplant and tissue donations and blood transfusions from certain high-risk groups.
• Infection control guidance for CJD patients undergoing surgery have been drawn up by ACDP (available via HPA website).
• Pentosan polysulphate is under evaluation as a potential post-exposure prophylactic.

Surveillance

• In the UK, suspected cases of CJD (including vCJD) should be reported to the national CJD Surveillance Unit (NCJDSU) in Edinburgh. This unit is responsible for surveillance, advising on diagnosis, and identification of certain control measures, e.g. to withdraw any blood donations made by the case. Surveillance is based on direct referral from targeted professionals (e.g. neurologists), unsolicited referrals from other professionals and review of death certificates with certain causes of death coded.
• European-level surveillance occurs through two EU-funded schemes, 'EUROCJD' and 'NEUROCJD'.

Response to a case in the UK

• Neurologists should report to local CCDC or equivalent. CCDC to report to national CJD Surveillance Unit. (Guidance available on NCJDSU website.)
• Investigate patient's medical history, especially recent surgery or organ or tissue donation. NCJDSU and National Blood service will normally investigate for blood donations. If there is a possible risk of transmission as

result of these procedures, report to CJD Incident Panel via CDSC (see HPA website).
- Advise on infection control measures.
- A look back exercise should be considered in any case of vCJD who has undergone an invasive procedure, particularly if involving nervous or lymphoid tissue. This should be based upon a risk assessment considering the type of exposure and how long previously the exposure occurred. Advice is available from the CJD Incident Panel. Those at highest risk are probably those exposed to instruments on the first few occasions of use after the potential contamination.

Investigation of a cluster

- Seek advice from National Steering Group (contact via CDSC). Guidance also available on HPA and NCJDSU websites.
- The uncertain and prolonged incubation period make the identification and investigation of clusters difficult. For vCJD, look for common exposures over a wide period of time, particularly common sources of beef and bovine products since 1980, and consider the possibility of iatrogenic transmission.

Suggested case definition

Definite: progressive neuropsychiatric disorder and neuropathological confirmation of vCJD on post-mortem.

Probable: progressive neuropsychiatric disorder, lasting more than 6 months, with routine investigations not suggesting an alternative diagnosis and no history of iatrogenic exposure *and* either (a) or (b).

(a) Four from following list:
- Early psychiatric symptoms; persistent painful sensory symptoms; ataxia, myoclonus *or* chorea *or* dystonia; dementia.
- *And* EEG does not show changes typical of sporadic CJD.
- *And* bilateral pulvinar high signal on MRI scan.

(b) Positive tonsil biopsy.

3.13 *Clostridium difficile*

Clostridium difficile (CD) was identified as the cause of pseudomembranous colitis (PMC) in the 1970s. CD-associated disease (CDAD) is a spectrum of disease triggered by antibiotic exposure that comprises colonisation, toxin-production, diarrhoea and severe colitis. CD causes 25% of cases of antibiotic-associated diarrhoea and a greater proportion of more severe disease. CDAD is an important healthcare-associated infection (HCAI). In 1996, CDAD was estimated to cost £4000 per case due to prolonged hospital stay and additional treatment costs.

Suggested on-call action

- Hospital outbreaks will be managed by the infection control doctor. Local health protection team should be prepared to participate in meetings of the outbreak control group.
- Local health protection team may be called upon to investigate and manage incidents involving CDAD in community nursing homes.

Epidemiology

Laboratory reports of CD increased from 20,556 in 2000 to 28,819 in 2002. Part of this increase is due to increased investigation and reporting. Elderly, hospitalised patients are at greatest risk. There is a background rate of CD infection in most hospitals, and outbreaks occur from time to time.

Clinical features

In a typical case of CDAD, diarrhoea starts within a few days of commencing antibiotics, although antibiotics taken 1–2 months previously may still predispose to infection. There may be abdominal pain and fever.

Laboratory confirmation

Laboratories test specimens for CD toxin, using either an immunoassay detecting both toxin A and toxin B or a neutralised cell cytotoxicity assay. Culture is required if typing is to be performed to establish which strains are present in a ward or hospital and for antibiotic sensitivity testing.

Transmission

CD is present in the in faeces of 3% of healthy adults, 7% of asymptomatic care-home residents and 20% of elderly patients on long-stay wards. CD is transmitted from patients with symptomatic CDAD either directly, via the hands of healthcare workers, through the accumulation of spores in the environment or on contaminated fomites such as commodes. Spread does not occur from an asymptomatic carrier in the absence of diarrhoea. Transmission to medical and nursing staff has been reported, although this is unusual and the disease is usually mild and short-lived. Community-acquired CDAD does occur and is probably under diagnosed.

Acquisition

CDAD occurs when a pathogenic strain of CD colonises the gastrointestinal tract of a susceptible patient. Once established, CDAD is a toxin-mediated condition. Risk factors that predispose to CDAD are age, antibiotic treatment, cytotoxic agents, intensive care, nasogastric intubation, concurrent illness and alteration in gut motility.

Prevention

• Control of antibiotic usage. In hospitals there should be strict antibiotic policies.
• Standard infection control procedures.
• Any patient with diarrhoea should be isolated with enteric precautions and faecal samples should be submitted for toxin testing.
• A high level of environmental cleanliness should be maintained.

Surveillance

• Clinicians should send faecal specimens whenever patients present with diarrhoea of potentially infectious aetiology.
• Laboratories should test diarrhoeal specimens for CDAD from all patients aged 65 years and over.
• Include in surveillance of hospital-acquired infection. In the past, surveillance of CD infection in England and Wales was through voluntary laboratory reporting of isolates of the organism and detection of toxin. However, mandatory surveillance of CDAD started in 2004.

Response to a case

• Involve hospital infection control team.
• Side room isolation with enteric precautions, use of gloves and aprons and attention to handwashing by all staff.
• Treatment should be based on the advice of a medical microbiologist.
• Moniter susceptible contacts.
• Thorough environmental cleaning, but use of environmental disinfectants unnecessary.
• Exclusion of high-risk groups (Box 2.2.1) until 48 hours after first normal stool.

Investigation of a cluster

• All patients with diarrhoea should be identified, risk factors should be documented and faecal samples submitted for toxin tests and culture.
• In a hospital outbreak, typing may help to determine whether all patients are infected with the same strain, whether relapses are due to the original outbreak strain and whether patients are infected with more than one strain at a time.
• Routine environmental sampling is not recommended but may form part of an investigation, especially if isolates can be typed.
• Community outbreaks are uncommon.

Control of an outbreak

• Strict adherence to antibiotic policies.
• Case finding through enhanced surveillance.

- Side room isolation.
- Enteric precautions and handwashing.
- Restricting movements and transfers of patients.
- Environmental cleaning.
- Disinfection and sterilisation of equipment.
- Correct handling of infected linen.
- Screening for and treatment of asymptomatic patients who are CD carriers is unnecessary.
- There is no need to screen asymptomatic staff for carriage of CD. Staff who are asymptomatic carriers do not present a risk to patients and they can continue in their normal duties.
- Staff who are on antibiotics can remain at work, even if CD is affecting patients.

Suggested case definitions

CD diarrhoea: diarrhoea not attributable to any other cause at the same time as a positive toxin assay (with or without a positive CD culture) and/or endoscopic evidence of PMC.

Outbreak of CD diarrhoea: two or more related cases satisfying the above criteria with dates of onset in a given time period that is determined locally, based on knowledge of the background rate. Genotyping may be helpful in determining whether cases are linked.

3.14 *Clostridium perfringens*

Clostridium perfringens (formerly *C. welchii*) is primarily a food-borne pathogen, which causes a mild gastrointestinal illness due to an enterotoxin. It is a cause of outbreaks, usually associated with mass catering.

Suggested on-call action

If you or the reporting laboratory/clinician is aware of other potentially linked cases, consult local outbreak plan.

Epidemiology

The incidence of *C. perfringens* food poisoning presenting to general practice in England is about 1.3 per 1000 person per year. *C. perfringens* is identified as the cause of 1.4% of all gastroenteritis outbreaks reported in the UK, but this rises to 8% of those thought to be food-borne. There is little known variation by age, sex, ethnicity, occupation and geography. Reported cases are higher in autumn and winter months (especially December) than in summer, perhaps because of seasonal consumption of the types of foods often associated with infection. The association of infection with institutions or large gatherings likewise probably reflects patterns of food preparation. Outbreaks often have a high attack rate.

A much more serious disease (enteritis necrotans) is caused by different strains and is rare in Europe. *C. perfringens* is also the major cause of gas gangrene .

Clinical features

The main features of *C. perfringens* food poisoning are watery, often violent, diarrhoea (>90% of cases) and colicky, often severe, abdominal pain (80%). Nausea (25%) and fever (24%) may occur, but vomiting is rare (9%). Most cases recover within 24 hours, although elderly or debilitated patients may be more severely affected and occasional deaths are reported.

Laboratory confirmation

C. perfringens can be isolated from anaerobic culture of stool samples. They are divided into five types (A–E) on the basis of toxin production. Those most frequently associated with food poisoning are the A2 strains, which form markedly heat resistant spores. A1 strains, whose spores are relatively heat sensitive, may also cause illness.

As asymptomatic carriage of *C. perfringens* is extremely common in healthy humans and carriage of heat-resistant organisms not uncommon, isolation of the organism from sporadic cases is of little value. However, serotyping (75 serotypes plus a number of untypable strains), which allows cases to be linked to each other and to strains from potential food vehicles, is a powerful tool in outbreak investigation. Other factors that may help separate cases from carriers are a quantitative culture of organisms (over 10^6/g faeces usually significant) or the demonstration of enterotoxin in faeces. Several colonies should be sent for serotyping as more than one serotype can be present in the same specimen; failure to do this may confuse epidemiological investigation of an incident.

Transmission

C. perfringens is ubiquitous in soil and in the gastrointestinal tracts of mammals and birds. Many opportunities exist for spores to contaminate food, particularly meat and meat products, but provided contamination remains low, illness does not result. *C. perfringens* can grow at temperatures between 20 and 50°C with optimal growth at 43–45°C, when a generation time of 10 minutes can be achieved. Spores, particularly those of the A2 strains, can survive normal cooking, including boiling for longer than 1 hour. These 'heat-activated' spores will then germinate in the protein-rich environment as the food cools: the longer the food remains at the organism's preferred temperature, the larger the number of resulting organisms. If the food is not then reheated to at least 70°C for 2 minutes throughout its bulk to kill the vegetative cells before eating, then a potentially infectious dose is ingested. The ingested organisms sporulate in the gut and (probably as a result of the initial heat shock) produce as a by-product the enterotoxin, which causes disease. Bulk cooking of meat/poultry stews, roasts, pies and gravies appear to be particularly vulnerable to this chain of events.

Acquisition

The incubation period is usually 8–18 hours, although a range of 5–24 hours has been reported. *C. perfringens* gastroenteritis is not spread from person to person, and asymptomatic food handlers are not thought to be infectious to others. The infectious dose in food is usually greater than 10^6 organisms. There is no evidence of effective immunity postinfection.

Prevention

• Prevention is dependent upon adequate temperature control of food after (initial) cooking. Meat dishes should be served whilst still hot from initial cooking *or*, if not served immediately
  (i) refrigerate to below 10°C within 2 hours of end of cooking.
  (ii) reheat with a method known to achieve 70°C for at least 2 minutes throughout the bulk of the food. Microwaves, in particular, may not be able to achieve this.
  (iii) cook and reheat as small a quantity of food as is practicable. A maximum portion of 3 kg of meat was suggested after one large outbreak.
• Take particular care in large functions, or if consumers likely to include elderly or debilitated people.

Surveillance

Report to local public health authorities (notifiable as 'food poisoning' in the UK) and to national surveillance systems.

Response to a case

• As with all cases of diarrhoea, hygiene advice should be given and it is best if the case does not attend work or school until he/she has normal stools.
• Occupational details should be sought: cases in risk groups 1–4 (see Box 2.2.1) should be excluded until 48 hours after the first normal stool. No microbiological clearance is necessary.
• No action is necessary with asymptomatic contacts of cases.

Investigation of a cluster

A laboratory-identified cluster is currently a rare event. Should one occur in a group of individuals with a compatible clinical illness, then analysis of person/place/time variables should be followed by a semistructured questionnaire aimed at identifying common foods, especially cooked meat/poultry products and meals eaten outside the home.

Control of an outbreak

• As secondary spread from cases is unlikely, the aim of the outbreak investigation is to discover how it happened so that lessons can be learnt. In practice this means trying to identify how an infectious dose resulted in a food presented for consumption.
• The vehicle of infection is identified by microbiological analysis of remaining food to find the same serotype as the cases (make sure you know how the food was stored after serving but before sampling) or by an analytical epidemiological study to show that cases were statistically significantly more likely to have eaten the food than controls.
• The environmental investigation will concentrate on how the food was cooked, stored and reheated. It is worth remembering that type A1 spores should not survive adequate initial cooking.

Suggested case definition for analytical study of *C. perfringens* outbreak

Clinical: diarrhoea or abdominal pain with onset between 8 and 18 hours of exposure.
Confirmed: Clinical case with isolate of outbreak serotype and/or demonstration of enterotoxin in faeces.

3.15 Coxsackievirus infections

Coxsackieviruses are enteroviruses that cause a range of clinical syndromes, including hand, foot and mouth disease (HFMD).

Suggested public health on-call action

None generally needed.

Epidemiology

Infection may be sporadic or epidemic. In recent years annual laboratory reports in England and Wales of group A isolates have varied between 72 and 453 and of group B between 207 and 1231. Most isolates are from faecal samples or throat swabs, with fewer from CSF. Isolation rates for all enteroviruses were highest among infants aged 1–2 months. Sixty per cent of patients were aged under 5 years. The clinical conditions associated with virus isolation are typically meningitis and other more serious infections. Milder clinical syndromes do not normally merit laboratory diagnosis. Laboratory data must be treated cautiously as some groups of patients will be investigated more vigorously, and only certain serotypes are detected by the cell culture method used by most laboratories. Predominant serotypes were similar to those reported in other countries. Most reports were made between July and mid-December. Viral activity peaks at intervals of 2–5 years. There is evidence of spread of epidemic serotypes across Europe in certain years. Outbreaks of A9 were reported in the UK in 1976 and 1985 and A16 was epidemic in 1981. An outbreak of viral meningitis due to B5 was reported in Cyprus in 1996.

The GP data from England and Wales show a mean weekly incidence of HFMD in 2003 of 0.57 per 100,000 population compared with 1.29 in 2002. The incidence was 8 in those aged 1–4 years and 5 in those aged 0–11 months.

Clinical features

Infection may be clinical (see Table 3.15.1) or subclinical. HFMD is usually due to coxsackievirus A16 and is a mild illness with fever and a vesicular rash in the mouth and on the palms,

Table 3.15.1 Clinical syndromes caused by Coxsackievirus infection

Acute haemorrhagic conjunctivitis	Subconjunctival haemorrhages and lid oedema. Often due to serotype A24.
Epidemic myalgia (Bornholm disease)	Chest or abdominal pain, aggravated by movement and associated with fever and headache. Outbreaks have been reported.
Hand, foot and mouth disease	A mild infection with ulcers in the mouth and a maculopapular or vesicular rash on the hands, feet and buttocks. Often due to serotype A16. Systemic features and lymphadenopathy are absent and recovery is uneventful.
Herpangina	Fever, painful dysphagia, abdominal pain and vomiting with vesicles and shallow ulcers on tonsils and soft palate.
Meningitis	Fever with signs and symptoms of meningeal involvement Encephalitic signs may be present.
Myocarditis	Starts with non-specific symptoms such as fever and aches then progresses to breathlessness, palpitations and chest pain. Heart muscle necrosis varies in extent and severity. Heart failure may follow. Serum cardiac enzymes may be elevated; there may be ECG and chest X-ray abnormalities. Most patients with viral myocarditis recover fully. Treatment is largely supportive.
Pericarditis	Presents with retrosternal chest pain, aggravated by movement, fever and malaise. A pericardial rub may be present.
Skin rashes	Rashes are common including a fine pink rubella-like rash or petechial, purpuric, vesicular, bullous or urticarial rashes.

soles and buttocks. HFMD due to a closely related virus, enterovirus 71, has been reported from several Asian countries and was associated with occasionally fatal neurological involvement in Taiwan in 1998.

Laboratory confirmation

Coxsackieviruses may be isolated in tissue culture from faeces or other clinical specimens. Serological tests and PCR are also available. Coxsackieviruses are small RNA viruses that belong to the enterovirus genus of the picornaviridae family. Two groups are recognised, group A (23 serotypes) and group B (6 serotypes), which are now classified in three species along with other enterovirus and echovirus serotypes.

Transmission

Human clinical and subclinical cases are the reservoir of infection. Spread is by direct contact with faeces, blisters and respiratory droplets. Enteroviruses may also spread indirectly via environmental water and sewage.

Acquisition

The incubation period is 3–5 days and a person will be infectious during the acute illness and while the virus persists in the faeces.

Infection generally leads to immunity although infection with different serotypes may occur.

Prevention

• Standard and enteric precautions particularly handwashing and hygienic disposal of faeces will reduce exposure.
• Pregnant women may wish to avoid exposure, as a possible risk of abortion has been suggested.

Surveillance

Sporadic cases will not normally be reported to public health authorities, but clusters of cases and outbreaks should be reported.

Response to a case

Children with HFMD may attend school or nursery when well enough.

Response to a cluster and control of an outbreak

The local public health team may wish to alert local schools and general practitioners if an outbreak of HFMD occurs.

Case definition
Characteristic clinical appearance with or without laboratory confirmation.

3.16 Cryptosporidiosis

Cryptosporidium parvum is protozoan parasite, which usually causes an acute self-limiting diarrhoeal illness. Its' main public health importance lies in the severe illness caused in immunocompromised individuals, the lack of specific treatment and the potential to cause outbreaks, including large water-borne outbreaks.

Suggested on-call action
• If case in risk group for onward transmission (Box 2.2.1), exclude from work or nursery. • If you or reporting laboratory/clinician is aware of other potentially linked cases, consult local outbreak plan.

Epidemiology

Cryptosporidium is the fourth most commonly identified cause of gastrointestinal infection in the UK, with around 5500 isolates reported a year. Evidence of past infection is common with seroprevalence rates of 20–35% reported in Europe. Diagnosed infection rates are highest in children aged 1–5 years and low in those over 45 years (Table 3.16.1), although in Finland most cases are reported as occurring in adults, due to travel abroad. Males and females are affected equally.

Cryptosporidiosis has a marked seasonal pattern: in Western Europe peaks occur in the spring and late autumn (Fig 2.2.2), although one or both may be absent in some localities or in some years. Groups at particular risk of infection include animal handlers, travellers abroad (particularly to developing counties), contacts of cases, homosexual men and the immunosuppressed. Rates may also be higher in rural areas. The reported incidence of cryptosporidiosis in some AIDS centres is as high as 20%, although this is not universal. The age profile of cases in immunosuppressed patients is higher than that shown in Table 3.16.1.

Clinical features

The main presenting symptom is diarrhoea, which in immunocompetent individuals may last from 2 days to 4 weeks, with an average

Table **3.16.1** Age distribution of sporadic cryptosporidiosis

Age group (years)	% of total cases
Under 1	6
1–4	39
5–14	17
15–24	13
25–34	13
35–44	7
45–54	3
55–64	1
65 plus	2

Source: PHLS study group, 1990.

of 2 weeks. The diarrhoea may contain mucus but rarely blood, may be profuse and may wax and wane. The diarrhoea is often preceded by anorexia and nausea, and accompanied by cramping abdominal pain and loss of weight. Headache, myalgia, fever or vomiting may occur in a proportion of cases.

Immunosuppressed patients have difficulty in clearing the infection, particularly HIV infected individuals with CD4 T lymphocyte counts below 200 cells/mm^3. Many such individuals have a prolonged and fulminant illness which may contribute to death.

Laboratory confirmation

The mainstay of diagnosis is microscopy of stool samples to detect cryptosporidia oocysts. It is important that such microscopy be undertaken by experienced personnel, both to maximise ascertainment and because a wide variety of microscopic structures (e.g. yeasts) can be confused with *Cryptosporidium* oocysts. Repeat sampling may improve ascertainment. Individual cases are sometimes diagnosed by intestinal biopsy. Serological methods have been used in epidemiological studies, including the huge Milwaukee outbreak.

Genotyping is now available in the UK and splits *C. parvum* into 'genotype 1' (also known as *C. hominis*), which is found only in man and accounts for approximately one-third of cases, and 'genotype 2', found in animals and humans (two-thirds). About 1% of human cases are caused by cryptosporidia other than *C. parvum*; these may be indistinguishable on mioroscopy but can be identified by genotyping.

Transmission

Cryptosporidium parvum has been demonstrated in a wide variety of animals including cattle, sheep, goats, horses, pigs, cats, dogs, rodents and humans. Clinical disease and most oocyst excretion are thought to occur mainly in young animals. Transmission to humans is by faeco–oral spread from animals or other humans. The main routes of spread are as follows:

Person to person

Cryptosporidiosis can be transmitted by cases to family members, nursery contacts, carers and sexual partners. Spread can be direct faeco–oral or via contaminated items such as nappies. Aerosol or droplet spread from liquid faeces may also occur. Secondary spread in households is common and may occur after resolution of clinical symptoms in the index case. Many outbreaks have been reported in nurseries.

Animal to person

Human infection with genotype 2 may occur from contact with farm or laboratory animals and, occasionally, household pets. In addition to agricultural and veterinary workers, those at risk include children visiting farms on educational or recreational visits where they may handle lambs or calves. A number of outbreaks associated with such visits have been reported.

Drinking water

Contamination of drinking water may occur from agricultural sources or human sewage contamination. Oocysts passed in faeces can survive in the environment for months. They are resistant to chlorination and their removal relies on physical methods of water treatment such as filtration, coagulation and sedimentation. Over 20 drinking water related outbreaks have been reported in the UK, but the largest such outbreak occurred in Milwaukee, USA in 1993 when an estimated 400,000 people became ill. A review of the UK outbreaks found a common thread of an inadequacy in the treatment provided or of the operation of the treatment process.

Other

Infection has been reported via food and milk. Many swimming pool outbreaks have been reported, usually as a result of faecal contamination of water and inadequate pool maintenance. Transmission has been reported from healthcare workers to patients (both immunosuppressed and immunocompetent) and between patients. The source of much cryptosporidiosis in the UK remains unclear. Genotype 1 may be associated with travel abroad.

Acquisition

The incubation period is unclear: 7–10 days would seem to be average, but a range spanning 1–28 days has been reported. The infectious period commences at onset of symptoms and may continue for several weeks after resolution. Asymptomatic infection has also been reported.

The infective dose appears to be very small, perhaps as low as 10 oocysts in some cases (thus enabling autoinfection) with an ID_{50} of 130 oocysts. The UK Expert Group found it was not possible to recommend a health-related standard for *Cryptosporidium* in drinking water. In immunocompetent individuals the immune response successfully limits the infection. AIDS patients are at increased risk of acquisition and increased severity. Relative immunosuppression due to chickenpox and malnutrition has also been associated with infection, but renal patients do not appear to be at increased risk. Oocyst excretion may be very high in the immunosuppressed.

Prevention

• Handwashing after contact with faeces, nappies and animals (take particular care in contact with these if immunosuppressed).
• Safe disposal of sewage, taking particular care to avoid watersources.
• Risk assessment for water supplies, protection against agricultural contamination, adequate water treatment (e.g. coagulation aided filtration) and monitoring of water quality, particularly turbidity.

• Enteric precautions for cases (Chapter 1.2) and exclusion of those in at-risk groups (Box 2.2.1).
• Immunosuppressed patients to boil water (both tap and bottle) before consumption and avoid contact with farm animals and infected humans.
• Guidelines for farm visits by children have been developed and can be adapted for local use (Health and Safety Executive, UK). Guidelines have also been developed for swimming pools (Pool Water Advisory Group, UK).
• *Cryptosporidium* is resistant to many common disinfectants. Ammonia, sodium hypochlorite, formalin, glutaraldehye and hydrogen peroxide may be effective. Heating to 72°C for 1 minute inactivates the parasite.

Surveillance

• All clinically significant infections should be reported to local public health authorities (notify as suspected food poisoning in UK) and to national surveillance systems.
• The most important function of surveillance of cryptosporidiosis is the detection of outbreaks, particularly water-borne outbreaks. All diarrhoeal samples should be examined for oocysts and all positives reported. Home postcode should be collected on all cases to be plotted on water supply zone maps, which can provided by water providers and need regular updating. Trigger levels can be calculated for districts and regions. A seasonal baseline can be set based on historical data with 95% or 99% confidence intervals calculated from Poisson distribution tables. High figures for 1 week only may be the result of reporting delay (look at dates of onset). The age distribution of cases should also be monitored.
• Water providers should also undertake appropriate monitoring of water quality and inform the local public health authorities of potentially significant failures, e.g. levels of one oocyst per 10 L of water (see Box 3.16.1).

Response to case

• Enteric precautions for case (see Chapter 1.2).

Box 3.16.1 Response to detection of oocysts in water supply

The relationship between oocyst counts and the health risk to those who drink the water is unclear. However, the water companies in the UK will inform public health authorities of breaches in water quality standards. An appropriate response would be (based on Hunter, 2000):

Collect information for risk assessment:
- When and where sample taken.
- Number of oocysts detected and results of any viability testing.
- Results of repeat testing (should be done urgently).
- Source and treatment of affected water supply.
- Any recent changes in source or treatment.
- Distribution of water supply.
- Any treatment failure or high turbidity identified
- How long water takes to go through distribution system.
- History of *Cryptosporidium* sampling and results for this supply.
- Any previous outbreaks associated with this supply.

For a low oocyst count in a supply in which oocysts frequently detected and not associated with previous outbreaks, further action may not be necessary.

Call Incident Management Team if significant exposure likely, e.g.
- unusually high oocyst count or demonstration of viability
- evidence of treatment failure or increased turbidity.
- groundwater source.
- association with previous outbreaks.

Possible actions:
- None.
- Advice to particular groups.
- Enhanced surveillance for human cases.
- Provision of alternative water supply.
- Boil water notice to affected area.

Boil water notices are issued if risk is thought to be ongoing, e.g.
- repeat samples positive.
- treatment or turbidity problems continue.
- contaminated water not yet cleared from distribution system.

- Exclude from work/school if in risk group (Box 2.2.1) until 48 hours after first normal stool. No microbiological clearance necessary.
- Cases should not use swimming pools until 2 weeks after first normal stool.
- Investigate illness in family or other contacts.
- Obtain history of raw water consumption (including postcodes of premises on which consumed and any consumption from private water supplies), contact with other cases, contact with animals, nurseries, swimming pools, travel and milk consumption in previous 14 days.

Investigation of cluster

- Check to see if neighbouring areas, particularly those sharing a water supply, have an increase.
- Check age-range of affected cases: an increase in cases in adults could suggest water-borne infection or link with immunosuppressed patients. If most cases are in school-aged children, consider visits to farms or swimming pools or, if under 5 years, links to nurseries.
- Epidemic curve may suggest point source, continuing source or person to person spread.

Box 3.16.2 Selected recommendations of Bouchier report

1.2.6 Water providers to develop local liaison arrangements with Health and Local Authorities for rapid appraisal of potential health risk.

1.2.8 Water utilities to provide CCDC with water supply zone maps. HA to make early contact with water provider if outbreak of cryptosporidiosis suspected.

1.2.9 Human cryptosporidiosis to be laboratory reportable disease.

1.2.10 HA to make postcode of cases available to water providers for mapping.

1.2.40 Criteria should be in place for identifying outbreaks and activating control teams.

1.2.55 All parties to simulate incident/outbreak events to rehearse emergency procedures.

1.2.61 Outbreak Control Team to use guidance on Epidemiological Investigation of Outbreaks of Infection (Appendix A4 of report).

1.2.63 All water to be used by immunocompromised persons should be boiled first.

Further reading: Bouchier IT (Chairman). *Cryptosporidium in water supplies. Third report of the group of experts to: Department of Environment, Transport, and the Region and the Department of Health.* London: DETR, 1998.

• Check with water provider whether any recent evidence of increased contamination or failure of treatment.

• Plot cases by water supply zones. Check with water provider how cases relate to water sources (e.g. reservoirs, treatment centres) during relevant period: supply zones are not fixed and some areas may also receive water from mixed sources.

• Collect and review risk factor details from individual cases for hypothesis generation and further investigation as appropriate (see Chapter 4.3). Case finding may also be necessary.

• Organise confirmatory testing and genotyping by reference laboratory. If genotype 1, look for potential humans sources; if genotype 2, consider animal and human sources.

Control of an outbreak

• If a water-borne outbreak likely then
(i) issue 'boil water' notice if contamination likely to be ongoing. A communications plan should already exist for public information. Water needs only to be brought to the boil: prolonged boiling is not necessary.
(ii) organise Outbreak Control Team to include relevant water company specialists/managers and Local Authority. If potentially serious, add appropriate experts (e.g. CDSC, public health microbiologist and

Environment Agency in England and Wales). The addition to the team of an individual who has dealt with such an outbreak before should be considered.
(iii) consult Bouchier report (see Box 3.16.2) for more detailed advice.

• Exclude symptomatic cases in risk groups (Box 2.2.1).

• Advise public on how to prevent secondary spread.

• Institute good practice guidelines at any implicated nursery, farm, swimming pool or hospital.

Suggested case-definition for analytical study of outbreak

(a) Cohort study (e.g. nursery, school class):
    Clinical: diarrhoea within 2–14 days of exposure.
Confirmed: diarrhoea and oocysts seen in faecal specimen.
(b) Case-control study (e.g. general population):
Diarrhoea plus oocysts (of correct genotype, if known) in faeces, with no other pathogen isolated, no previous cases of diarrhoea in family in last 14 days and date of onset since commencement of increase in cases.

3.17 Cyclosporiasis

Cyclospora cayetanensis is a protozoan that causes human gastroenteritis.

Epidemiology

Infection occurs worldwide. In the UK about 60 cases are reported annually, the major risk factor being travelling abroad; risk areas include the Americas (Mexico, Guatemala, Peru), the Caribbean, China, the Indian subcontinent (including Nepal), Indonesia, south-east Asia, Turkey and Yemen. A probable food-borne outbreak has occurred in Germany, but the large outbreaks seen in North America have not been reported in Europe.

Diagnosis

Cyclosporiasis presents with watery diarrhoea, often associated with weight loss, nausea, abdominal cramps, gas, anorexia and fatigue. Diarrhoea may be prolonged but is self-limiting. Diagnosis is confirmed by detection of oocysts in faeces. If *Cyclospora* is suspected, inform the laboratory so that stool concentration can be carried out. Laboratories with little experience of *Cyclospora* should refer putative positives to more experienced laboratories for confirmation, as pseudo-outbreaks have occurred.

Transmission and acquisition

Humans are so far the only host species identified for *C. cayetanensis*. Oocysts are excreted in a non-infective unsporulated form; sporulation takes about a week in the environment and infection results from ingestion of mature sporulated oocysts. Spread is therefore indirect via vehicles such as drinking water, swimming pools and food. Outbreaks have been associated with fresh raspberries, basil and lettuce. The incubation period is 1–12 days (median 7 days).

Control

Prevention and control in developed countries relies on sanitary disposal of faeces and advice to travellers. Should a cluster of cases occur within Europe, ask each case about travel abroad: if no history of travel, then take a food history asking specifically about raw fruit, salad and vegetables and imported food.

3.18 Cytomegalovirus

Cytomegalovirus (CMV), a herpes virus, causes a variety of infections. Its major impact is in the newborn and the immunocompromised.

> **Suggested on-call action**
>
> No person-to-person spread under normal conditions, therefore no need for urgent action.

Epidemiology

Approximately half the adult population in developed countries, virtually all gay or bisexual men with AIDS and 75% of other HIV risk groups have been infected with CMV.

Clinical features

Congenital infection may cause stillbirth, perinatal death, present as cytomegaloviruria in an otherwise normal infant or as a disease with fever, hepatitis, pneumonitis and severe brain damage. Infection acquired postnatally or later in life is often asymptomatic, or an acute febrile illness, cytomegalovirus mononucleosis, may occur.

CMV is a major cause of morbidity in immunocompromised patients. Disease may result from reactivation of latent infection. There may be pulmonary, gastrointestinal (GI) or CNS involvement; CMV causes retinitis and ulcerative disease of the GI tract in the terminal phase of AIDS. A post-transfusion syndrome, which resembles infectious mononucleosis, can develop following transfusion with blood containing CMV.

Laboratory confirmation

Virus particles may be excreted by individuals without active disease, and a positive culture must be interpreted with caution. The demonstration of active disease may require biopsy: histologic findings of viral inclusion bodies in colonic, esophageal or lung tissue, as well as identification of virus by special stains or culture, are necessary. Periodic assessment of CMV-DNA load in peripheral blood by quantitative PCR may be useful for identification of patients at high risk of developing CMV disease and for monitoring the effects of antiviral therapy. CMV retinitis, however, is typically diagnosed by ophthalmologic findings alone in high-risk patients. A diagnosis of CMV encephalitis can be made by brain biopsy or by detection of CMV-DNA in CSF.

Transmission

CMV is transmitted through body fluids, blood or transplanted organs. In the newborn, infection may have been acquired transplacentally or during birth.

Acquisition

The incubation period for transfusion CMV mononucleosis is 2–4 weeks.

Virus excretion is irregular and the virus may remain latent for long periods.

Prevention

• Screening of transplant donors for active disease.
• Ganciclovir has been proposed for the prophylaxis of CMV disease in transplant recipients at risk of CMV disease and the prevention of CMV disease in HIV +ve individuals.

Surveillance

No need to report individual cases, other than through routine laboratory surveillance.

Response to a case

• No public health response usually necessary.

Investigation of a cluster and control of an outbreak

• Investigate to ensure that it is not caused by exposure to contaminated blood or blood products.

Suggested case definition

Neonatal: clinically compatible disease with isolate or PCR positive.
Adult: clinically compatible disease with isolate or CMV-DNA detection or antigen detection or specific IgM-positive or four-fold rise in antibody titre.

3.19 Dengue fever

Dengue is a febrile disease caused by a flavivirus with four distinct serogroups and is transmitted by the bite of *Aedes* mosquitoes.

Suggested on-call action

None usually necessary.

Epidemiology

Endemic throughout the tropics and subtropics. Almost half the Dengue imported into

Europe comes from Asia. Dengue haemorrhagic fever is most common in children less than 10 years old from endemic areas.

Clinical features

Dengue presents with an abrupt onset of fever, chills, headache, backache and severe prostration. Aching in the legs and joints occurs during the first hours of illness. Fever and symptoms persist for 48–96 hours, followed by rapid defervescence, and after about 24 hours a second rapid temperature rise follows (saddleback temperature). Typical dengue is not fatal.

In dengue haemorrhage fever (DHF) bleeding tendencies occur with shock 2–6 days after onset. Mortality for DHF ranges from 6 to 30%; most deaths occur in infants less than 1 year old.

Laboratory confirmation

Serologic diagnosis may be made by haemagglutination inhibiting and complement fixation tests using paired sera.

Transmission

Spread by mosquito bites (e.g. *Aedes aegypti*). No person-to-person spread.

Acquisition

The incubation period is 3–15 days.

Human-to-human spread of dengue has not been recorded, but people are infectious to mosquitoes during the febrile period.

Prevention

• Avoidance of mosquito bites, e.g. with bed nets and insect repellent.
• Control or eradication of the mosquito vector.
• To prevent transmission to mosquitoes, patients in endemic areas should be kept under mosquito netting until the second bout of fever has abated.

Surveillance

Public health officials should be informed of individual cases.

Response to a case

• Isolation not required.
• Specimens should be taken using universal precautions and the laboratory informed.

Investigation of a cluster and control of an outbreak

Not relevant to European countries.

Suggested case definition

A clinically compatible case confirmed by
• growth from or demonstration of virus in serum and/or tissue samples by immunohistochemistry or by viral nucleic acid detection; *or*
• demonstration of a fourfold or greater rise in IgG or IgM antibody titres to one or more dengue virus antigens in paired serum samples.

3.20 Diphtheria

Diphtheria is an infection of the upper respiratory tract, and sometimes the skin. It is caused by toxin-producing (toxigenic) strains of *Corynebacterium diphtheriae*, and occasionally by toxigenic *C. ulcerans*. It is a rare infection, although when a case does occur it tends to generate significant work for the public health team, as it is potentially fatal if untreated.

Suggested on-call action

• Obtain full clinical details, travel and vaccination history.
• Liaise with both local and reference labs to ensure rapid diagnosis and toxogenicity testing.
• Prepare list of close contacts.
• If diagnosis strongly suspected, arrange for immediate swabbing, chemoprophylaxis and vaccination of close contacts.
• Ensure case is admitted to specialist unit.

Epidemiology

Diphtheria is rare in countries with well-established immunisation programmes. In the UK, where immunisation was introduced in 1940, there are about four cases a year. Most of these are imported from the Indian subcontinent and many are mild cases in vaccinated individuals. The case fatality rate is 5–10%. Indigenous cases are very rare, although there are a few UK-acquired cases every year due to toxigenic *C. ulcerans*. There has been a rise in infections due to nontoxigenic strains of *C. diphtheriae* in recent years; these cases have presented with a mild sore throat only.

The epidemiology is similar in other countries of Western Europe, although there was a small outbreak among alcoholics in Sweden during the 1980s. A large epidemic of diphtheria occurred in countries of the former USSR during the 1990s; at its peak in 1995 there were approximately 52,000 cases and 1700 deaths. By 2002 there were less than 1000 cases, most in Russia, although a small number of cases still occur every year in the Baltic states.

Clinical features

Diphtheria is rarely recognised on clinical grounds, as many cases are in vaccinated individuals. In classical respiratory diphtheria there is sore throat, fever, enlarged cervical lymph nodes and swelling of the soft tissues of the neck—the 'bull neck' appearance. The pharyngeal membrane, which is not always present, is typically grey, thick and difficult to remove. There may be hoarseness and stridor. Nasal diphtheria usually presents with a blood-stained nasal discharge. Cutaneous diphtheria causes small ulcers, often on the legs. The disease is caused by a toxin that particularly affects the heart and nervous system. The effects of this toxin are irreversible and so late treatment (with antitoxin) is ineffective.

Laboratory confirmation

It is usually the identification of a *Corynebacterium sp.* from a nose or throat swab or skin ulcer that alerts the public health physician to the possibility of diphtheria. Any isolate of a potentially toxigenic *Corynebacterium* should be referred promptly to the national reference laboratory for confirmation and toxigenicity testing. Where the diagnosis seems likely, an acute serum specimen should be obtained before giving antitoxin, and any skin lesions should be swabbed.

Transmission

Man is the only reservoir and carriers are rare in vaccinated populations, so an infectious case is the usual source. Transmission is usually by air-borne droplets or direct contact with infected respiratory discharges or skin ulcers; rarely from contact with articles contaminated by discharges from infected lesions. Diphtheria is not highly infectious, although exposed cutaneous lesions are more infectious than nasopharyngeal cases.

Acquisition

The incubation period is 2–5 days, occasionally longer. Cases are no longer infectious after 3 days of antibiotic treatment. Untreated cases are infectious for up to 4 weeks. The infectious dose is not known. Natural immunity usually (although not always) develops after infection.

Prevention

• Vaccinate with diphtheria toxoid (usually combined with tetanus, pertussis, polio and Hib). The UK schedule is three doses at 2, 3 and 4 months of age, with boosters at 3–5 years and 13–18 years (N.B.: the second booster is with a low-dose adult formulation).
• Boosters also recommended for travellers to countries where diphtheria is endemic or epidemic.

Surveillance

• All forms of the disease notifiable in most European countries, including the UK.
• Report immediately to the public health authorities on suspicion.
• Laboratory reporting should specify whether the organism is a toxin producer

Response to a case

• Secure confirmation from reference laboratory.
• All cases must be assessed by a suitably experienced physician. Unless there is strong clinical suspicion, other control measures can await confirmation as a toxin producer (this can be done urgently, e.g. at HPA Colindale).
• No control measures required for infections due to nontoxigenic strains. Confirmation of toxigenicity can be obtained within a few hours by PCR.
• For confirmed or strongly suspected toxigenic infections, action is outlined below for case and contacts:

Measures for the case

• Arrange strict barrier nursing until microbiological clearance demonstrated (minimum two negative nose and throat swabs, at least 24 hours apart, the first at least 24 hours after stopping antibiotics).
• Secure microbiological clearance with a 7-day course of erythromycin (or other macrolide antibiotic).
• Give a booster or primary vaccination course (depending on vaccination status).
• The effects of diphtheria toxin are irreversible, so early diagnosis and treatment with antitoxin is vital. It is important to know how to access supplies of diphtheria antitoxin, including out of hours.

Measures for close contacts

• Close contacts include household and kissing contacts; this may be extended further, e.g. to school contacts if many of these less close contacts are unvaccinated.
• Obtain swabs from nose and throat, and any skin lesions, for culture.
• Monitor for 7 days from last contact with case (daily measurement of temperature and examination of throat).
• Exclude foodhandlers and those with close contact with unvaccinated children from work until all swabs shown to be negative.
• Give a 7-day course of erythromycin (or other macrolide antibiotic).
• Obtain further nose and throat swabs after course of antibiotics, and repeat course if still positive.
• Give a booster or primary vaccination course (depending on vaccination status).
• Infections due to toxigenic *C. ulcerans* should be treated the same as *C. diphtheriae*, as there is some evidence that person-to-person transmission may occur.
• No public health action required for infections due to nontoxigenic *C. diphtheriae*, although the patient should be treated with penicillin or erythromycin if symptomatic.

Investigation of a cluster

Obtain travel history or links to travellers.

Response to an outbreak

As for an individual case, but in addition consider the need for a community-wide vaccination programme.

Suggested case definition for an outbreak

Laboratory evidence of infection due to toxigenic *C. diphtheriae* or *C. ulcerans*, in a patient with compatible symptoms. Sore throat only in a vaccinated individual is a compatible symptom.

3.21 Encephalitis, acute

Suggested on-call action

The causes of acute encephalitis are unlikely to cause outbreaks and do not require public health action unless rabies is suspected.

Acute encephalitis is inflammation of the brain, caused by a variety of viruses. The commonest cause in western Europe is herpes simplex type 1 (about 30 cases a year in the UK), which is a severe infection mainly affecting adults; the case fatality rate may be as high as 70%. Herpes simplex encephalitis is intrinsically acquired, so no public health action is required in response to a case.

Tick-borne encephalitis (see Chapter 3.76) occurs in many European countries, and there are several mosquito-borne encephalitides in the USA. Other causes of acute encephalitis are Japanese B encephalitis (Chapter 3.39), West Nile Virus (chapter 3.86) and rabies (Chapter 3.61). Encephalitis also occurs as an acute complication of measles and chickenpox. Acute encephalitis is notifiable in England, Wales and Northern Ireland.

3.22 Enterococci, including glycopeptide-resistant enterococci

Enterococci, including the species *E. faecalis* and *E. faecium*, are normally present in the gastrointestinal tract. They are of low virulence but can cause a range of infections in immunocompromised hospital patients, including wound infection, urinary tract infection, septicaemia and endocarditis. Enterococci may also colonise open wounds and skin ulcers. Enterococci readily become resistant to antibiotics. By the mid-1980s resistance to commonly used antibiotics was widespread, leaving only glycopeptides (vancomycin and teicoplanin) available for treatment. In 1987 vancomycin-resistant enterococci (VRE) were reported and have since spread to many hospitals. Vancomycin resistance may be coded by transferable plasmids and there is concern that it may transfer to other more pathogenic bacteria. Transfer to MRSA has been reported.

Suggested public health on-call action

The local health protection team should be prepared to assist the infection control doctor to investigate and control nosocomial outbreaks of glycopeptide-resistant enterococci.

Epidemiology

There were 4568 reports of enterococcal bacteraemia from laboratories in England during 2002 and of these 256 were vancomycin resistant. Glycopeptide-resistant enterococci (GRE) are becoming more common in hospitals throughout the world, there are different strains of GRE and hospital outbreaks have been reported from dialysis, transplant, haematology and intensive care units.

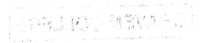

Clinical features

Enterococcal infection should be suspected in any case of sepsis in critically ill hospitalised patients, particularly those with severe underlying disease. GRE bacteraemias may be associated with a poorer clinical prognosis compared with non-GRE bacteraemia.

Laboratory diagnosis

Appropriate microbiological investigation is essential to accurately identify enterococci and detect glycopeptide resistance. Enterococci are often detected in mixed culture where the clinical significance is unclear. Typing of strains is available.

Transmission

• The lower gastrointestinal tract is the main reservoir: most infection is endogenous.
• Spread can occur from infected or colonised patients, either directly or indirectly via the hands of medical and nursing staff, contaminated equipment or environmental surfaces.
• Animal strains of GRE may colonise the gastrointestinal tract of humans via contaminated food.

Acquisition

• Most infection is endogenous.
• Stool carriage may persist for months or years.
• Risk factors include prior antibiotic therapy (glycopeptides or cephalosporins), prolonged hospital stay, admission to intensive care or other specialist units.

Prevention

• Prudent use of antibiotics in medical and veterinary practice.
• Prompt diagnosis of GRE by the microbiology laboratory (routine screening for vancomycin resistance among clinical isolates).
• Implementation of appropriate control of infection measures (standard precautions and source isolation).

• Selective screening for VRE in intensive care units, etc.
• Periodic antibiotic sensitivity surveys.

Surveillance

• Cases should be reported to national surveillance schemes and isolates may be submitted to the appropriate Antibiotic Reference Unit.
• In the UK, national surveillance of *Staphylococcus aureus* positive blood cultures has been extended to include enterococci (GRE and non-GRE).

Response to a case

• Treatment is with a combination of antibiotics guided by sensitivity testing (colonisation is more frequent than infection).
• Removal of catheters and drainage of abscesses may be necessary.
• Attempted clearance of carriage by oral therapy is usually unsuccessful and is not recommended.
• Screening staff for stool carriage is of no value.
• Emphasise hand hygiene and ward cleaning.
• Implement infection control measures based on clinical risk assessment.
• Patients with GRE (especially where there is diarrhoea or incontinence) should be isolated in single rooms or cohorted in bays on the open ward.
• When a patient with GRE is transferred to another institution, inform clinical and infection control staff.

Investigation of a cluster

Isolates from both infected and colonised patients should be typed: hospital outbreaks can involve a single strain whereas community strains are usually of multiple types.

Control of an outbreak

• Reinforce measures for a single case.
• Screening to identify colonised patients (faecal sample most useful screening specimen).

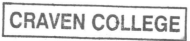

3.23 Epstein–Barr virus

Epstein–Barr virus (EBV), a member of the herpesvirus family, is the cause of infectious mononucleosis (glandular fever). EBV is also associated with Burkitt's lymphoma in African patients, and other neoplasias.

Epidemiology

In countries where there is overcrowding and poor hygiene, 90% of children have serological evidence of EBV infection by the age of 2 years. In developed countries, infection is delayed until adolescence and early adult life.

Clinical features

The clinical features of infectious mononucleosis (IM) are fever, tonsillitis, lymphadenopathy, splenomegaly and hepatitis. Treatment with ampicillin leads to a temporary erythematous maculopapular skin rash. Young children generally have a mild non-specific illness.

Laboratory confirmation

Diagnosis is confirmed by the finding of atypical mononuclear cells in the peripheral blood. Heterophile antibody tests such as the Paul Bunnell or Monospot tests are often used as first line tests. Test for IgM and IgG to EBV-viral capsid antigen and tests for EBV nuclear antigen are also available.

Transmission

Most cases are spread from asymptomatic carriers by oro–pharyngeal route as a result of contact with saliva, either directly during kissing or indirectly on hands or fomites. Attack rates may be as high as 50%. EBV can also be spread in blood transfusions.

Acquisition

The incubation period is 4–6 weeks. After recovery a person may remain infectious for several months because EBV persists in the lymphoid tissue of the oropharynx and is excreted in saliva. Lifelong immunity follows infection, although latent infection can reactivate.

Prevention

Health education and hygienic measures where practical may reduce exposure to saliva, especially from infected persons.

Surveillance

Reporting of cases is not generally required.

Response to a case

Exclusion of cases is not necessary. Splenic enlargement is common in IM and spontaneous splenic rupture is a rare, potentially fatal complication occurring in 0.1–0.5% of patients. Although evidence is lacking, it is prudent to recommend that strenuous physical exercise is avoided for 3–4 weeks after the onset of illness and that contact sports are avoided until there is no evidence of splenomegaly.

3.24 *Escherichia coli* O157 (and other *E. coli* gastroenteritis)

Many different strains of *E. coli* are associated with gastrointestinal illness, which can be classified into seven main syndromes. The most serious illness is that caused by verocytotoxic *E. coli* (VTEC), also known as enterohaemorrhagic *E. coli* (EHEC), which has the potential to cause haemolytic uraemic syndrome, HUS, (the commonest cause of acute renal failure in children) and death. The other syndromes are summarised in Table 3.24.1.

The most common VTEC strain in most European countries is *E. coli* O157:H7 (others are given in Table 3.24.2). It may be food-borne and can cause large outbreaks with the potential for secondary spread.

Suggested on-call action

1 If *E. coli* O157 or other VTEC:
  • Exclude if in high risk group (Table 2.2.1).
  • If other cases known to you or reporting clinician or laboratory, implement outbreak plan.
  • If no other cases known, ensure risk factor details collected on next working day.
2 If other *E. coli* gastroenteritis: exclude if in high-risk group (Table 2.2.1).

Epidemiology

VTEC have become recognised as major infective causes of bloody diarrhoea a in Europe. Around 900 laboratory-confirmed cases of *E. coli* O157 infection are reported annually in the UK, including around 20 outbreaks. The highest age specific incidence of diagnosed infection is in children under 5 years, and there is a slight male preponderance. Infection is more common in summer and early autumn (Fig 2.2.2). Reported rates in Europe for 1996 varied from 0.1 per million inhabitants in Spain to 20 per million in the UK, although there was also marked variation in ascertainment. There is marked regional variation within the UK, with the highest rates in rural areas, particularly in Scotland.

Approximately 80% of reported cases in the UK are sporadic, but a large outbreak in central Scotland associated with contaminated meats from a butcher's shop caused 17 deaths in elderly people in 1996. An outbreak in Japan in the same year, associated with bean sprouts in mass-produced lunches for schoolchildren, led to 8000 identified cases. About 10% of UK cases acquire their infection abroad.

HUS has an incidence of about 0.8 per 10,000 children under 5 years, of which 90% are 'typical' (diarrhoea associated, Table 3.24.2). *E. coli* O157 is the most common cause of typical HUS in most countries studied.

Clinical features

Infection with *E. coli* O157 may cause no symptoms; a diarrhoeal illness; haemorrhagic colitis with bloody diarrhoea and severe abdominal pain but usually no fever; haemolytic uraemic syndrome with renal failure, haemolytic anaemia and thrombocytopaenia, particularly in children; and thrombocytopenic purpura, particularly in adults, which may add neurological complications to the features of HUS. The case fatality rate of severe infection (HUS or TTP) is reported as 3–17%.

HUS may occur 2–14 days after the onset of diarrhoea (usually 5–10 days). It affects 2–8% of all reported cases and is more common if diarrhoea is bloody. VTEC causes the more common glomerular ('typical') form of HUS (Table 3.24.2).

Laboratory confirmation

Diagnosis is usually based on stool culture. Because most *E. coli* O157 differ from the majority of *E. coli* in not fermenting sorbitol,

Table 3.24.1 *E. coli* causing diarrhoea (other than VTEC)

Designation	Epidemiology	Illness	Incubation	Sources	Main 'O' serogroups
Enteropathogenic (EPEC)	Sporadic cases and outbreaks in children, usually aged less than 2 years, especially in developing countries.	Watery diarrhoea, often mucus but usually no blood. Also fever and possibly vomiting or respiratory symptoms. Lasts up to 2 weeks.	9–12 hours	Faeco–oral, e.g. via fomites and hands in nurseries and hospitals. Contaminated infant foods in developing countries.	18, 25, 26, 44, 55, 86, 111, 114, 119, 125, 126, 127, 128ab, 142, 158, 608
Enterotoxigenic (ETEC)	Major cause of travellers' diarrhoea. Dehydrating diarrhoea in children in developing countries.	Watery diarrhoea, abdominal pain, nausea, low-grade fever. Lasts 1–5 days, may be prolonged.	10–72 hours	Food and water contaminated by humans. Nosocomial and hotel outbreaks reported.	6, 8, 11, 15, 20, 25, 27, 63, 78, 80, 85, 114, 115, 128ac, 148, 149, 153, 159, 167, 173.
Enteroinvasive (EIEC)	Occasional cause of travellers' diarrhoea or outbreaks in developed countries. Serious infection common in children in developing world.	Watery diarrhoea, often with blood and mucus. Abdominal pain, fever. Lasts up to 2 weeks.	10–18 hours.	Probably contaminated food.	28ac, 29, 52, 112ac, 115, 124, 136, 143, 144, 145, 147, 152, 159, 164, 167

Enteroaggregative (EaggEC)	Common in developing countries (including Indian subcontinent) and a risk for travellers. Children more commonly affected. Outbreaks reported in Western Europe.	Diarrhoea, usually watery. May be blood or mucus. Often chronic in children or AIDS. Often vomiting and dehydration in children.	20–50 hours.	Probably contaminated food and water.	3, 15, 19, 44, 62, 73, 77, 86, 98, 111, 113, 127, 134
Diffuse-adherence (DAEC) or diarrhoea-associated haemolytic (DHEC)	Preschool children in developing countries.	Diarrhoea (mucoid and watery). Fever, vomiting. Lasts about 8 days.	Unclear	Unclear	–
Cytolethal distending toxin-producing (CDT-producing)	Importance as yet unclear.	Diarrhoea	Unclear	Unclear	–

Control

Enteric precautions for cases, personal hygiene.
Exclude risk groups until 48 hours after first normal stool.
Advice to travellers abroad.
Handwashing and environmental cleaning in nurseries.

Table 3.24.2 Causes of haemolytic uraemic syndrome

Typical ('post-diarrhoeal', 'epidemic', 'D+'):
- *E. coli* O157:H7 and O157:H
- Other *E. coli* (e.g. O26, O55, O91, O103, O104, O111, O113, O116, O119, O128, O130, O145, O157)
- Viruses, e.g. coxsackie
- *Shigella* dysentery
- *Campylobacter*
- *Streptococcus pneumoniae*
- Influenza

Atypical ('sporadic', 'D-'):
- Inherited disorders
- SLE
- Cancer
- Drugs, e.g. mitomycin C, cyclosporin, quinine, crack cocaine
- Pregnancy
- Oral contraceptives
- Idiopathic

they show up as pale colonies when plated on sorbitol-McConkey agar. This plate should be used as a routine screen for all diarrhoeal specimens, irrespective of history of blood in stool. Biochemical and serological tests can then confirm the isolate as O157. However, if clinical suspicion of VTEC is high, the possibility of a sorbitol fermenting VTEC should be considered. VTEC strains produce one or both of two verocytotoxins (VT1 and VT2): tests for these toxins are available at reference laboratories. Phage typing and genotyping are available to aid epidemiological investigations. Twenty-nine different phage types were identified from human cases in a European study, with the predominant type varying by country of origin: two-thirds of cases in the UK were due to three phage types (PT2, PT21/28 and PT8), PT2 and PT8 predominated in Germany, PT4 and PT8 in Sweden, PT32 in Ireland and PT2 in Finland. Genomic typing may also be available if indicated. Serology can be used for retrospective diagnosis, and salivary testing may be available. Methods exist for examining food, water, environmental and animal samples for *E. coli* O157.

Transmission

The natural reservoir of *E. coli* O157 is the gastrointestinal tract of animals, particularly cattle, but also sheep, goats, deer, horses, dogs, birds and flies. Humans are infected via following:

- Contaminated foods: carcasses may become contaminated through contact with intestinal contents at slaughter. Mincing beef compounds the problem as the contaminating organisms may be introduced into the interior of foods such as beefburgers where they will survive inadequate cooking. Other food vehicles may be cross-contaminated in the kitchen from raw food (e.g. cooked meats) or in the field by animal faeces (e.g. 'windfall apples' and radish sprouts). Milk (and other dairy products), either unpasteurised, inadequately pasteurised or contaminated postpasteurisation, has been implicated in some outbreaks. The organism is relatively resistant to acid, fermentation and drying.
- Direct contact with animals, e.g. at farm visitor centres. Excreting animals are usually asymptomatic. Soil and water contaminated by animal faeces has led to outbreaks in campers and is also linked to sporadic infection.
- Secondary faeco–oral spread from infected cases is common, particularly in families and institutions, as a result of sharing personal items such as towels and via food. Asymptomatic excretion is common in family contacts of cases.
- Other routes: drinking and bathing in contaminated waters have both been liked with incidents of infection. Nursing and laboratory staff have acquired infection through occupational exposure.

Acquisition

The incubation period ranges from 1 to 9 days between exposure and onset of diarrhoea, with a median of 3–4 days.

The infectious period is unclear. One-third of children under 5 years of age excrete the organism for at least 3 weeks, but prolonged asymptomatic carriage appears to be unusual. Microbiological clearance is usually viewed as two consecutive negative faecal samples, taken at least 48 hours apart. The infectious dose is low, probably under 100 organisms. The role of immunity is not clearly understood. Children under 5 and the elderly are at particular risk of serious infection, such as HUS.

Prevention

• Minimise contamination of carcasses at slaughter.
• Adopt the hazard analysis critical control point (HACCP) approach in both food processing and food service industries to prevent survival of or contamination by *E. coli* O157.
• Good kitchen practices including separation of raw and cooked foods and storage of foods below 10°C.
• Cook beef, lamb and venison products so that any contaminating organisms are subjected to minimum of 70°C for 2 minutes. Cook beefburgers until juices run clear and no pink bits remain inside.
• Pasteurise all milk.
• Adequate hygiene and toilet facilities in nurseries and schools. Supervised handwashing in nurseries and infant schools.
• Precautions during farm visits by children, including the following:
    (i) Handwashing after touching animals.
    (ii) Avoid eating and drinking whilst visiting animals.
    (iii) Keep face away from animals.
    (iv) Do not put hand to mouth.
    (v) Do not touch animal droppings.
    (vi) Clean shoes after visit.
• Keep animals off fields for 3 weeks before allowing their use for recreation or camping.

Surveillance

• All cases of *E. coli* O157 infection or unexplained HUS should be reported to the local public health authority as a matter of urgency. VTEC is statutorily notifiable in Austria, Finland and Sweden. In the UK, cases should be notified as 'suspected food poisoning'.
• Laboratories should test all samples from cases of diarrhoea or bloody stools for *E. coli* O157 and report positives to the appropriate surveillance system on the same day.
• Clinicians should report individual cases of unexplained 'typical' HUS and any cluster of bloody diarrhoea to local public health departments as a matter of urgency, even if the causal agent is unknown.

Response to a case

The severity of disease, particularly in children and the elderly, the small infectious dose and the ability to spread person to person and via contaminated food means that even single cases require prompt investigation.
• National guidelines are available in the UK (see Appendix 2).
• If in high-risk group, for avoiding further transmission (Box 2.2.1), exclude from work or nursery until asymptomatic and two consecutive negative faecal specimens taken at least 48 hours apart.
• Consider cases in infant school children as risk group 4 (Box 2.2.1) and exclude until microbiological clearance.
• Household contacts in high-risk groups to be screened. Exclude those in all high-risk groups (Box 2.2.1) until two negative faecal specimens obtained from the contact and, for risk groups 3 and 4 only, until the index case becomes asymptomatic.
• Enteric precautions during diarrhoeal phase.
• Hygiene advice to cases and contacts, particularly handwashing. Suggest remaining off work/school until normal stools for 48 hours for those in non-high-risk groups.
• Food and water history from all cases covering all 10 days before onset.

- Prompt referral to hospital at first sign of complications.

Investigation of a cluster

- Organise phage typing, toxin typing and, if possible, genotyping with reference laboratory.
- Undertake hypothesis generating study to cover all food and water consumed in 10 days before onset of illness, and all social, school and work activities and visits undertaken. Include exposure to farm animals, pets and cases of gastroenteritis. Ask specifically about minced beef or lamb products, cooked meats and milk.
- Investigation of social networks may reveal potential for person-to-person spread via common (possibly asymptomatic) contacts.

Control of an outbreak

An outbreak of VTEC is a public health emergency and requires a prompt and thorough response. Particular actions include the following:
- Hygiene advice to all cases and contacts.
- Exclude cases as detailed above.
- Enhanced cleaning in all institutional outbreaks.
- Supervised handwashing for children in affected nurseries and infant schools.
- Exclude all cases of diarrhoea from affected (non-residential) institutions, until normal stools and two consecutive negative samples taken at least 48 hours apart received.
- In day-care establishments for children under 5 years of age (high risk of HUS and poor hygiene) screen all attenders. Exclude all positives until microbiological clearance achieved. Adopt similar approach for confused or faecally incontinent elderly attending day-care facilities.
- In residential accommodation for children under 5 or the elderly, screen all residents.

Maintain enteric precautions for all positives until microbiological clearance achieved. Preferably nurse in private room with own washbasin and exclusive use of one toilet whilst diarrhoea continues.
- Institute *urgent* withdrawal of any implicated food. If local supplier involved, ensure personally that this is done, e.g. in UK use local authority powers under Food Safety Act (1990) to seize food. If national or regionally distributed food, contact relevant government department, e.g. Food Standards Agency in UK.
- Issue 'boil water notice' for contaminated drinking water.
- Ensure adequate precautions taken at any implicated farm open to public (HSE guidance available in UK).
- Monitor cases at increased risk of HUS or TTP to ensure prompt referral.
- Antibiotic prophylaxis not generally recommended.

> **Suggested case definition for outbreak**
>
> *Confirmed*: diarrhoea with demonstration of *E. coli* O157 of outbreak strain in stools.
> *Presumptive*: HUS occurring after diarrhoea with no other cause identified.
> *Clinical*: diarrhoea in person epidemiologically linked to outbreak (e.g. onset within 9 days of consuming vehicle) with further investigations awaited.

3.25 Giardiasis

Giardia lamblia, also known as *G. intestinalis* or *G. duodenalis*, is a protozoan parasite that causes intestinal infection throughout the world. In developed countries the illness is particularly associated with water-borne outbreaks, nurseries and other institutions and travel abroad.

Epidemiology

Prevalence rates (including asymptomatic excretion) of between 2 and 7% have been demonstrated in developed countries, although a study in England and Wales found an annual community incidence of disease of only 0.5 per 1000, of which about one-fifth were reported to national surveillance. Reports in Britain have fallen over the last decade to 3520 in 2003. The most commonly affected age groups are children under 5 years and adults aged 25–39 years. A seasonal peak in July–October is reported. Groups with higher rates of infection include residents of institutions, travellers abroad, gay men and the immunocompromised.

Clinical features

About a quarter of acute infections are asymptomatic excretors. Symptomatic diarrhoea may be accompanied by malaise, flatulence, foul-smelling greasy stools, abdominal cramps, bloating, nausea and anorexia. Prolonged diarrhoea, malabsorption and weight loss are suggestive of giardiasis.

Laboratory confirmation

Giardia infection is usually confirmed by microbiological examination of fresh stool samples for cysts. A single stool sample will identify only about 60% of those infected but three samples (preferably taken on non-consecutive days) will identify over 90%. Cysts may not yet be present at the onset of disease. Antigen assays are reported to be highly sensitive and specific, although they are not yet universally available. They may have a role in cohort screening during outbreaks.

Transmission

Giardiasis results from faeco–oral transmission of *Giardia* cysts. This can occur directly or via food or water. Humans appear to be the main reservoir for *G. lamblia* infection. Other animals including dogs, cats, rodents and domesticated ruminants are commonly affected by *G. lamblia*, but whether they are important reservoirs for humans is not clear. *Giardia* cysts are environmentally resistant and survive well in cold water. Giardiasis is the most frequently diagnosed water-borne disease in the United States, and water-borne outbreaks have been reported from Europe. Recreational contact with water may also be a risk. Person-to-person spread is increasingly recognised as important, both in institutions and from children in the community and within families.

Acquisition

The median incubation period is 7–10 days but extremes of 3–25 days have been reported. Cyst excretion may persist for up to 6 months and may be intermittent. As few as 25 cysts may cause infection. Breastfeeding has a protective effect; but there is increased susceptibility in those who have had gastric surgery or who have reduced gastric acidity.

Prevention

Prevention of giardiasis is dependent on
- adequate treatment of water supplies; standard chlorination is not sufficient to destroy cysts and should be supplemented by filtration, flocculation or sedimentation.
- adequate control of infection and food hygiene practices in institutions, especially those dealing with children.

- handwashing after toilet use and before preparing food.
- advice to travellers abroad on safe food and water.

Surveillance

Diagnosed cases should be reported to local public health departments (notify as 'food poisoning' in UK) and to national surveillance centres.

Response to a case

- Hygiene advice should be given. Ideally, the case should not attend work or school until he/she has normal stools.
- Cases in risk groups 1–4 (Table 2.2.1) should be excluded until 48 hours after the first normal stool. Microbiological clearance is not necessary before return. Schoolchildren should ideally not attend school until they have had no diarrhoea for 24 hours.
- Treatment of symptomatic cases.
- Screening of symptomatic household contacts may identify individuals needing treatment.

Investigation of a cluster

Enquiries should include water consumption (compare to water supply zones), food sources, swimming pools, contact with day centres (especially for children) or other institutions, travel and (if cases mainly adult men) sexual contact.

Control of an outbreak

- Water-borne outbreaks are usually due to use of untreated surface water, inadequate water treatment (e.g. ineffective filtration) or sewage contamination. Geographic mapping of cases will help the local water company identify areas for further investigation.
- Outbreaks in nurseries and other institutions are controlled by enhanced infection

control, especially supervised handwashing for all children, and exclusion and treatment of all symptomatic children. Some would also recommend treatment of asymptomatic carriers: while this will help control the outbreak and prevent spread to community and family contacts, the benefit to the asymptomatic individual is unclear.

Suggestion case definition for an outbreak

Demonstration of cysts plus either
- diarrhoea *or*
- link to outbreak group.

3.26 Gonorrhoea, syphilis and other acute STIs

Sexually transmitted infections (STIs) are defined by their route of transmission: they are transmitted by direct sexual contact. For HIV infection, see Chapter 3.37 and for genital Chlamydia infection, see Chapter 3.10.

Suggested public health on-call action

The public health team may be alerted to clusters of cases of STI (e.g. syphilis or gonorrhoea) and should be prepared to initiate or assist with an investigation.

Epidemiology

In recent years in the UK, annual totals of diagnoses of STIs including syphilis have increased. Similar increases have been seen in other Western European countries and there have been spectacular increases in Eastern Europe and the former Soviet Union. There is evidence of a substantial burden of STI morbidity particularly among men who have sex with men, young men and women, those of black ethnic origin and those living in urban areas. Diagnoses of chancroid and granuloma inguinale, while common in subtropical and tropical countries, are rare in the UK but outbreaks of lymphogranuloma venereum have occurred in the Netherlands. More detail is given in Table 3.26.1.

Diagnosis

See Table 2.7.1.

Transmission

STIs are spread by direct, usually sexual, contact with infectious discharges or lesions. Syphilis may also be spread *in utero* and via blood transfusions.

Acquisition

Incubation periods vary, see Chapter 2.7.

Prevention

The prevention of STIs depends on
• health and sex education to discourage multiple sexual partners and casual sexual activity and to promote correct and consistent use of condoms.
• early detection of cases and prompt effective treatment.
• identification, examination and treatment of the sexual partners of cases.
• opportunistic or routine screening and treatment of certain subgroups of the population who may be at increased risk of STIs or their complications. An example is the routine use of

Table 3.26.1 Epidemiology of acute STIs in England and Wales

Chlamydia infection	Genital chlamydia infection is the most commonly diagnosed STI seen in GUM clinics. There were 89,818 diagnoses in 2003, a 9% increase compared with 2002. These increases reflect not only increased prevalence but also increasing opportunistic and demand-led screening.
Gonorrhoea	Compared with 2002, gonorrhoea diagnoses at GUM clinics decreased by 3% from 25,065 to 24,309. The peak reached in 2002 contrasts with 12,829 in 1998.
	There is a disproportionately high incidence of gonorrhoea in young men and women, homosexual and bisexual men, those of black-Caribbean ethnic origin and those living in urban areas.
	The number of isolates that are resistant to penicillin is declining but there has been an increase in strains that are resistant to ciprofloxacin. It is possible that a rise in treatment failures could enhance transmission of gonorrhoea. Most resistant strains are in persons of white ethnic origin and are acquired in the UK.
Infectious syphilis	Between 2002 and 2003 diagnoses of syphilis at GUM clinics increased by 28% (from 1232 to 1575).
	In the past most cases of infectious syphilis were acquired abroad, notably in Eastern Europe, and many were acquired homosexually.
	Recently there have been outbreaks of syphilis in several UK cities amongst homosexual men and heterosexual men and women.
Genital herpes simplex virus infection and genital warts	Compared with 2002, diagnoses of genital herpes at GUM clinics decreased by 2% (from 18,432 to 17,990) in 2003.
	Genital warts increased by 2% in 2003 (from 69,569 to 70,883).
	The long-term increases in genital warts and genital herpes simplex infection are due to changes in health seeking behaviour as well as changes in incidence.

syphilis serological tests in pregnancy, to prevent congenital syphilis.

Surveillance

See Chapter 2.7.

Response to a case

- Individual cases of STIs are not generally reported to the local health protection team.
- The case should receive prompt effective treatment and should refrain from sexual intercourse until treated.
- Sexual contacts should be identified, examined and treated as appropriate.

Investigation of a cluster and control of an outbreak

An STI outbreak has been defined as
- observed number of cases greater than expected over a defined time period;

- linked cases of STIs;
- the need for reorganisation of services or identification of additional resources to manage cases;
- any case of congenitally acquired infection.

The underlying principles of outbreak investigation are applicable to STIs. However STIs have particular features:
- STIs are associated with some degree of stigma.
- Confidentiality concerns may restrict the availability of patient data.
- Effective control involves treating patients and sexual contact(s).
- Sustained behavioural change may be required to reduce spread in sexual networks.

Special features of STI outbreaks:
- Identification and initial investigation of outbreaks is usually multiagency involving the local GUM physician, sexual health advisers at GUM clinics, the local health protection team and a local microbiologist.

Table 3.26.2 Managing STI outbreaks at local level

Increase in number of cases in local area	Review local clinical surveillance data
	Discuss with other local colleagues
	Compare with national disease trends
Is there a problem?	Confirm local increase
Is there an outbreak?	Inform local public health authorities
	Undertake descriptive epidemiology using routine surveillance data
	Epidemic curve
	Age/sex/sexuality distribution
	Establish Outbreak Control Group
Characterise outbreak and institute control measures	Active case surveillance
	Analytic epidemiology
	Focused research
	Implement control measures based on evidence
	General measures:
	Health education
	Partner notification
	Targeted strategies:
	Peer-led interventions
	Review GUM service provision
	Venue outreach and screening
Evaluate control measures	Review processes and outcomes
	Audit interventions
	Monitor surveillance data
	Outbreak report
	Key lessons

- Intervention will require the identification of sexual contacts and sexual networks and the dissemination of health promotion messages.
- Compared with other outbreaks of infection, STI outbreaks will usually take longer to investigate and control.

The local health protection team should be prepared to initiate or assist with an epidemiological investigation in collaboration with others. Guidelines on investigating STI outbreaks have been published (Table 3.26.2).

3.27 Hantavirus

Hantavirus infection is an acute zoonotic viral disease.

Suggested on-call action
None usually required.

Epidemiology

Hantavirus infections are found where there is close contact between people and infected rodents. In Europe foci are recognised in the Balkans, the Ardennes and Scandinavia. Sweden reports approximately 200 cases, Finland 1000 and Russia more than 10,000 cases annually, and more than 1000 cases have been documented in the former Yugoslavia. Cases have also been documented in other European countries (France, Belgium, Germany, Greece, Netherlands).

Clinical features

The clinical picture depends upon the subtype causing the infection and is characterised by haemorrhagic fever with renal syndrome (HFRS), or acute pulmonary oedema (HPS). HFRS manifests as fever, thrombocytopenia and acute renal failure, and HPS as fever with respiratory difficulty. A number of different subtypes exist, each of which is associated with a particular rodent species. Of the two European subtypes, Puumala tends to cause milder disease (nephropathia epidemica), but Dobrava HFRS is often severe (Table 3.27.1).

Laboratory confirmation

Demonstration of specific antibody (IgM or IgG) by ELISA or IFA. IgM is often present on hospitalisation. PCR for specific RNA may be available.

Transmission

Usually aerosol transmission from rodent excreta. Human-to-human transmission has been reported in South American (AndesVirus) HPS.

Acquisition

The incubation period is 1–6 weeks.
The infectious period for HPS is unclear.

Table 3.27.1 Main hantavirus serotypes

Syndrome	Serotype	Geography
HFRS	Dobrava	Balkans
	Puumala	Northern Europe
	Hantaan	Asia
	Seoul	Worldwide
HPS	Sin Nombre	North America
	Various other serotypes	North and South America

Prevention

In areas that are known to be endemic, rodents should be excluded from living quarters.

Response to a case

- HFRS is not transmitted person to person and there is no need for urgent public health action.
- In view of the possibility of person-to-person spread in HPS suspected cases should be nursed in isolation.

Suggested case definition

HFRS or HPS confirmed by IgM or PCR.

3.28 Head lice

Head lice (*Pediculus humanus capitis*) are wingless insects that live close to the scalp where they feed by biting and sucking blood. The female head louse lives for 3–4 weeks and lays on average 10 eggs per day. The eggs are tear-shaped, 1 mm in length and are securely glued to the hair shaft close to the scalp. The eggs hatch after 7–10 days and the emerging nymphs moult three times before reaching maturity in 6–12 days when mating occurs. The full-grown louse is 2–3-mm long. Empty egg sacks are white and shiny, and may be found some distance from the scalp as the hair grows out. Although there may be large number of lice on an affected head, the average number is about 10.

Suggested on-call action

Not generally applicable.

Epidemiology

Questionnaire surveys suggest a prevalence of 2% and an annual incidence of 37% in UK primary school children. Primary care data from the UK give a rate of 28 per 1000 patient years at risk. Anyone with head hair can get head lice but children aged 3–12 years are particularly affected.

Clinical features

Head lice infestation is associated with little morbidity but causes high levels of anxiety amongst parents. Many early infestations are asymptomatic. Itching and scratching of the scalp may occur after 4–6 weeks due to sensitivity to louse saliva. Occasionally secondary bacterial infection may occur.

Confirmation

Diagnosis depends on finding live lice on the head. Empty egg shells (nits) are not proof of active infestation. Lice move rapidly away from any disturbance, and examination of dry hair is unreliable. Lice can only be reliably detected by combing wet lubricated hair with a 'detector' comb. If lice are present they fall out or are stuck to the comb. If necessary, lice and nymphs can be examined with a magnifying glass or low-power microscope to confirm their presence.

Transmission and acquisition

Transmission is by direct contact with the head of an affected person. Lice cannot jump or fly but move readily through dry hair and cross from person to person when heads touch. Transmission occurs in schools, at home and in the wider community. Indirect spread when personal items are shared is possible, but head lice do not survive for more than 48 hours away from the scalp. A person will remain infectious for as long as there are adult lice on the head. Anyone with hair can be affected and re-infestation may occur. Humans are the only source of head lice, which are host-specific and do not spread from or to animals.

Prevention

- It is probably impossible to completely prevent head lice infestation.

• A number of preventative measures have been promoted including repellents such as piperonal, regular brushing and electronic combs but evidence for their effectiveness is limited.

• Reducing head lice infestation depends on case finding by regular diagnostic wet combing followed by prompt treatment of cases if active infestation is found.

• Contacts of cases must also be examined and treated if appropriate.

Surveillance

• Surveillance data may be available from primary care, e.g. Weekly Returns Service of the Royal College of General Practitioners and the General Practice Research Database (GRPD). In the UK Prescribing Analysis and Cost (PACT) data provides additional insights into insecticide prescribing patterns.

• If head lice are causing particular problems in community settings. such as schools, the local public health team should be informed.

Response to a case

• There are two main methods of treatment (see Box 3.28.1).

• The role of other agents such as 'natural' products and flammable or toxic substances is unclear. Some success has been reported with newer occlusive agents.

• No treatment method is 100% effective. In one study the overall cure rate for wet combing was 38% compared with 78% for malathion lotion.

• Treatment may fail because of misdiagnosis, non-compliance, re-infestation, pediculocide resistance or use of an ineffective preparation.

• Contacts of a case should be examined for head lice by wet combing and treated if necessary.

• It is not necessary to exclude children with head lice from school or nursery (see Table 3.28.1).

Investigation of a cluster

• Clusters of cases of head lice may be reported from schools or other institutional settings.

• The school health nurse is usually the most appropriate person to investigate and advise on control measures.

Control of an outbreak

• Parents should be alerted and asked to carry out case finding by wet combing.

• They should be advised to treat their child promptly if live lice are discovered, using one of the two treatment options.

• Accurate information, explanation and sympathetic reassurance will be required.

Box 3.28.1 Treatment of head lice

Chemical pediculocides	A number of chemical pediculocides are available including carbaryl, malathion and the pyrethroids (permethrin and phenothrin). Lotions and liquids are preferred and contact time should be 12 hours. A single application may not kill unhatched eggs and a second application is advised after 7 days. After treatment, wet combing should be carried out to check for lice. Pediculocides should only be used if live lice are confirmed, and should never be used prophylactically.
Mechanical removal	Lice and larvae as they hatch can be mechanically removed by wet combing well-lubricated hair with a detector comb every 4 days for 2 weeks. This process which must be carried out meticulously breaks the life cycle of the head louse.

Table 3.28.1 Head lice: suggested responsibilities

Parents	Brush or comb their children's hair each day.
	Use detector comb to detect infestation.
	Inform contacts of infested family members about the infestation.
	Advise school, nursery or playgroup if infection discovered.
	Ensure recommended treatment has been carried out.
Health visitors and school health nurses	Education of parents about head lice.
	In case of outbreaks in schools and nurseries ensure policy is being correctly followed.
	Advise families with recurrent problems and consider further measures.
Head teacher	Inform the parents of pupils about any outbreaks of head lice and advise on treatment and contact tracing incorporating the advice of the school nurse, a standard letter may be sent.
	There is no need to send children home from school on the day when an infestation is found, treatment should be started that evening and the child may continue at school.
Consultant for Communicable Disease Control and Community	Receive reports of particular head lice problems in community settings and advise on management.
	Involve other carers, such as community nurses, GPs and teachers as appropriate.
Infection Control Nurses	Make available information on head lice for the public and professionals.
General practitioners and practice staff	Explain the use of a detection comb and wet combing to confirm active infestation.
	Discuss the two treatment options.
	Make available patient information leaflet.
	Prescribe pediculocides when appropriate:only those with confirmed infestations should be treated.
Pharmacists	Explain the use of a detection comb and wet combing to confirm active infestation.
	Discuss the two treatment options.
	Offer for sale of wet combing materials including detector combs or pediculocides as appropriate.
	Shampoos should not be offered for sale.
	Patient information leaflet should be provided with all prescriptions and sales of head lice treatment

3.29 *Helicobacter pylori*

Helicobacter pylori causes a chronic infection associated with chronic upper gastrointestinal disease.

Epidemiology

Infection occurs worldwide. Prevalence in developed countries is 20–50% (up to 75% in socially deprived areas) and, in general, increases with age, with acquisition rates higher in children. However, there is also a cohort effect of decreasing incidence with time.

Diagnosis

Most infection is asymptomatic, but it may cause gastritis and both gastric and duodenal ulceration. Infection is also associated with gastric adenocarcinoma. The annual incidence of peptic ulcer disease is 0.18%, and over 90% of these patients will have *H. pylori* infection. Diagnosis is by serology, breath testing with urea, culture from gastric biopsy/aspirate, or antigen testing of faeces. Treatment is with a mix of antibiotics and antisecretory drugs.

Transmission and acquisition

Transmission is unclear but probably by ingestion of organisms, most likely faeco–oral, but perhaps by oral–oral or gastro–oral routes. Spread via contaminated gastric tubes and endoscopes is recorded and endoscopists have increased risk. Infectivity is assumed to be lifelong and higher in those with achlorhydria.

Control

Other than routine hygiene and disinfection, there is insufficient evidence at present to recommend further preventative interventions. Eradication of infection is associated with remission of gastritis and peptic ulceration.

3.30 Hepatitis A

Hepatitis A virus (HAV) is an enterically transmitted acute infection of the liver, which is primarily spread faeco-orally.

Epidemiology

The incidence of hepatitis A has been decreasing in developed countries over the last 50 years. A cyclical pattern with peaks every 6–10 years is demonstrable in many countries; however, the last such peak in the UK was in 1990 when over 7500 laboratory confirmed cases were reported in England and Wales. By 2000–2003 reports had fallen to around 1000 per annum. Incidence of HAV is less in Scandinavia (where the cyclical pattern has disappeared) and higher in Mediterranean countries (Table 3.30.1). The incidence of confirmed cases in the Western Europe is highest in those aged 15–34 years, although younger cases are more likely to be asymptomatic and therefore less likely to be diagnosed. A marked

Table 3.30.1 General patterns of HAV infection in European countries

Endemicity	Countries	Age of cases	Most common transmission
Very low	Scandinavia	Over 20	Travel abroad
Low	Germany Netherlands Switzerland UK	5–40	Common source outbreaks, person to person, travel abroad
Intermediate	Austria Belgium France Southern Europe Eastern Europe	5–24	Person to person, common source outbreaks, contaminated food/water, travel abroad

excess of males has become apparent in the last few years. A significant minority of cases have travelled abroad, most commonly to Mediterranean countries or the Indian subcontinent. Other groups at increased risk include those in contact with a case of HAV (e.g. household or nursery), homosexually active men, intravenous drug users, haemophiliacs and residents and workers in institutions for the mentally handicapped.

Clinical features

The clinical picture may range from no symptoms to fulminant hepatitis and is greatly influenced by age. Less than 10% of those aged under 6 years develop jaundice but 40% have fever and dark urine and 60% have symptoms such as nausea/vomiting, malaise and diarrhoea. Around half of older children and three quarters of adults develop jaundice after a 2–3 day prodrome of malaise, anorexia, nausea, fever and dark urine. Overall case fatality is around 0.5% but increases with age to over 10% in those over 70 years. Chronic infection does not occur.

Laboratory confirmation

Confirmation of acute HAV is dependent upon demonstration of specific IgM antibodies, which are usually present at onset of symptoms and persist for around 3 months. IgG antibody persists for life and so in the absence of IgM, a fourfold rise in titres in paired samples is required for diagnosis, although patients rarely present in time for this to this to be demonstrable. Persistent IgG may be taken as evidence of immunity due to past infection (or vaccination). Salivary IgM (and IgG) testing is available at specialist laboratories and may be useful in outbreak investigations. HAV-RNA can be detected in blood and stool early in the infection. Subtyping may also be available.

Transmission

HAV infection is spread primarily by the faeco–oral route from other humans. Up to 10^8 infectious units per millilitre are excreted in faeces during the late incubation period and the first week of symptoms. Viraemia also occurs during the prodromal phase of the illness but at much lower levels than in stool. Saliva and urine are of low infectivity.

Faeco–oral spread is likely to be responsible for secondary transmission to household (average secondary attack rate about 15%) and nursery contacts, perhaps aided by transmission via fomites. HAV can spread rapidly but silently among mobile, faecally incontinent children in nurseries and then cause illness in their contacts. Infection in illicit drug users has been reported in several European countries and is likely to be due to poor hygiene, although contamination of drugs and needle sharing may contribute. Travellers to endemic countries risk exposure via food or water: this includes children of immigrants from such countries. HAV can survive for 3–10 months in water, suggesting that even in Europe, shellfish harvested from sewage contaminated waters are a potential source; shellfish concentrate viruses by filtering large quantities of water and are often eaten raw or after gentle steaming, which is inadequate to inactivate HAV. Infected food handlers with poor personal hygiene may also contaminate food. Imported fruit and salad vegetables have also caused outbreaks.

Many cases of HAV do not have a recognised risk factor: it is likely that many of these contracted their infection from an undiagnosed or asymptomatic child case in their household. Such cases may be a factor in community outbreaks that evolve slowly over several months.

Acquisition

The incubation period is reported as 15–50 days (mean 28 days) and appears to be less for larger inocula of the virus. The infectious period is from 2 weeks before onset of symptoms until 1 week after, although some, particularly children, may excrete a week longer. Infectivity is maximal during the prodromal period.

Immunity to previous infection is lifelong, but because of the decreasing incidence over the last half-century, a majority of those under 50 years of age are susceptible. Those at increased risk of severe disease include those with chronic liver disease or chronic hepatitis B or C infection and older people.

Prevention

• Personal hygiene, including handwashing; ensuring toilet hygiene in nurseries and schools; care with food and water during travel to less-developed countries; and careful hygiene after anal sex.
• Sanitary disposal of sewage and treatment of water supplies.
• Vaccination of travellers (aged 5 years or above) to countries outside of Northern or Western Europe, North America or Australasia, at least 2 weeks before the date of departure. If time permits those over 50 years of age or born in high endemicity areas or with a history of jaundice can be tested for immunity before vaccination.
• Vaccine can be given up to day of travel. Immunoglobulin (HNIG) may be available for immunocompromised travellers.
• Vaccination of other risk groups, including patients with chronic liver disease or haemophilia, those with chronic hepatitis B or C, sexually active homosexual men, intravenous drug users and certain laboratory staff. Local risk assessment may suggest that vaccine should be offered to staff and residents of certain institutions where good hygiene standards cannot be achieved. Sanitation workers who come into direct contact with untreated sewage may also be considered for vaccine.
• Shellfish should be steamed for at least 90 seconds or heated at 85–90°C for 4 minutes before eating.
• Sodium hypochlorite, 2% glutaraldehyde and quaternary ammonia compound with 23% HCI are effective on contaminated surfaces.

Surveillance

• Confirmed or suspected cases of hepatitis A should be reported to local public health authorities (notifiable as 'viral hepatitis' in Great Britain).

• All laboratory confirmed acute cases (e.g. IgM positive) should be reported to national surveillance systems.

Response to a case

• Clinicians and microbiologists to report all acute cases to local public health authorities.
• Enteric precautions until 1 week after onset of jaundice (if no jaundice, precautions until 10 days after onset of first symptoms).
• Exclude all cases in groups with increased risk of further transmission (Box 2.2.1) until 7 days after onset of jaundice.
• Exclude household and sexual contacts with symptoms as for cases.
• Personal hygiene advice to case and contacts. Asymptomatic contacts that attend nursery or infant school should have handwashing supervised.
• Vaccination should be offered to relevant household, sexual and other close contacts. The best prophylactic strategy is as yet unclear, but we would suggest the following:
  (i) Presenting within 7 days of exposure: give vaccine.
  (ii) 7–14 days: give HNIG if available, otherwise give vaccine (can give both together, especially if at higher risk of serious disease).
  (iii) 2–4 weeks: give HNIG to adults and others at risk of severe disease.
• People who have recently eaten food prepared by the case may benefit from immunisation.
• Collect risk factor data for 2–5 weeks before onset: contact with case, travel abroad, institute for mentally handicapped or other institution, seafood, meals out of household, blood transfusion, occupation.

Investigation of a cluster

• Confirm that cases are acute (clinical jaundice and/or IgM positive).
• Describe by person, place and time. Does epidemic curve suggest point source, ongoing person-to-person transmission (or both) or continuing source? Are there cases in neighbouring areas?

• Collect risk factor data as for individual case and interview cases sensitively regarding sexuality, sexual activity, illicit drug use and imprisonment. Obtain full occupational and recreational history, e.g. exposure to faeces, nappies, sewage, untreated water, etc. Obtain as full a food history as patient recall allows for 2–5 weeks before onset.

• Discuss with microbiologist use of salivary testing for case finding and availability of genotyping to confirm cases are linked.

Control of an outbreak

• Try to define population at risk suitable for immunisation, e.g. staff and pupils at a nursery.

• Hygiene advice to cases, contacts and any implicated institution. Ensure that toilet and hygiene facilities are adequate.

• For community outbreaks, re-inforce hygiene measures in nurseries and schools and vaccinate contacts of cases.

• For prolonged community outbreaks with disease rates of over 50 per 100,000 per annum, consult with relevant experts on appropriateness of vaccination of affected population.

Suggested case definition for an outbreak

Confirmed: demonstration of specific IgM in serum or saliva.
Suspected: case of acute jaundice in at risk population without other known cause. (Confirmation important in groups at risk of other hepatitis viruses, e.g. drug users).

3.31 Hepatitis B

Hepatitis B is an acute viral infection of the liver. Its public health importance lies in the severity of disease, its ability to cause long-term carriage leading eventually to cirrhosis and hepatocellular cancer, its transmissibility by the blood-borne route and the availability of vaccines and specific immunoglobulin.

Suggested on-call action (next working day)

• Arrange for laboratory confirmation.
• Identify likely source of infection for acute cases.
• Arrange for testing and vaccination of close household/sexual contacts.

Epidemiology

The incidence of acute hepatitis B varies considerably across Europe. In most countries the incidence is low (less than 5 per 100,000), with a few notable exceptions, mainly in the Baltic States, where the incidence may be as high as 35 per 100,000 (see Table 3.31.1). The true incidence is higher, as about 70% of infections are subclinical and may not be detected. Most cases are in adults at high risk of infection (see Table 3.31.2), although horizontal transmission within families also occurs in the higher incidence countries. The carriage rate is below 1% in most countries, although there is considerable geographical variation within countries, with higher rates in inner cities amongst those of black and minority ethnic origin. Some ethnic groups have high rates of carriage, notably those from countries in south-east Asia and the Far East. The UK and Scandinavian countries have among the lowest rates of acute infection and carriage in the world.

Clinical features

Hepatitis B is clinically indistinguishable from other causes of viral hepatitis. After a non-specific prodromal illness with fever and malaise, jaundice appears and the fever stops. The course of the disease is very variable and

Table 3.31.1 Hepatitis B in Europe

Country	Incidence of acute disease per 100,000	Prevalence of HBsAg	Immunisation programme
Austria	<5	n/a*	universal, infant
Belgium	<5	<1%	universal, infant + adolescent
Cyprus	n/a	n/a	universal, infant
Denmark	n/a	n/a	selective
Czech Republic	<5	<1%	universal, infant + adolescent
England and Wales	<5	<1%	selective
Estonia	30–35	<1%	universal, newborn + adolescent
Finland	n/a	n/a	selective
France	n/a	n/a	universal, infant + adolescent
Germany	5–10	<1%	universal, infant + adolescent
Greece	<5	2%	universal, infant + child (6 years)
Hungary	<5	<1%	universal, adolescent
Ireland	n/a	n/a	selective
Italy	<5	1%	universal, infant + adolescent
Latvia	30–35	2%	universal, newborn
Lithuania	10–15	1%	universal, newborn + adolescent
Luxembourg	15–20	n/a	universal, infant
Malta	<5	n/a	universal, child (9 years)
Netherlands	<5	<1%	selective
Poland	5–10	n/a	universal, newborn + adolescent
Portugal	n/a	n/a	universal, newborn + adolescent
Slovakia	<5	1–2%	universal, infant
Slovenia	<5	<1%	universal, child (7 years)
Spain	n/a	n/a	universal, infant + adolescent
Sweden	n/a	n/a	selective

Source: Surveillance of vaccine-preventable hepatitis in the EU countries and associated states (www.eurohep.net).
*n/a = Data not yet available (collection is ongoing).

jaundice may persist for months. Liver failure is an important early complication.

Table 3.31.2 Risk groups for hepatitis B in Europe

Intravenous drug users
Homosexual and bisexual men who frequently change sex partners
Close family and sexual contacts of cases and carriers
Haemophiliacs
Renal dialysis patients
Healthcare workers
Staff and residents of mental institutions
Morticians and embalmers
Prisoners
Long-term travellers to high and medium prevalence countries
Babies born to acutely infected or carrier mothers

Laboratory confirmation

The diagnosis and stage of infection can be determined from the antigen and antibody profile in the blood (Fig 3.31.1). Patients with detectable hepatitis B antigen at 6 months (surface antigen (HBsAg) and/or e antigen (HBeAg)) are considered to be carriers.

Transmission

Man is the only reservoir. Transmission is from person to person by a number of blood-borne routes, including sharing of drug-injecting equipment, transfusions of blood and blood products, needlestick injuries, skin

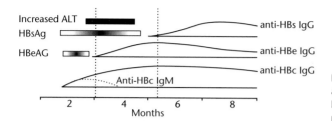

Fig. 3.31.1 Occurrence of hepatitis B virus markers and antibodies in the blood of infected patients.

piercing with inadequately sterilised equipment, mother to baby transmission during or soon after childbirth and sexual intercourse.

In low-prevalence countries transmission occurs mainly through shared syringes, needlestick injuries, sexual contact, bites and scratches. In high-prevalence countries, perinatal transmission is the most important route; ulcerating skin disease and biting insects also play a role in developing countries.

Acquisition

The incubation period is 3–6 months. Carriers of hepatitis B surface antigen who are also e antigen positive and/or e antibody negative are much more infectious than those who are e antibody positive. Patients who do not become carriers and develop natural immunity are immune for life.

Approximately 10% of patients with acute hepatitis B become chronic carriers. Long-term complications of being a carrier include cirrhosis and hepatocellular carcinoma.

Prevention

• Ensure that all blood and blood products are screened and not derived from donors at risk of infection.
• Adopt universal procedures for the prevention of blood-borne virus transmission in hospitals and all other situations where needles and other skin-piercing equipment are used (e.g. acupuncture clinics, tattoo parlours, ear/body-piercing).
• Prevent infected healthcare from performing exposure-prone procedures.
• Promote condom use.
• The above general measures for the

prevention of blood-borne virus infections are covered in more detail in Chapter 2.10.
• Hepatitis B vaccination, of infants and/or older children, is recommended in most EU countries (see Table 3.31.1), except for the UK and a few other countries, where selective vaccination is recommended only for high-risk groups (see Table 3.31.2).
• The schedule is three injections at 0, 1 and 6 months. Where more rapid protection is required (e.g. for travellers or for post-exposure prophylaxis) this schedule can be accelerated to 0, 1 and 2 months (or to 0, 7 and 21 days), in which case a fourth dose should be given at 12 months. The vaccine should not be given in the buttock as efficacy may be reduced.
• Protection is probably lifelong in a healthy adult who responds to the primary course. Healthcare workers and babies born to hepatitis B carrier mothers should, however, have their antibody status checked 4–6 months after immunisation. Poor responders (anti-HBs 10–100 mIU/mL) should receive a booster dose and in non-responders (anti-HBs < 10 mIU/mL) a repeat course should be considered. Adults over 40 years of age and those with immunodeficiency are more likely to be non-responders.
• Screen all women in pregnancy. Babies born to mothers who are HBsAg-positive and anti-HBe-positive (i.e. low infectivity) should receive an accelerated course of vaccine. Babies whose mothers are e antigen-positive, or who have had acute hepatitis B in pregnancy, or who have no e markers, or whose e markers are not known, should in addition to a course of vaccine receive hepatitis B-specific immunoglobulin (HBIG) 200 IU intramuscularly as soon as possible after birth.
• Offer post-exposure prophylaxis for significant exposures to a known or suspected HBsAg source (see Table 3.31.3). A significant exposure

Table 3.31.3 HBV prophylaxis for reported exposure incidents

HBV status of person exposed	Significant exposure			Non-significant exposure	
	HbsAg positive source	Unknown source	HbsAG negative source	Continued risk	No further risk
≤1 dose HB vaccine pre-exposure	Accelerated course of HB vaccine* HBIG × 1	Accelerated course of HB vaccine*	Initiate course of HB vaccine	Initiate course of HB vaccine	No HBV prophylaxis. Reassure
≥2 doses HB vaccine pre-exposure (anti-HBs not known)	One dose of HB vaccine followed by second dose 1 month later	One dose of HB vaccine	Finish course of HB vaccine	Finish course of HB vaccine	No HBV prophylaxis Reassure
Known responder to HB vaccine (anti-HBs ≥10 mIU/mL)	Booster dose of HB vaccine	Consider booster dose of HB vaccine	Consider booster dose of HB vaccine	Consider booster dose of HB vaccine	No HBV prophylaxis Reassure
Known non-responder to HB vaccine (anti-HBs <10 mIU/mL 2–4 months post-vaccination)	HBIG ×1 Consider booster dose of HB vaccine	HBIG ×1 Consider booster dose of HB vaccine	No HBIG Consider booster dose of HB vaccine	No HBIG Consider booster dose of HB vaccine	No HBV prophylaxis Reassure

From S. Handysides, *Exposure to Hepatitis B Virus: Guidance on Post-Exposure Prophylaxis*, CDR Review, PHLS Communicable Disease Surveillance Centre, 1992, with permission.

*An accelerated course of vaccine consists of doses spaced at 0, 1 and 2 months or 0, 7 and 21 days. A booster dose is given at 12 months to those at continuing risk of exposure to HBV.

is one in which HBV transmission may occur. This may be an injury involving a contaminated needle, blade or other sharp object or blood contaminating non-intact skin or eyes. HBV does not cross intact skin. Exposure to vomit, faeces and sterile or uncontaminated sharp objects poses no risk. Transmission is not known to have occurred as a result of spitting or urine splashing.

• The dose of HBIG is 200 IU for children aged 0–4 years, 300 IU for children aged 5–9 years and 500 IU for adults and children aged 10 years or more.

Surveillance

• Acute hepatitis B is notifiable in most European countries.
• Surveillance should ideally be based on laboratory reports, as the disease is clinically indistinguishable from other causes of viral hepatitis. IgM and e-antigen/antibody results should be included with notifications to facilitate public health action.

Response to a case

• Obtain laboratory confirmation, assess whether acute (IgM and/or clinical history) and how infectious (HBeAg, anti-HBe, HbsAg).
• If acute, determine possible source of infection: history of i.v. drug abuse, sexual orientation, occupation, recent surgery/blood transfusion/dialysis, acupuncture/tattoo/ear-piercing and travel.
• If infectious, give advice to case to limit infectivity to others and identify sexual and close household contacts: arrange to have their hepatitis B markers checked to see if they have already been infected before vaccinating them. Contacts who are HBsAg, anti-HBs or anti-HBc positive do not need to be vaccinated, although for sexual partners the first dose of vaccine should be given while awaiting test results and the use of condoms advised until immunity is established.

Investigation of a cluster and response to an outbreak

• Look for a common source and take appropriate action.
• If an infected healthcare worker is the source, a look-back investigation should be conducted to identify other cases associated with the healthcare worker (see Chapter 4.6).

> **Suggested case definition for an outbreak**
>
> Jaundice plus presence in serum of HBsAg, or HBeAg, or anti-HBc IgM.

3.32 Hepatitis C

Hepatitis C is a worldwide public health problem. Large numbers of people are chronically infected with hepatitis C virus (HCV) and a substantial proportion will develop chronic liver disease in the future.

> **Suggested on-call action**
>
> Only rarely will HCV cases, clusters or incidents be notified outside normal office hours. Local circumstances will determine what immediate action should be taken.

Epidemiology

HCV was first identified in 1989 and an antibody test became available in 1990. Laboratory reports of HCV infection are influenced by the availability and extent of testing and reporting of results. Current tests do not differentiate between present and past infection and since most acute infections are asymptomatic it is difficult to distinguish incident from prevalent cases.

In England and Wales, there were 6512 reports of positive anti-HCV tests in 2003 compared with 5898 in 2002. Of the reports that included risk factor information over 90%

identified injecting drug use as the main route of transmission. In England the overall seroprevalence of anti-HCV is 0.5% suggesting that 200,000 persons may be chronically infected. Most of these will be undiagnosed. Infection is more prevalent in subgroups that have been exposed to the virus in the past, such as injecting drug users and those who have had multiple transfusions including haemophiliacs. Overall seroprevalence in France is 1.2% and in Italy it is 3%. Higher prevalence rates are seen in many other countries and worldwide it is estimated that 170 million people may be infected with HCV.

Clinical features

Acute hepatitis C is often asymptomatic. There may be elevated liver enzymes but jaundice is uncommon and serious liver disease is rare. Following infection 20% will clear the virus in 2–6 months. Of those that are chronically infected 75% will have some degree of active liver disease and of these 25% will progress to cirrhosis over the ensuing 20 years of whom 1–4 % will develop liver cancer each year. In the UK around 100 people die each year where the underlying cause of death on the death certificate is hepatitis C, but HCV also contributes to a proportion of the 5000 deaths each year from chronic liver disease, cirrhosis and hepatocellular carcinoma. Fifteen per cent of liver transplant recipients have hepatitis C.

Laboratory confirmation

HCV is a small enveloped single-stranded RNA virus. Anti-HCV IgG antibody tests are normally positive within 3 months of infection. To indicate whether the virus is still present quantitative and qualitative PCR tests for HCV-RNA are used. Test are available to distinguish between the six different HCV genotypes.

Transmission

HCV is spread by contact with blood or body fluids from an infected person. Those at greatest risk are current and past injecting drug users, those who received blood products before heat treatment in 1986 and recipients of blood transfusions before testing was introduced in 1991. Other less efficient routes of transmission are vertical spread from mother to infant, unprotected sex with an infected partner, through medical and dental procedures abroad with contaminated equipment; during tattooing or skin piercing with blood-contaminated equipment, horizontal spread in households as a result of sharing contaminated toothbrushes or razors and from patient to healthcare worker and vice versa. In the UK there have been five incidents involving spread of HCV from health care workers involving a total of 15 patients.

Acquisition

The incubation period is 6–9 weeks. A person will remain infectious for as long as they are infected with the virus.

Prevention

Unlike hepatitis A and hepatitis B, no vaccine is available for hepatitis C. In the UK, a Hepatitis C Strategy was published in 2002 followed by an Action Plan in 2004. It is envisaged that hepatitis C will be controlled by
- improved surveillance,
- raising public and professional awareness,
- case finding by more testing of those at risk,
- better treatment and care,
- preventing transmission amongst injecting drug users, young people and in prisons by needle exchanges and targeted education and
- promoting infection control measures in community and healthcare settings.

Surveillance

- Hepatitis C is a statutory notifiable disease in the majority of EU countries. In UK, viral hepatitis (unspecified) is notifiable.
- Cases of chronic HCV infection detected as a result of serological testing should be reported to national surveillance.

Table 3.32.1 Target groups for particular HCV prevention measures

Injecting drug users	Needle exchange schemes
	Supply of other injecting equipment such as spoons, filters, water and tourniquets
	Methadone maintenance programmes
	Health education targeted at younger drug injectors and people injecting drugs for the first time
	Promote hygienic injecting practices
	Encourage other drug administration routes such as smoking and snorting
	Consider alcohol and hepatitis B (co-factors in development of liver disease)
	Established IDUs and ex-IDUs should have access to appropriate services
People with HCV infection, their sexual partners and household contacts	Access to information, counselling, testing and referral
	Adopt measures to reduce the risk of further transmission (see Chapter 2.10, precautions for blood-borne infections)
Healthcare and social care workers including staff of alcohol and drug agencies	Ensure good knowledge of HCV and other blood-borne viral infections
	Implement infection control measures
	Guidelines on occupational aspects of HCV have been published
	Guidelines are available for staff in drugs services and renal dialysis centres
Prisoners, prison staff and Probation Service staff	Access to information and professional advice, including counselling, testing and referral
	Supply injecting equipment in prisons
General population, particularly young people	Ensure awareness of HCV and transmission
	Implement precautions to manage bleeding and blood spillages in the community
	Follow infection control guidelines for skin piercing, tattooing, etc
Blood, organ and tissue donation	People with HCV and those who may have been exposed to HCV should not donate blood or carry a donor card
	Screening and heat treatment should be used where appropriate
HCV infection in mothers and infants	Universal antenatal screening for HCV is not recommended
	Pregnant women at risk of HCV infection should be offered hepatitis C testing
	Breastfeeding should be discouraged only if the mother is viraemic

• Rarely acute cases are diagnosed and these should be reported to the local health protection teams for investigation.

• In the UK details of cases where the date of infection is known should be reported to the National Hepatitis C Register.

Response to a case

• The cases should receive information about the infection and advice on preventing further spread. Patient advice leaflets are available.

Table 3.32.2 Hepatitis C case definitions

Suggested case definition

Clinical
An acute illness with
(a) discrete onset of symptoms (such as nausea, vomiting, abdominal pain and diarrhoea) *and*
(b) jaundice or abnormal serum aminotransferase levels.
Laboratory
(a) Elevated serum AST/ALT level and anti-HAV IgM negative *and*
(b) anti-HBc IgM negative, or if not done, HBsAg negative *and*
(c) anti-HCV screening-test-positive verified by an additional more specific assay (e.g. RIBA for anti-HCV or HCV RNA)

• For acute cases, enquire about the circumstances of exposure and the possibility of infection as a result of healthcare, acupuncture, other alternative therapy and blood transfusion.
• The case should be referred for further investigation and possible treatment if indicated and longer-term support and counselling.
• The UK National Institute for Clinical Excellence has published treatment guidelines. Following treatment with interferon alpha and ribavarin, 38–43% remain free of virus after 6 months.

Investigation of an HCV incident or outbreak

• All those who have potentially been exposed should be identified and offered testing. Those with evidence of infection will need counselling and follow-up by a liver specialist who can advise on treatment options.
• If a healthcare worker who has performed exposure prone procedures is found to have HCV infection, a look back exercise may be required (see Chapter 4.6).

3.33 Delta hepatitis

Delta hepatitis is caused by a satellite virus that infects patients only during the antigen-positive stages of acute hepatitis B or long-term HBsAg carriers. The epidemiology is thus similar to that of hepatitis B (see Chapter 3.31), although less common; worldwide about 5% of HBsAg carriers are infected with delta hepatitis. Transmission is by the same routes as that of hepatitis B. The incubation period is 2–8 weeks. General control measures for blood-borne viruses will prevent spread of delta hepatitis. There is no specific vaccine or immunoglobulin.

3.34 Hepatitis E

Hepatitis E virus (HEV) is the main cause of enterically transmitted non-A non-B hepatitis worldwide.

Epidemiology

Although rare in north-west Europe (an average of 30 cases per annum are reported in the UK), HEV is responsible for around half of acute sporadic hepatitis in many developing countries and outbreaks have occurred in Asia, including the Indian subcontinent, Africa and Central America. Most clinically reported cases occur in young or middle-aged adults.

Diagnosis

HEV causes an illness similar to hepatitis A (abdominal pain, anorexia, dark urine, fever, hepatomegaly, jaundice, malaise, nausea and vomiting) without chronic sequelae or carriage. The severity of hepatitis is dose-dependent. Case-fatality is low, except in women infected in the third trimester of pregnancy, when it may reach 20%. Specific IgM testing is available in specialist laboratories, although a positive result should be treated with caution in those without risk factors.

Transmission and acquisition

HEV is transmitted faeco-orally, with most outbreaks linked to contaminated drinking water. Food-borne transmission also occurs. Person-to-person spread is inefficient (1–2% secondary attack rate), but nosocomial spread is described. Virus excretion in stools probably occurs before clinical onset and lasts up to 14 days afterwards. The incubation period is reported as 15–60 days (mean 30–40 days).

Control

Prevention relies primarily on provision of safe water supplies: European travellers, particularly if pregnant, to developing countries should take care with food and water. Confirmed or suspected cases in Europe should be notified to local public health authorities.

3.35 Herpes simplex

Infection with herpes simplex viruses (HSV) is characterised by a localised primary infection, latency and recurrence. HSV 1 is typically associated with gingivostomatitis and HSV 2 with genital infection (see Chapter 3.26). However, either may affect the genital tract and HSV 2 can cause primary infection of the mouth.

Suggested public health on-call action
Usually none required.

Epidemiology

The incidence of HSV 1 infection peaks first in pre-school aged children. There is a second lower peak in young adults. It is rare in infancy because of passive maternal antibody. In large seroprevalence studies, HSV-1 seroprevalence ranges from 52% in Finland, to 57% in the Netherlands, 67% in Belgium, 81% in Czech Republic, and 84% in Bulgaria. Seropositivity increases with age. A large proportion of teenagers and young adults remain HSV-1 susceptible, particularly in northern Europe. UK General Practitioners reported a mean weekly incidence of herpes simplex in 2003 of 6 per 100,000 population, similar to previous years.

Clinical features

Primary infection produces a painful gingivostomatitis. As a result of autoinoculation lesions may affect other sites such as the eye and finger (herpetic whitlow). The illness resolves after 10–14 days. Complications include eczema herpeticum, Bell's palsy, encephalitis, meningitis, ocular herpes and erythema multiforme. Following primary infection, HSV persists in the dorsal root ganglia of the trigeminal nerve. A range of trigger factors including upper respiratory tract infections, fatigue, emotional stress, physical trauma, exposure to sun, dental extraction, menstruation and drugs such as corticosteroids may lead to reactivation of the virus leading to herpes labialis (the cold sore). Reactivation may affect 45% of persons who have had a primary infection.

Laboratory confirmation

HSV are typical large DNA herpes viruses. The diagnosis is usually made clinically, but vesicle fluid or scrapings can be examined for virus particles by electron microscopy. Monoclonal antibodies or viral culture are required to distinguish HSV from varicella-zoster virus infection.

Transmission

Humans are the only reservoir of infection and spread is by direct contact with oral secretions during kissing and contact sports (herpes gladiatorum). Air-borne transmission is unlikely. The virus does not survive for long periods in the environment and cannot penetrate intact skin. HSV is highly infectious, especially in young children and attack rates approach 80% in non-immune subjects.

Acquisition

The incubation period is 1–6 days. The virus may be shed in the saliva for 1–8 weeks after primary infection and for about 3 days in recurrent infection. At any one time 20% young children may be shedding virus. Patients with impaired cellular immunity, skin disorders and burns are at risk of severe and persistent HSV infections.

Prevention

• Health education and attention to personal hygiene may reduce exposure.
• Gloves should be available for health and social care staff in contact with potential infection.
• Patients with HSV infection should avoid contact with infants, burns patients, and people with eczema or impaired immunity.
• Sunscreen and oral antivirals may be considered to prevent reactivation.

Response to a case/ cluster/outbreak

• Treatment is symptomatic and supportive.
• Oral antivirals may be considered for primary infection and reactivation particularly when there is severe disease.
• Topical antivirals may be used for reactivation.
• Ocular herpes simplex disease is the commonest cause of corneal blindness in high-income countries and should be treated as an ophthalmic emergency.
• Patients with extensive infection should be nursed with source isolation.
• Children with cold sores do not need to be excluded from school.

Case definition

Characteristic lesions with or without laboratory confirmation by electron.

3.36 *Haemophilus influenzae* type b

Haemophilus influenzae type b (Hib) is a bacterial infection of young children, which causes meningitis and other bacteraemic diseases including pneumonia, epiglottitis, facial cellulitis and bone and joint infections. Its importance lies in the high rate of disease complications and the availability of a vaccine.

Suggested on-call action

• Seek laboratory confirmation.
• Obtain vaccination history.
• Arrange for chemoprophylaxis and vaccination of contacts.

Epidemiology

The disease is commonest in children under 5 years. Before vaccination was introduced in the UK, Hib was the second most common cause of bacterial meningitis overall, and the commonest in young children. One in 600 children developed invasive Hib disease before the age of 5. The case fatality rate is 4–5% (higher in infants) and up to 30% of survivors have permanent neurological sequelae, including deafness, convulsions and mental impairment.

Hib is now rare throughout Europe, although an increase has been reported in recent years in the UK and the Netherlands. The increase has been observed in both vaccinated children and unvaccinated adults. The reasons for this increase include reduction in herd immunity, absence of a booster dose and the use of an acellular pertussis-containing combination vaccine causing Hib interference. In the UK, the number of cases rose from an all-time low of 37 in 1998 to 269 in 2002. Following a mass vaccination campaign in children aged 6–48 months, the disease incidence has declined again.

Other serotypes of *H. influenzae* occasionally cause invasive disease and non-encapsulated *H. influenzae* sometimes cause ear infections or acute exacerbations of chronic bronchitis.

Clinical features

Hib meningitis typically has a slower onset than meningococcal meningitis, with symptoms developing over 3 or 4 days. There is progressive headache, drowsiness and vomiting with intermittent fever. Photophobia may be present. A haemorrhagic rash can be present, but is unusual. In soft tissue, bone and joint infections there is swelling of the affected area. Hib epiglottitis presents with acute respiratory obstruction.

Laboratory confirmation

This is important as the clinical features are variable and non-specific; this is also to ascertain vaccine failures. A positive culture may be obtained from blood or CSF. Alternatively Hib antigen can be demonstrated by latex agglutination or PCR. All strains should be sent to the national reference laboratory for confirmation and typing.

Transmission

Man is the only reservoir. Transmission is by droplet infection and direct contact with nose and throat secretions. In unvaccinated populations carriage is common in young children; about 4–5% of unvaccinated 3-year-olds are carriers. Vaccination prevents carriage.

Acquisition

The incubation period is not known, but is probably only 2–4 days. Cases are non-infectious within 48 hours of starting effective antibiotic treatment. Disease usually results in lifetime immunity, although repeat infections have been described. Immunity is also derived from carriage, from infection with cross-protective antigens, such as *Escherichia coli*, and from vaccination.

Prevention

Routine vaccination of infants with protein-polysaccharide conjugate vaccines. Three doses required in infants; children over 12 months require only a single dose. Booster dose in the second year of life recommended in most countries (still under consideration in the UK at the time of writing). Only contraindication is a severe reaction to a previous dose.

Surveillance

• Hib meningitis notifiable in most countries of Europe (including UK); this does not apply to other forms of invasive Hib disease.
• Should always be based on laboratory reports.
• Report any case in a vaccinated child to the national surveillance unit.

Response to a case

• Laboratory confirmation must be sought.
• Check vaccination status of the case and of household contacts.

Box 3.36.1 Chemoprophylaxis for invasive Hib disease

Rifampicin, orally, 20 mg/kg daily for 4 days (maximum 600 mg daily).

- Household contacts do not require chemoprophylaxis if all children in the household have been vaccinated.
- If there are any unvaccinated children under 5 years of age in the household, they should be vaccinated and all household members (including adults, who may be the source of infection) should be given chemoprophylaxis (Box 3.36.1). The case should also receive chemoprophylaxis and vaccine.
- Warn patients of the adverse effects of rifampicin (red staining of urine, sputum, tears and contact lenses, interference with the oral contraceptive pill).
- No need to exclude siblings or other close contacts of cases from nursery or school.

Investigation and control of a cluster

- Give chemoprophylaxis (and vaccine, if unvaccinated) to nursery contacts if there are two or more cases within 120 days.
- In addition to the measures described for a case, may be a need to conduct a local vaccination programme if coverage is low.

Suggested case-definition for an outbreak

Confirmed: clinically compatible illness with an isolate or antigen detection of Hib from a normally sterile site.
Clinical: meningitis or epiglottitis with no other cause in
- an unvaccinated child under 5 years of age *or*
- an unvaccinated individual with links to confirmed case(s).

3.37 HIV

Acquired immune deficiency syndrome (AIDS), first described in 1981, is the result of advanced infection with human immunodeficiency virus (HIV-1). There is a second human immunodeficiency virus, HIV-2, which is endemic in western Africa. It causes a spectrum of disease similar to that produced by HIV-1.

Suggested public health on-call action

- Most cases do not require an on-call response.
- Advise on the management of HIV-related incidents, particularly exposure incidents (see Box 3.37.1).

Epidemiology

It is estimated that worldwide in 2003 there were 38 million people living with HIV, with five million new HIV infections and three million deaths. Some countries are more affected than others and within countries there are often wide variations between different geographical areas and subsections of the population. In Eastern Europe and Central Asia injecting drug use (IDU) is the main route of transmission and 1.3 million people mainly aged under 30 years are now infected. Estonia, Latvia, the Russian Federation and Ukraine are the worst-affected countries. In Western Europe, in 2003, 580,000 people were living with HIV compared to 540,000 in 2001. The majority of these have access to antiretroviral therapy and so are staying healthy and living longer than infected persons elsewhere. In the UK a range of different sources of surveillance data are available (Table 3.37.1). Similar surveillance data sources are used in other European countries.

Compared with some its European neighbours (Table 3.37.2) the UK has a low prevalence of HIV infection, although this is

Table 3.37.1 Main sources of UK surveillance data: HIV and AIDS

Clinicians' reports of diagnoses of HIV, AIDS and deaths

Laboratory reports of new HIV infections

Survey of prevalent HIV infections diagnosed (SOPHID)

Death reports

Laboratory reporting of CD4 counts

Results of voluntary HIV testing

Unlinked anonymous HIV prevalence monitoring

GUM clinic attenders

Injecting drug users

Antenatal patients

Reports of occupational HIV exposure

Reporting of HIV infection in pregnancy and in children

increasing due to continuing transmission in homosexual and bisexual men and migration of HIV-infected heterosexual men and women from Africa. In 2002, there were 50,000 persons with HIV infection. The current epidemiology of HIV infection in the UK is summarised in Table 3.37.3.

Clinical features

HIV-1 binds to CD4 receptors on lymphocytes or macrophages. The virus is internalised and integrated into the host cell genome leading to permanent infection. Virions may bud from the cell surface to infect another cell or infection may be spread when cells divide. Eventually the infected cells are killed by the virus. The CD4 count is normally 600–1200 cells/mm^3

Table 3.37.2 New diagnoses of HIV and rates per million population by country and year of report (1996–2003) and cumulative totals (data reported by 31 December 2003)

Country	2001		2002		2003		Cumulative total
	No.	Rate	No.	Rate	No.	Rate	
Austria	402	49.6	442	54.5	423	52.1	2347
Belgium	962	93.6	987	95.9	1032	100.0	15762
Czech Republic	51	5.0	50	4.9	61	6.0	662
Denmark	319	59.8	290	54.2	241	44.9	3929
Estonia	1474	1089.7	899	671.9	541	–	3400
Finland	128	24.7	130	25.0	134	25.7	1625
France	–	–	–	–	1714	–	1714
Germany	1342	16.3	1867	22.7	1823	22.1	21608
Greece	428	39.1	403	36.7	431	39.3	6706
Hungary	82	8.2	80	8.1	63	6.4	1104
Ireland	299	77.4	364	93.1	399	100.9	3408
Italy	1136	69.5	1202	73.5	–	–	4720
Latvia	807	343.3	542	232.7	403	174.7	2710
Lithuania	72	20.7	397	114.6	110	31.9	845
Luxembourg	41	92.9	33	73.8	47	103.7	592
Malta	11	28.1	12	30.6	9	22.8	210
Netherlands	–	–	3335	207.6	834	–	8419
Poland	564	14.6	574	14.9	610	15.8	8495
Portugal	2465	245.7	2546	253.4	2298	228.4	23374
Slovakia	8	1.5	11	2.0	13	2.4	192
Slovenia	16	8.0	22	11.1	14	7.1	220
Sweden	270	30.5	286	32.3	382	43.0	6306
United Kingdom	4289	72.8	6024	102.0	6953	117.3	61179

WHO European Region data (where available).

Table 3.37.3 Summary of the current epidemiology of HIV infection in the UK

Sex between men and women	In the UK in 2003 there were 3801 reports of heterosexually acquired HIV infection (1336 men, 2465 women). Over 80% were infected abroad, mostly in Africa. Few infections were acquired in Asia, Latin America or the Caribbean. Few cases in the UK are infected by a high-risk partner such as a bisexual man or IDU. In other European countries there has been more heterosexual spread from IDU. Nearly half of HIV infections acquired heterosexually are currently undiagnosed and when diagnosed two-thirds have low CD4 counts. High-risk behaviour is increasing among heterosexuals.
Homosexual and bisexual men	In the UK in 2003 there were 1735 new diagnoses of HIV in men who have sex with men (MSM). This group remains at greatest risk of acquiring HIV infection and there is no evidence of a decline in incidence. About a third of newly diagnosed MSM have a low CD4 count suggesting late diagnosis. The incidence of other STIs has increased amongst MSM indicating behaviour associated with increased HIV risk. The de-tuned assay laboratory technique, which identifies recent infections, suggests there has been little change in HIV incidence. Over 60% of infected MSM live in London.
Mother and child	By mid-2004, the cumulative total of HIV cases in the UK was 64,599 and of these 16,783 (25%) were women. In 2003 there were 2947 new diagnoses of which 84% were due to heterosexual exposure. In 2002 there were 8750 prevalent cases in females. In the UK over 300 HIV infected pregnant women give birth each year. Two-thirds of these births are in London where the level of HIV infection amongst women giving birth is now 1 in 250 but the proportion of undiagnosed infections has fallen to 25% as a result of antenatal screening. Women who are aware of their infection can benefit from interventions to reduce the risk of mother to child transmission to under 5%. In UK , by mid-2004, a total of 4615 infants had been born to HIV-infected mothers. There have been reports of 1506 children with HIV infection; vertical transmission and blood factor receipt are the main routes of exposure.
Injecting drug users	Around 7% of UK cumulative HIV diagnoses are due to injecting drug use (IDU) a smaller proportion than in other European countries due to the introduction of harm reduction measures such as needle exchange programmes in the mid 1980s. The average age at diagnosis is rising suggesting that recent infections remain at low levels in this group. However rates of equipment sharing are increasing indicating the potential for further spread of HIV and other blood-borne viruses in this group. Elsewhere in Europe IDU remains an important route of transmission.
Blood or tissue transfer	In total 1764 people in the UK have been infected by this route nearly all before the introduction of heat inactivation and donor screening in 1985. There have been two instances of blood being accepted for transfusion in the UK when the donor was in the 'window period' when recent HIV infection was not detected by the screening antibody test.

but in HIV infection it may fall to less than 200 cells/mm^3, leading to severe immunosuppression, which is associated with opportunistic infections, neoplasia and full-blown AIDS. Following exposure to HIV there is a period of viraemia during which the individual is very infectious and may experience fever and rash. Antibodies to HIV develop and the infection may then remain dormant for many years. The clinical manifestations of HIV infection range

Table 3.37.4 Clinical manifestations of HIV infection

Acute retroviral syndrome	About 1–6 weeks after exposure, fever, sweats, malaise, myalgia, rash. HIV (p24) antigen is usually detectable in serum, and EIA antibody test is often negative.
AIDS-related complex (ARC)	ARC includes persistent generalised lymphadenopathy (PGL), immune thrombocytopenic purpura (ITP), oropharyngeal candidiasis, herpes zoster, chronic diarrhoea, hairy leukoplakia and the constitutional wasting syndrome.
AIDS infections	• *Pneumocystis carinii* pneumonia • Oesophageal or bronchial candidiasis • Cytomegalovirus infection • Extrapulmonary cryptococcosis • *Mycobacterium avium-intracellulare* infection • Coccidioidomycosis, disseminated • Cryptosporidiosis of more than 1 month's duration • Herpes simplex • Histoplasmosis, disseminated or extrapulmonary • Isosporiasis, chronic intestinal • Toxoplasmosis
AIDS neoplasms	• Kaposi's sarcoma • Non-Hodgkin's lymphoma • Invasive cervical cancer • Brain lymphoma
Other conditions	• Tuberculosis • Perianal and genital condyloma acuminata • Seborrhoeic dermatitis • Psoriasis • Molluscum contagiosum • HIV encephalopathy • Peripheral neuropathies

from the initial acute retroviral syndrome to full-blown AIDS (Table 3.37.4).

Laboratory confirmation

Diagnosis is usually made with a fourth generation ELISA test that detects both anti-HIV-1, anti-HIV-2 and p24 HIV antigen. Simple/rapid assays based on agglutination or immuno-dot techniques and available in a variety of formats and are becoming more widely used. A positive test should be confirmed by two further tests such as Western blot or line immunoassay. Quantification of plasma HIV-1 RNA is used to predict disease progression and monitor response to anti-viral treatment. Genetic analysis can identify subtypes of HIV suggesting connections between individuals sharing the same strain and anti-viral resistance testing is also available.

Transmission

HIV is spread from person to person as a result of exposure to infected blood or tissues, usually as a result of sexual contact, sharing needles or syringes or transfusion of infected blood or blood components. Normal social or domestic contact carries no risk of transmission. Transmission is especially efficient between male homosexuals in whom receptive anal intercourse and multiple sexual partners are particular risk factors. In countries where heterosexual spread is common, STIs causing genital ulceration and multiple partners are associated with the highest rates of transmission. HIV is present in saliva, tears and urine but transmission as a result of contact with these secretions is uncommon. HIV infection is not thought to be transmitted by biting insects. Between 15 and 30% of infants born to HIV

Table 3.37.5 HIV preventative measures

- Sexual transmission can be reduced by promoting sexual abstinence or completely monogamous relationships between two uninfected partners or by reducing the number of sexual partners and minimising exposure to body fluids during intercourse by using condoms.
- Services for diagnosing and treating STIs including voluntary confidential testing for HIV infection and HIV counselling.
- Health education and treatment programs for IDU including needle exchange schemes and drug substitute prescribing programmes.
- Counselling and testing for HIV infection for all pregnant women as part of antenatal care combined with interventions to reduce the risk of vertical transmission from mother to infant including anti-viral treatment, caesarean section and advice to refrain from breastfeeding.
- Healthcare workers and others should be advised to take particular care when handling blood or sharp instruments and to adopt infection control measures for the prevention of blood-borne viral infections when caring for any patient with HIV infection. Treatment with anti-viral drugs may be appropriate following occupational exposure to HIV-contaminated material.
- Transmission by tissues, blood and blood products can be prevented by serological testing of blood and by heat treatment of blood products. Persons at increased risk of HIV infection should be advised to refrain from donating blood, organs or tissues.

infected mothers are infected with HIV as a result of vertical transmission either before, during or shortly after birth due to breastfeeding.

Acquisition

Following exposure HIV nucleic acid sequences may be detected in the blood within 1–4 weeks and HIV antibodies can be detected within 4–12 weeks. Untreated half of those with HIV infection will develop AIDS within 7–10 years and of these 80–90% will die within 3–5 years. Highly active antiretroviral therapy (HAART) reduces disease progression. A person with HIV infection will be infectious to others from shortly after the onset of the HIV infection throughout the rest of his or her life. Infectiousness increases with the degree of immunosuppression, viral load and the presence of STIs. Susceptibility to HIV infection is universal.

Prevention

- The variability of HIV-1 makes the development of an effective vaccine unlikely in the near future.
- Most HIV prevention programmes rely on public health education to reduce activities

that carry a risk of HIV transmission, particularly high-risk sexual activity and injecting drug use. The main HIV preventative measures are summarised in Table 3.37.5.

Surveillance

- Not notifiable in the UK but AIDS is statutorily notifiable in the majority of European countries and HIV is notifiable in many.
- Anonymised reporting of cases to local and national surveillance schemes. In the UK the CCDC may maintain a confidential, anonymised database of local residents with HIV infection for epidemiological and service planning purposes. Data on local cases are sought from the microbiologist and the GUM, infectious disease and haematology consultants and should be updated at least every year. The data can be compared with central databases held by CDSC.

Response to a case

- There is no cure for HIV infection but a large number of anti-viral drugs are available that slow the progression of disease. Treatment guidelines and standards are available. Treatment is aimed at reducing the plasma viral load and is started before the immune system is irreversibly damaged. Hospital patients with HIV infection should be nursed with infection control precautions for blood-borne viral infections (see Chapter 2.10). Side room isolation is unnecessary unless there is a risk of haemorrhage.

• The person with HIV infection should be offered advice on preventing further spread and should be encouraged to identify sexual and needle sharing contacts so that counselling and HIV testing can be arranged.

Investigation and control of an HIV incident or cluster

• Clusters of cases of HIV infection may be detected when contact tracing is carried out in sexual or drug using networks. Occasionally a local increase in the incidence of HIV infection may occur. Standard outbreak investigation methods should be adopted. Particular care is needed to preserve patient confidentiality. Colleagues in the local GUM clinic or drug team should be able to assist with case finding, interviews and blood tests.

• HIV-related incidents occur more commonly and may include a healthcare worker with HIV infection, a percutaneous injury involving exposure to material from an HIV-infected person (Box 3.37.1) or a person with HIV infection who will not reliably follow advice to prevent further spread. Guidelines on how to respond to many of these incidents are available (see Appendix 2). Generally public health legislation has not proved to be helpful in controlling spread from a person with HIV infection.

Box 3.37.1 HIV post-exposure prophylaxis

• The risk of acquiring HIV infection from a patient with HIV infection following a needlestick injury is 3 per 1000 injuries and less than 1 per 1000 following mucous membrane exposure. Risks are greater with hollow needles, needles that are visibly blood-stained or which have been in an artery or vein, deep injuries and injuries from source patients who are terminally ill. Risk of infection can be reduced by 80% by post-exposure prophylaxis (PEP) with antiretroviral drug combinations.

• PEP may also be considered following HIV exposure in non-occupational settings.

Action following an HIV exposure
• A risk assessment should be carried out by someone other than the exposed person. It may be appropriate for the exposed person to take the first dose of PEP pending the outcome of a more thorough risk assessment.

• A significant exposure would be percutaneous exposure, exposure of broken skin or mucous membrane exposure. High-risk body fluids are blood, semen, vaginal secretions, amniotic fluid, human breast milk, CSF, fluid from body cavities and joints, blood-stained saliva, tissues and organs. Urine, vomit, saliva and faeces are low-risk materials unless visibly blood-stained. The HIV status of the source patient may be known. If not, a designated doctor should approach the patient and ask for their informed agreement to HIV testing. This course of action should be universally adopted with all significant exposures.

• With unknown sources the risk assessment will be informed by consideration of the circumstances of the exposure and the epidemiological likelihood of HIV in the source. In most such exposures in the UK it will probably be difficult to justify the use of PEP.

• Most exposures requiring PEP will take place in an acute hospital setting, particularly in hospitals that regularly care for people with HIV infection. Starter packs containing a 3-day course should be readily available at strategic locations. Counselling and support should be available.

Box 3.37.1 *(Continued)*

• PEP should ideally be started within an hour and continued for 4 weeks. However, it may still be worth considering starting PEP even if up to 2 weeks have elapsed since the exposure. There should be weekly follow-up by an experienced occupational health practitioner.

• All healthcare workers occupationally exposed to HIV should have follow-up counselling, post-exposure testing and medical evaluation whether or not they have received PEP. All should be encouraged to seek medical advice about any acute illness that occurs during the follow-up period. Pending follow-up, and in the absence of seroconversion, healthcare workers need not be subject to any modification of their working practices. They should, however, be advised about safer sex and avoiding blood donation during the follow-up period. At least 6 months should elapse after cessation of PEP before a negative antibody test is used to reassure the individual that infection has not occurred.

UK healthcare workers seconded overseas
• Of the eight probable occupationally acquired HIV infections reported in the UK, seven were associated with exposure in high-prevalence areas abroad.

• Employers should consider making 7-day starter packs of PEP drugs available to workers and students travelling to countries where antiretroviral therapy is not commonly available. In circumstances where it has been considered necessary to start PEP, expert advice by phone will be required to help the student or healthcare worker to decide whether or not PEP needs to be continued for four weeks and if so, whether urgent repatriation is required.

Exposure outside the healthcare setting
• Exposure outside the healthcare setting may include sexual exposure, sharing drug-injecting equipment and significant exposure to HIV-infected material in other circumstances.

• Such exposures may give rise to request for PEP or the need to consider it. There is insufficient evidence at present to make a recommendation either in favour of the use of PEP in these circumstances, or against its use. Benefit is more likely when the risk of transmission is considered high, such exposure is considered unlikely to be repeated, PEP can be started promptly and good adherence to the regime is considered likely.

Pregnancy
PEP can be used in pregnancy; however, expert advice should be sought.

The choice of drugs for PEP
PEP currently (2004) comprises
• Zidovudine 200 mg tds or 250 mg bd;
• plus lamivudine 150 mg bd;
• plus nelfinavir 750 tds or 1250 bd (or soft-gel saquinavir).

Suggested case definition

HIV infection is defined by positive laboratory tests for HIV. In addition AIDS is defined by the development of one or more of the specific marker infections or neoplasms.

3.38 Influenza

Influenza virus is a highly infectious cause of acute respiratory infection. It is a major cause of morbidity during epidemics and can be life-threatening in the elderly and chronically unwell. It also has the potential to cause devastating pandemics.

> ### Suggested on-call action
>
> • Suggest case limits contact with non-vaccinated individuals who are at risk of severe disease.
> • If linked to other cases in an institution, activate Outbreak Control Plan.

Epidemiology

Influenza causes both annual winter epidemics of varying size and severity, and occasional more severe pandemics. All age groups are affected, with highest incidence in children, but most hospitalisations and deaths are in the elderly. Between 3000 and 30,000 excess winter deaths per year are attributed to influenza in the UK depending on the size of the epidemic. Community outbreaks occur at variable times between November and March and tend to last 6–10 weeks, peaking at around the fourth week of the outbreak.

Influenza A and B viruses may alter gradually ('antigenic drift'): every few years this will result in a significant epidemic with rapid spread and a 10–20% attack rate. Influenza A may also change abruptly ('antigenic shift') leading to the circulation of a new subtype to which there is little existing population immunity and causing a major pandemic, usually with severe disease in all ages: these have occurred in 1918 (causing 20–40 million deaths worldwide), 1957 and 1968. Despite the huge impact of pandemics, more deaths result from the steady accumulation associated with yearly non-pandemic influenza activity.

Clinical features

About half of cases will have the classic flu picture of a sudden onset of fever, chills, headache, muscle aches, myalgia and anorexia. There may also be a dry cough, sore throat, or runny nose. Up to 25% of children may also have nausea, vomiting or diarrhoea if infected by influenza B or A (H1N1). The illness lasts 2–7 days and may include marked prostration.

Up to 10% of these cases progress to tracheobronchitis or pneumonia. Those at particular risk of complications are those with underlying chronic chest, heart or kidney disease, diabetes or immunosuppression, smokers and pregnant women.

Twenty per cent of infections are asymptomatic and 30% have upper respiratory symptoms but no fever. Influenza A (H_3N_2) may cause more severe disease than H_1N_1 or Influenza B, particularly in the elderly.

Laboratory confirmation

Confirmation of diagnosis is dependent upon laboratory tests, usually by direct immunofluorescence (DIF), virus isolation or serology. The virus may be detected from nasopharyngeal aspirates, nasal swabs or throat swabs: these must be collected early in the disease and require special transport media. Results can be available in 2–3 days, although 1 week is usual for routine samples. Serology requires two specimens, 10–21 days apart, and is about 80% sensitive: it is useful for retrospective diagnosis. In outbreaks, PCR testing (highly sensitive in early infection) or same day DIF or ELISA results may be available.

Influenza virus has three types (A, B, C) of which influenza C produces only sporadic infections. Subtyping of influenza A is based on a combination of H antigen (15 subtypes) and N antigen (9 subtypes), e.g. HIN1 or H3N2. All recent common human pathogens are combinations of H1, H2 or H3 with N1 or N2. Strains may be further differentiated by serology and named after the place and years of their identification (e.g. A/Sydney/97); these can be compared to current vaccine strains.

Transmission

Influenza in humans is transmitted via the respiratory secretions of cases, mainly by air-borne droplet spread, but also via small particle aerosols. Coughing and sneezing particularly promote spread. Transmission is facilitated by overcrowding and enclosed spaces, particularly by the number of susceptibles sharing the same room as the case. Spread in such circumstances is usually rapid and attack rates high.

Transmission may also occur via direct or indirect contact. This may occasionally cause a slowly evolving outbreak with low attack rates. Many outbreaks have occurred in hospitals.

The reservoir for influenza A is zoonotic, particularly aquatic fowl. Transmission to humans is rare but new strains may be spread directly or via intermediaries such as pigs (see Box 3.38.1). Influenza B only affects humans.

Acquisition

The incubation period is short, usually 1–3 days, occasionally up to 5 days. The infectious period lasts from 1 day before until 3–5 days after onset of symptoms in adults. Studies in children have found virus excretion from 3 days before onset to up to 9 days after; in practice, they can return to school when clinically well. Those with severe illness may also excrete for longer periods and at higher levels. The infectious dose is low.

Box 3.38.1 Avian influenza: why all the fuss?

In recent years there has been much international concern over reports of human infection with avian influenza strains such as H5N1, H9N2 and H7N7. Some avian viruses cause serious infections in humans (H5N1 disease in Hong Kong in 1997 had 33% mortality) but fortunately they do not spread easily, if at all, between humans. However, influenza viruses have the ability to undergo genetic reassortment and co-infection with both avian and human influenza strains in humans or pigs could produce a new strain with the increased virulence of the avian strain and the ability to spread easily from person to person like human influenza. Transmission of this highly pathogenic virus could then occur to a population with no existing immunity and, as yet, no vaccine to protect them. Although such a virus is most likely to arise in China or Southeast Asia, modelling suggests that it would only take 2–4 weeks to spread from Hong Kong to the UK (and presumably the rest of Europe) because of modern patterns of international travel. Rapid containment of incidents where avian strains infect humans is therefore essential to reducing the risk of future pandemics.

Although most containment activities will take place in the source area, European countries can limit the risk to their population by measures aimed at early detection of cases and minimising their contact with others. Exact measures would depend on the current risk but might include:
- information distributed at ports of entry;
- detection of symptomatic cases on entry to the country;
- high index of clinical suspicion in recent travellers, appropriate microbiological testing and reporting to public health authorities;
- voluntary home isolation of infected cases;
- effective infection control measures in hospitalised cases;
- general education messages;
- particular information for ethnic minorities with links to affected area of world;
- in addition, if person-to-person spread reported for this strain: identification of contacts of cases, voluntary home isolation and prompt prophylaxis may be considered.

Possible case definition:
- Clinical illness compatible with influenza (e.g. unexplained respiratory illness with fever and cough) *and*
- Travel in last 7 days to country or area reporting avian influenza *and*
- Contact with domestic fowl, wild birds, swine or confirmed human case or suspected human case (death from unexplained respiratory illness)

Immunity develops and protects against clinical illness with the same strain for many years. Cross immunity to related strains occurs. It is not clear why outbreaks often cease before exhausting the pool of susceptibles.

Prevention

• Basic personal hygiene to reduce transmission by coughing, sneezing or contaminated hands.
• Immunisation reduces the risk of hospital admissions and death and has a good safety record. Annual immunisation with WHO recommended vaccines should be offered to all those with an increased risk of serious illness from influenza ('at risk'). Current UK recommendations, which are similar to most European countries, are that this should include all those aged 65 years or more, plus those aged 6 months or more, with any of the following:

chronic respiratory disease, including asthma, or
chronic heart disease, or
chronic renal disease, or
immunosuppression due to disease or treatment, or
diabetes mellitus.

• In addition, people in long stay residential care homes should also be vaccinated because of the risk of rapid spread and the potentially severe consequences of infection. As efficacy in elderly people may be lower than the 70–90% in younger adults, indirect protection in this group may also be valuable.
• Immunisation is offered to healthcare workers in the UK both to protect patients and maintain staffing levels, and it is recommended that social care providers should also offer vaccination to their staff.
• Some European countries also immunise household contacts of 'at-risk' individuals (in line with WHO recommendations), children on long-term aspirin and pregnant women.
• Uptake of immunisation in disease-based risk groups has been poor in some European countries, including the UK. Primary care staff can increase uptake by compiling an at-risk register from chronic disease, computerised patient or prescription records, or as patients are seen during the year. A letter should be sent to each of these patients, preferably from their family doctor, recommending vaccination. Education on the benefits of vaccination is required both for the target population and for healthcare workers. Health authorities should appoint a co-ordinator to lead on improving influenza immunisation uptake locally.
• The antiviral drug, oseltamivir can be prescribed when influenza A or B virus is circulating in the community for the prevention of influenza in those aged 13 years and over who

belong to an 'at-risk' group, and
have not had an influenza immunisation this season, or who had one within the last 2 weeks, or have had an influenza immunisation but the vaccine did not match the virus circulating in the community, and
have been in close contact with someone with influenza-like symptoms, (includes being a resident in residential care establishment where a resident or staff member has influenza-like illness), and
can start taking oseltamivir within 48 hours of being in contact with the person with influenza-like symptoms.

• National and local planning prior to occurrence of a pandemic (see Box 3.38.2 for local plan). Both WHO and the EU have recommended that member states construct such plans.

Surveillance

• Influenza activity can be monitored via a combination of clinical surveillance for 'influenza-like illness' and laboratory data.
• At the international level, WHO co-ordinates a global network covering 83 countries and publishes information in the

Box 3.38.2 Main features of a district pandemic influenza plan

Assumptions
1 Attack rates will be higher than normal (perhaps 25% of population clinically infected) disrupting most services.
2 Case-fatality rates will be higher. This may cause perhaps a 50% increase in the total number of deaths from all causes at the height of the pandemic.
3 All sectors of the population may be at risk of severe disease, including younger adults and children.
4 A new vaccine will take 4–8 months to produce and even then, may be in short supply.
5 There will be insufficient supplies of antivirals, hospital beds (potentially a 25% or greater increase in total hospital admissions) and intensive care facilities to meet all needs.

Objectives
1 Reduce mortality and morbidity.
2 Care for large numbers at home, in hospital and dying.
3 Maintain essential public services.
4 Provide up to date reliable information to staff and public.

Administrative steps in advance
1 Multiagency pre-pandemic planning.
2 Constitution for Pandemic Co-ordinating Committee.
3 Roles and responsibilities for individuals/agencies.
4 Arrangements for updating plans.

Calculate vaccine requirements
1 Frontline healthcare staff.
2 Other essential public services.
3 Individuals at high risk of severe disease.
4 Residents of long stay facilities.
5 Rest of population by age-bands.

Contingency plans
1 Communications.
2 Surveillance.
3 Immunisation services.
4 Antiviral dispensary services.
5 Local outbreak plans (hospital and community).
6 Maintaining health services:
    6.1 increased workload and disruption to treatment of other conditions;
    6.2 staff absence and disruption to normal supplies, utilities and transport;
    6.3 increased need for high dependency care and infection control facilities;
    6.4 care in the community options.
7 Mortuary arrangements.
8 Maintaining essential public services, including social services.
9 Port health measures.

Weekly Epidemiological Record. Twenty-three countries participate in the European Influenza Surveillance Scheme. Weekly updated bulletins are available at www.eiss.org.

- At the national level, data are available from:

  telephone helplines for patients (e.g. NHS Direct diagnostic algorithms).

  general practice consultations (e.g. sentinel surveillance systems).

  illness in schoolchildren (e.g. Medical Officers of Schools Association).

  death certification (e.g. Office of National Statistics).

  emergency admissions to hospital (e.g. via NHS systems).

  collaborative studies (e.g. surveillance samples collected from primary care patients with influenza-like illness).

  laboratory surveillance of routine samples. However, these samples are heavily biased in terms of age (particularly children) and severity (hospitalisation).

UK data from these sources are available on the HPA website (www.hpa.org.uk).

- Regional or district monitoring may also be useful. Clinical data can be obtained from computerised GPs or other primary care providers. Participating GPs and local laboratories should ideally co-operate to obtain representative virological surveillance data. Timely local feedback of interpreted data is particularly useful to local health service planners during the winter.
- Some countries set thresholds for clinical activity, indices. These vary according to baselines in each country, e.g. for the countries of the UK (Table 3.38.1).

Response to a case

- Although spread may occur before diagnosis, symptomatic cases should ideally not attend work or school until recovered.
- Avoid contact with those at increased risk of severe illness. In hospital, isolate or cohort during acute illness.
- Handwashing and safe disposal of respiratory secretions.

Response to a cluster

Only of concern if cases have links to institutions containing individuals at increased risk of severe disease and/or rapid spread.

Control of an outbreak

For outbreaks in institutions containing individuals at risk of severe disease

- if virological diagnosis of outbreak not confirmed, organise rapid testing.
- organise typing of virus to compare to vaccine.
- immunise anyone not yet protected.
- oseltamivir prophylaxis for at-risk patients for 2 weeks until vaccine induced protection present (influenza A or B). If not available, consider zanamivir (A or B) or amantadine or rimantadine (both A only) as alternatives.
- exclude staff and visitors with respiratory illness.
- isolate or cohort those with acute symptoms.

Table 3.38.1 Thresholds for primary care consultation rates for influenza-like illness

Level	General Practice consultation rate per 100,000 population		
	England	Wales	Scotland
Baseline	<30	<25	<50
Normal seasonal	30–199	25–100	50–600
Above average	200–399	>100–400	>600–1000
Epidemic	400+	>400	>1000

• reinforce hygiene measures.

• treat influenza-like illness in at-risk patients (irrespective of vaccine status) with zanamivir or oseltamivir, unless contraindicated or symptoms have been present for over 48 hours.

Suggested case definition

Confirmed: upper or lower respiratory tract infection with laboratory evidence of influenza infection.

Clinical:

1 Managing an institutional outbreak – upper or lower respiratory tract infection without other identified cause in person epidemiologically linked to a confirmed case.

2 Monitoring a community outbreak – syndrome of fever, muscle ache and cough occurring during a period of high influenza virus activity.

3.39 Japanese B encephalitis

This is a mosquito-borne viral encephalitis caused by a flavivirus. It occurs throughout south-east Asia and the Far East. Most infections are inapparent, although the illness can be severe with high mortality and permanent neurological sequelae in survivors. The reservoir is pigs, and occasionally birds. Transmission to man is via a mosquito that lives in rice-growing areas. Transmission rates are highest in the rainy season.

Travellers to endemic countries are only at risk if they spend long periods (more than a month) in rural areas where pig farming and rice growing coexist. An unlicensed, inactivated vaccine is available. The schedule is three doses at days 0, 7–14 and 28; two doses at days 0 and 7–14 gives short-term protection in about 80% of vaccines. Severe allergic reactions have

occasionally been reported with the vaccine. The usual precautions against mosquito bites should be taken (see Chapter 3.46).

3.40 Kawasaki syndrome

Kawasaki disease (KD), also known as Kawasaki syndrome or 'mucocutaneous lymph node syndrome', is a generalised vasculitis of unknown aetiology, possibly caused by an infectious agent. Twenty to twenty-five per cent of untreated children develop coronary artery abnormalities.

Suggested on-call action

None.

Epidemiology

KD has been reported throughout the world and is being increasingly recognised. KD occurs more often in boys than in girls (1.5:1); about 80% of cases are less than 5 years old. Incidence rates in North America are highest in children of East Asian (especially Japanese or Korean) ethnicity. The disease occurs year-round; a greater number of cases are reported in the winter and spring. Several regional outbreaks have been reported since 1976 in North America.

Clinical features

In the absence of a specific diagnostic test, Kawasaki disease is a clinical diagnosis based on the characteristic history and physical findings. Features may include conjunctivitis; swollen, fissured lips; strawberry tongue; cervical lymphadenopathy; erythematous rash; peeling of fingers and toes. Clinical criteria have been developed by the Japanese Kawasaki Disease Research Committee.

Consideration of measles is important, as appropriate control measures cannot be taken if measles is misdiagnosed as KD.

Risk factors for coronary artery aneurysms include male gender, age less than 1 year, recurrence of fever after an afebrile period of 24 hours and other signs, such as arrhythmias, of cardiac involvement.

Transmission

Unknown.

Acquisition

The incubation period and infectious period are both unknown.

Prevention

Currently based on secondary prevention: initial therapy is directed at reducing fever and other inflammatory features to prevent the development of coronary arthritis using intravenous immunoglobulin and oral acetylsalicylic acid.

Surveillance

Cases of KD should be reported to any specific KD reporting system, such as that run by the British Paediatric Surveillance Unit in the UK. Clusters should be reported to local public health departments.

Response to a case

Report to surveillance system.

Investigation of a cluster and control of an outbreak

Seek specialist advice. A cluster of KD cases should be used as an opportunity for detailed investigation to learn more about the aetiology.

Case definition
Seek advice from KD reporting system.

3.41 Legionellosis

Infection with *Legionella pneumophila* can cause a potentially life-threatening atypical pneumonia (Legionnaires' disease, LD) or a milder febrile illness (Pontiac fever, PF). Its public health importance lies in its ability to cause outbreaks, including large outbreaks in the community and hospital outbreaks with high case-fatality in particularly susceptible patients.

Suggested on-call action
• If linked to other cases, consult Outbreak Control Plan.   • If in hospital during incubation period, inform hospital infection control team.   • Otherwise, organise investigation of case on next working day.

Epidemiology

The true incidence of LD is not known: estimates range from 2 to 20/100,000. LD has been reported to be responsible for between 0.5 and 15% of community-acquired pneumonias, with the proportion increasing with severity of disease. Approximately 300 cases of LD are reported in the UK each year, of which over 70% are in males and over 95% aged over 30 years (age–sex differences are not obvious in PF). Cases peak from June to October, although there is usually a smaller secondary peak in spring.

Travel is a major risk factor for LD: 43% of reported UK cases are contracted abroad and a further 5% on trips within the UK. Within Europe those travellers most commonly affected are residents of northern European countries visiting southern Europe: the highest number of cases occur in travellers to Spain, followed by Turkey, France, Italy and Greece. The highest rate (per traveller) is in visitors to Turkey. About 12% of UK cases are linked to local outbreaks (predominantly due to 'wet cooling systems' or hot water systems) and about 6% are hospital-acquired. Many cases are, however, sporadic and often from an unidentified source. Large outbreaks have recently occurred in Spain, the Netherlands, Belgium and England.

Clinical features

Both LD and PF commence with non-specific flu-like symptoms such as malaise, fever, myalgia, anorexia and headache, often with diarrhoea and confusion. PF is self-limiting, but LD progresses to pneumonia which, in an individual patient, is difficult to differentiate clinically from other causes of atypical pneumonia. In an outbreak, diagnostic clues might be 25–50% of cases with diarrhoea, confusion, high fever, a lack of upper respiratory symptoms and poor response to penicillins or cephalosporins. About 12% of LD cases die, rising to about a third in nosocomial cases. Many individuals who seroconvert to *Legionella* will be entirely asymptomatic.

Laboratory confirmation

There are 41 named species of Legionella, comprising over 60 serogroups. Over 90% of legionellosis in immunocompetent individuals is due to *L. pneumophila*, which comprises 16 serogroups, of which serogroup 1 is responsible for the large majority of diagnosed infections. Legionellae are not usually identified in routine culture of sputum, although special media can be deployed. Serogroup 1 antibody may be tested for in most laboratories but takes 3–6 weeks to rise to diagnostic levels. Serogroup 1 antigen may be detected in urine samples at a much earlier stage of the illness (reference laboratories may also be able to test for the virulent 'mAb2+ve' subgroup in urine samples). Reference laboratories may be able to diagnose infection due to other serogroups, if routine samples are negative in epidemiologically suspected Legionnaires' clusters. Ideally all suspected cases of LD should have urine antigen testing (for rapid diagnosis of serogroup 1) and culture of appropriate respiratory secretions on selective media (for other species and serogroups and to allow subtyping) performed.

Legionellae are common contaminants of water and so routine environmental testing is not helpful. However, culturing is useful in investigating suspected water sources for identified cases: 5 L of water is necessary for culture. Biofilms are also worth culturing in outbreaks. Although some positive samples can be detected in 2–3 days, it may take 10 days to confirm a sample as negative. If cultures are available from both patient and suspected source, then subtyping is available for comparison of the organisms.

Transmission

The reservoir for the organism is environmental water, in which it occurs in low concentrations. Transmission to humans occurs via inhalation of aerosols or droplet nuclei containing an infective dose of the organism. Legionellae grow at temperatures between 25 and 45°C (preferably 30–40°C) and so the highest risk occurs with water systems that lead to the aerosolisation of water that has been stored at these temperatures. Such systems include hot water systems (especially showers), wet cooling systems (e.g. cooling towers and evaporative condensers), plastics factories, whirlpool spas, indoor and outdoor fountain/sprinkler systems, humidifiers, respiratory therapy equipment and industrial grinders. Wet cooling systems may contaminate air outside the building (up to 0.5–3 km away depending on conditions) and are a particularly frequent cause of outbreaks in Spain.

Legionellae can survive in water stored between 0 and 60°C. They survive normal levels of chlorination and are aided by sediment accumulation and commensal microflora in the water. Temperatures above 63°C are bactericidal, as are many common disinfectants (e.g. phenol, glutaraldehyde, hypochlorite).

Acquisition

The incubation period for LD is 2–10 days (average 5.5 days) and for PF is 5–66 hours (average 36 hours). Legionella is not communicable from person to person.

The infectious dose is unknown, but is certainly low. Attack rates are higher in PF (>90%) than in LD (<5%). Risk of disease may be related to amount of time exposed to the source. Cigarette smoking, advanced age, chronic lung or kidney disease, haematological malignancy, immunosuppression, diabetes and excess alcohol intake are risk factors for identified infection.

Prevention

- Design, maintenance and monitoring of water systems: store hot water above 60°C and deliver above 50°C; store and deliver cold water below 20°C. Eliminate stagnant water.
- New air-conditioning systems to be air-cooled.
- Maintenance and hygiene of wet cooling systems in line with national recommendations (e.g. Health and Safety Executive guidance). Drain when not in use.
- Disinfection, regular cleaning and changing of water in indoor fountains and whirlpool spas.
- Use sterile water for respiratory therapy devices.

Surveillance

- Notifiable in some countries, including Germany, the Netherlands and Belgium.
- Cases of laboratory confirmed legionellosis should be reported to local public health authorities on the day of diagnosis.
- Clusters of respiratory infection should be reported without waiting for confirmation.
- Confirmed cases should also be reported to the relevant national surveillance scheme.
- Legionellosis should be included in hospital infection surveillance schemes, especially for high-risk patients. Nosocomial pneumonia cases should be tested for *Legionella*.

- Cases associated with travel to other European countries are reported to the European Working Group for *Legionella* Infection (EWGLI) collaborator in the presumed country of infection by the project co-ordinating centre at HPA Colindale (UK).

Response to a case

- Ensure appropriate laboratory confirmatory tests undertaken.
- Report to local public health authority and national surveillance centre.
- Obtain risk factor history for 2–14 days (LD) or 0–3 days (PF) before onset of symptoms: details of places of residence and work; visits for occupational or leisure reasons; exposure to industrial sites, hotels, hospitals, leisure/sport/garden centres; air conditioning, showers, whirlpools/jacuzzis, fountains, humidifiers, nebulisers, etc.
- If recognised risk factor identified discuss inspection of possible source, examination of maintenance records and sampling with environmental health and microbiology colleagues. Enquire about respiratory illness in others exposed to potential source.
- Report travel outside district to relevant public health authority and travel outside country to national surveillance centre.
- If case likely to have acquired infection in hospital, convene incident control team. A single nosocomial case should lead to an environmental investigation, including the potable water supply. Isolation is unnecessary.
- If no risk factor identified, consider domestic water system as possible source. Also consider if possible nosocomial case spent part of incubation period at home.

Investigation of a cluster

- Undertake hypothesis generation exercise of risk factors as identified for individual cases including day-by-day analysis of movements in 14 days before onset.
- Further case finding: ensure all cases of community- or hospital-acquired pneumonia are tested for legionellosis. If serogroup 1 disease, encourage urine antigen testing for rapid

diagnosis. Where possible, also encourage culture so that typing may be performed. Alert colleagues in other areas to check whether cases visited your locality.

• Use geographical analysis of home, work and places visited of cases to look for links. Geographical information systems can be used to see if cases have been near each other and can also use weather data.

• If cases have been to same area, identify all potential sources. Consider identification, inspection and sampling of all cooling towers in area.

• In nosocomial outbreaks, test all water sources (hot and cold) and relevant environmental samples (e.g. showerheads) in suspect wards. Obtain specialist engineering advice on plumbing and heating systems.

• Compare typing results from cases and suspected source.

Control of an outbreak

• Shutdown of suspected source whilst expert engineering advice obtained.

• Drainage, cleaning, disinfection, maintenance and re-evaluation of suspected source. Occasionally major redesign or closure necessary.

• Warn clinicians of increase and of appropriate antibiotics.

• Rarely, temporary chemoprophylaxis in high-risk populations during a severe nosocomial outbreak may be considered.

Suggested case definition

Confirmed: case of pneumonia (LD) or flu-like illness (PF) with *Legionella* infection diagnosed by culture, urine antigen or fourfold rise in serum antibody titres.

Presumptive: pneumonia or flu-like illness with single high serum titre (1:64 by IFAT in outbreak; 1:128 in non-outbreak) or positive direct fluorescence (DFA).

Clinical: case of pneumonia epidemiologically linked to confirmed LD *or* case of flu-like illness linked to confirmed PF, awaiting final confirmation.

3.42 Leprosy

Leprosy is a chronic inflammatory disease caused by *Mycobacterium leprae*.

Suggested on-call action

No urgent action is required.

Epidemiology

Leprosy occurs in almost all the tropical and warm temperate regions. It becomes less common as living standards rise and is associated with overcrowding. All cases in North Europe are imported.

Clinical features

The organism has a predilection for the skin and nerves. Nerve involvement results in an area of anaesthesia and or muscle weakness/ wasting; tissue damage occurs secondarily to the anaesthesia.

The clinical appearance of the disease depends upon the degree of cell-mediated immunity (CMI). In tuberculoid (TT) disease there is a high degree of CMI and disease is localised, whereas in lepromatous (LL) there is little CMI and skin and nerves are heavily infiltrated with bacilli.

Immunologically mediated reactions usually occur during treatment as CMI returns. These may include erythema nodosum leprosum and tender enlarging nerves.

Laboratory confirmation

The diagnosis can usually be made following a careful examination. This is then confirmed by identifying mycobacteria in slit skin smears or histological preparations. In lepromatous patients, nodules should be biopsied and the nasal mucosa should be scraped. In tuberculoid patients the edge of a lesion should be biopsied.

Transmission

The major source of infection is patients with lepromatous leprosy who shed large numbers of bacilli in their nasal secretions. The portal of entry is probably the respiratory tract.

Acquisition

The incubation period varies from a few months to many years. Lepromatous patients may be infectious for several years.

Prevention

Identification and treatment of lepromatous patients is the mainstay of prevention.

Surveillance

• Leprosy is a notifiable disease in most countries.
• In the UK there is a leprosy register of all cases.

Response to a case

• Cases should be referred to a specialist unit for treatment.
• Lepromatous cases should be isolated until treatment has been initiated.

Investigation of a cluster

A cluster should be investigated for misdiagnosis or laboratory contamination.

Case definition

A clinically compatible case that is laboratory-confirmed by demonstration of acid-fast bacilli in skin or dermal nerve.

3.43 Leptospirosis

Leptospirosis is caused by the zoonotic genus *Leptospira*, which occurs worldwide.

Suggested on-call action

Person-to-person spread is rare so no urgent on-call action is required.

Epidemiology

Leptospirosis is an occupational hazard to those exposed to urine-contaminated water as a result of occupation or recreation, e.g. farmers, sewage workers, vets, miners, soldiers, swimmers, canoeists, divers and sailors, etc. Worldwide it is seen in areas of poverty, where there can be epidemics. In the UK the most commonly identified serovars are *L. hardjo* and *L. icterohaemorrhagiae*, associated with cattle and rats, respectively. Fewer than 50 cases a year have been reported in England and Wales during 1989–1999.

Clinical features

The clinical spectrum of disease is wide; any serovar can cause many clinical presentations. Classically there is an abrupt onset with headache, myalgia, conjunctival suffusion and fever. Following a week of illness the fever may settle only to rise again. During the later phase, meningism, renal and vasculitic manifestations may occur. The combination of leptospirosis with jaundice and uraemia is sometimes known as Weil's disease. Death is usually associated with renal failure; however, it may be due to myocarditis or massive blood loss.

Laboratory confirmation

The species *L. interrogans* comprises 130 serovars in 16 serogroups. During the first phase organisms may be visualised in (under dark field illumination) and cultured from blood, CSF or urine. The organism may persist in urine. As the immune response develops, a significant rise in IgM antibodies may be detected using ELISA. Confirmation is by high sensitivity microscopic agglutination test (MAT).

During the first phase of the illness there may be a leukopaenia, although jaundice may be associated with neutrophilia. About one quarter of cases will have an elevated urea.

Transmission

Leptospirosis affects many wild and domestic animals worldwide. Humans acquire the infection by contact with water, soil or other material contaminated with the urine of infected animals. Leptospires are excreted in the urine of infected animals and infection in man is due to contact with urine or urine-soaked soil. The organism probably enters through mucosa or broken skin. Leptospires can survive in fresh water for as many as 16 days and in soil for as many as 24 days.

Acquisition

The incubation period is usually 7–13 days (range 4–19 days). Patients continue to excrete leptospires for many months but person-to-person spread is rare. Previous infection protects against re-infection with the same serovar, but may not protect against other serovars.

Prevention

• Control rodent populations.
• Education of those at risk to avoid contaminated areas and cover cuts and abraded skin.
• Providing those at risk (e.g. sewage workers) with alert/information cards to ensure early intervention.

• Adequate occupational clothing.
• Immunisation of those with occupational exposure to specific serovars has been carried out in some countries (e.g. Italy, France and Spain).
• Some authorities recommend prophylaxis with doxycycline for those known to at high risk for limited periods (e.g. water sports in endemic areas)

Surveillance

Leptospirosis is notifiable in many countries, including the UK. Cases should be reported to public health authorities so that areas of risk can be identified.

Response to a case

• Treatment with intravenous antibiotics (e.g. benzyl penicillin) in the first 4 days probably reduces the severity of the attack, though the response may not be dramatic.
• Obtain risk factor information.

Investigation of a cluster

• Clusters should be investigated to determine areas of risk, such as particular water sports locations, so that the public can be informed.
• Laboratory typing may help identify risk factors.

Control of an outbreak

• Outbreaks usually occur in areas of poverty, particularly following flooding and disasters that have increased the rodent population.
• Rodent control is the main activity.
• Outbreaks resulting from occupational exposure e.g. to cattle, should be reported to the veterinary authorities.
• Antibiotic prophylaxis (e.g. doxycycline) may be considered.

3.44 Listeria

Infection by *Listeria monocytogenes* is usually food-borne but usually presents as septicaemia or meningitis. Although rare, infection in vulnerable groups has high case-fatality with fetuses, neonates, the elderly and the immuno-compromised particularly at risk.

Suggested on-call action

If you or reporting clinician/microbiologist know of associated cases consult Outbreak Control Plan.

Epidemiology

Approximately 150 cases of listeriosis are reported in the UK each year, a little higher than the typical incidence in Europe of 2 per million per annum. UK incidence was almost twice this level for a 3-year period in 1987–1999, and a food-borne outbreak affecting 1500 people occurred in Italy in 1997. Infection occurs worldwide. Reported infection is highest in those under 1 month of age, followed by those over 70 years. Approximately 15% of reported cases occur in pregnant women. These observations are likely to be due to ascertainment bias because of severity of infection. In contrast to the low reported incidence, the high case-fatality means that about 70 deaths are thought to be caused yearly in the UK. Human infection peaks in late summer and early autumn, whereas animal listeriosis peaks in spring.

Clinical features

Infection in immunocompetent adults is usually asymptomatic or a mild flu-like illness, although it may occasionally cause meningitis and/or septicaemia, particularly in the elderly or immunocompromised. Infection in pregnant women is also usually mild, but transplacental spread during the first trimester usually results in fetal death; fetal infection during the third trimester may result in stillbirth or neonatal septicaemia and/or meningitis within 48 hours of delivery. A red papular rash often accompanies this 'early onset' neonatal infection. Neonates are also susceptible to 'late onset' sepsis approximately 10 days after delivery. Case fatality is approximately 50% in early onset and 25% in late onset neonatal sepsis. Case-fatality is also high in those aged over 60 years. *Listeria* is now also known to cause febrile gastroenteritis and asymptomatic faecal carriage.

Laboratory confirmation

Diagnosis is usually by blood or CSF culture, which usually takes 48 hours, plus another 24 hours for confirmation. In *Listeria* meningitis, less than half of cases have organisms demonstrable on CSF microscopy, which also shows polymorphs or lymphocytes, increased protein and normal or decreased glucose. *Listeria* may also be identified in faecal, food and environmental samples, particularly after 'cold enrichment'.

There are 13 serovars of *L. monocytogenes*, of which 4b, 1/2a and 1/2b cause 90% of clinical cases. Serovar 4 was particularly associated with the increase and subsequent fall in cases in 1987–1999 (and most of the other large food-borne outbreaks) and is also associated with late-onset neonatal disease. Serovar 1/2 is particularly associated with early onset sepsis. Phage typing is also obtainable on 80% of serovar 4 and 37% of serovar 1/2 strains. Genotyping is also available in many countries.

Transmission

L. monocytogenes is widespread in the environment and can be found in soil, surface water, vegetation and a wide range of wild and domestic animals. It is extremely hardy and survives drying, freezing and thawing, remaining viable in soil or silage for more than 2 years.

The main route of infection for humans is consumption of contaminated food. The organism can grow at temperatures as low as $0°C$ (although optimum growth temperature is 30–37°C), is relatively tolerant of salt and nitrates and does not 'spoil' or taint food even at high levels of contamination. *Listeria* are endemic in food processing environments.

Many foods have been associated with transmission of infection but most have some or all of the following features: highly processed, refrigerated, long shelf life, near-neutral pH and consumed without further cooking. Implicated vehicles have included paté, unpasteurised soft cheese, butter, 'cook-chill' meals, sandwiches, cold meats, fish, hot dogs and salads. Some foods (e.g. those with high fat content) may also protect the organism against the neutralising effects of gastric acidity. Some outbreaks have been explained by long-term colonisation of difficult to clean sites in food processing facilities. Infected cattle can contaminate milk.

Other sources of infection include direct transmission from animals, which may cause cutaneous infection often with obvious occupational exposure; direct contact with the environment; transplacental transmission in pregnant women; exposure to vaginal carriage during birth or hospital cross-infection for late-onset neonatal sepsis; and nosocomial transmission in hospital nurseries and renal transplant units.

Acquisition

The incubation period has been variously reported from 1 day to over 3 months. Averages quoted for adults are 3 weeks, for neonates a few days and for intrauterine infection 30 days. Outbreaks of *Listeria* gastroenteritis may have much shorter incubation periods, perhaps averaging 24 hours or so.

Human excreters with normal hygiene are unlikely to be an important source of infection, except for neonates. The infectious dose is uncertain (possibly 100–1000/g food) and it is unclear what level is 'safe' for immunocompromised patients, leading many to suggest a 'zero tolerance' policy for food. Attack rates for food-borne outbreaks are generally very low.

In addition to fetuses, neonates and the elderly, those at risk of severe infection include patients with malignancy, cirrhosis, diabetes, prosthetic valves or joints, and impaired cell-mediated immunity including those on corticosteroid therapy. Low gastric acidity increases susceptibility.

Prevention

- Hazard analysis in food processing to reduce the risk of contamination and multiplication.
- Pasteurisation of dairy produce effectively kills *Listeria*.
- Limiting the length of storage of at-risk refrigerated food, e.g. cook-chill meals.
- Advice to pregnant women and immunosuppressed to avoid certain soft cheeses, paté and pre-packed salads.
- Thorough reheating of cook-chill/microwave foods, especially if served to vulnerable populations (e.g. hospital patients).
- Pregnant women to avoid contact with pregnant or newborn animals or silage.
- Thoroughly wash raw vegetables, fruit and salad before eating.
- Adequate infection control in delivery rooms and neonatal units.

Surveillance

• Listeriosis should be reported to local public health agencies: notify as 'suspected Food Poisoning' in UK. Meningitis is also notifiable in many countries.
• Laboratories should report all clinically significant infections to regional and national surveillance: these may detect outbreaks not apparent at local level.
• Consider as a cause of two or more cases of 'late onset' neonatal meningitis/septicaemia.

Response to a case

• Report to local and national/regional public health department to aid detection of clusters.
• Collect data on consumption of risk foods in last month.
• No exclusion required, although enteric precautions sensible for hospitalised patients.
• Send isolate to reference laboratory for typing.

Response to a cluster

• Discuss with microbiologist further investigation such as serotyping, phage typing or genotyping.
• Institute case finding with microbiologists and relevant clinicians to ensure adequate microbiological investigation of meningitis/septicaemia in neonates and elderly.
• Undertake a hypothesis-generating study to include all foods consumed, particularly those at increased risk of high level *Listeria* contamination, e.g. unpasteurised dairy produce, soft cheeses, paté, raw vegetables, salads, cold meats, highly processed foods and cook-chill or microwave products. The prolonged incubation will make accurate recall difficult; 'food preference' questions may also be useful. Consider direct exposure to animals (e.g. farms).
• If cases predominantly neonatal, look at age in days at onset: could this be nosocomial?

Control of an outbreak

• Product withdrawal of any implicated food.
• Obtain specialist Environmental Health advice to investigate and modify suspect food processes.

Suggested case definition
Flu-like illness, septicaemia or CNS infection, associated with isolate of the outbreak strain of *L. monocytogenes* from blood or CSF.

3.45 Lyme disease

Lyme disease (borreliosis, Bannwarth syndrome, erythema chronicum migrans) is a multisystem illness resulting from exposure to *Ixodes* ticks infected with *Borrelia burgdorferi*.

Suggested on-call action
No on-call action is required.

Epidemiology

Lyme disease is common in North America and Northern Europe in areas of heathland, affecting ramblers and campers. Geographic distribution of disease in Europe is associated with the known range of *I. ricinus*; the true incidence of disease is unknown as reporting is incomplete. Estimates of incidence/100,000 population are UK 0.3, France 16, Germany 25, Switzerland 30.4, Czech Republic 39, Sweden 69, Slovenia 120 and Austria 130.

Clinical features

Following a tick bite, which may be inapparent, a rash (erythema chronicum migrans) develops; the appearance is of an expanding erythematous circle with central clearing. Other manifestations include large joint polyarthritis (usually asymmetrical), aseptic meningitis, peripheral root lesions, radiculopathy, meningoencephalitis and myocarditis. These features may occur without the rash. The symptoms may persist over a prolonged period. The clinical manifestations seen in Europe and North America differ, with milder disease often reported in Europe.

Laboratory confirmation

Confirmation is by demonstrating elevated IgM antibody. The low sensitivity of serologic testing early in the disease means it is unhelpful; it may be more useful in later disease. Positive or equivocal results on an ELISA or IFA assay require confirmatory testing with a Western immunoblot. Some chronic patients may remain seronegative.

Transmission

Lyme disease is caused by a spirochete, *B. burgdorferi,* transmitted by the bite of *Ixodes* ticks. Deer are the preferred host for adult ticks in the USA; sheep in Europe. Other mammals (e.g. dogs) can be incidental hosts and may develop Lyme disease.

Acquisition

Erythema migrans, the best clinical indicator of Lyme disease, develops between 3 and 32 days after a tick bite. Lyme disease is not transmissible from person to person.

Prevention

• The main method of prevention is avoidance of tick bites through wearing long trousers.
• Transmission of *B. burgdorferi* does not usually occur until the tick has been in place for 36–48 hours; thus, screening and removing ticks after exposure can help prevent infection.
• A vaccine has been developed in the US; indications for use are uncertain, and it would not be effective against European variants.

Surveillance

• Cases should be reported to the public health authorities so that assessments of risk can be made.
• Statutory notifiable disease in many EU countries (not UK).

Response to a case

No public health response.

Investigation of a cluster and control of an outbreak

Clusters should be investigated to determine areas of high risk, so that those who might be exposed can be informed.

Suggested case definition
Clinical diagnosis: presence of erythema migrans in someone who has been exposed to tick bites.

3.46 Malaria

Malaria is a potentially fatal plasmodial infection. Increasing numbers of patients presenting to healthcare facilities in Europe will have travelled to places where they have been exposed to malaria. There is also a risk of airport and transfusion malaria.

<table>
<tr><td>

Suggested on-call action

None unless the case is thought to be trans-fusion related in which case other units from the same donor need to be identified and withdrawn urgently.

</td></tr>
</table>

Epidemiology

Malaria is endemic in more than 100 coun-tries throughout Africa, Central and South America, Asia and Oceania; more than two bil-lion people are exposed to the risk of malaria infection. *P. falciparum* and *P. vivax* are the most common species. *P. falciparum* is the pre-dominant species in Africa and Papua New Guinea. *P. vivax* dominates in South America and Asia; *P. malariae* is widely distributed but is much less common. *P. ovale* is mainly found in Africa. About 10,000 cases a year are reported in Europe, with a case fatality of about 0.5% in England and Wales.

There has been a recent fall in the number of imported cases in England and Wales, possibly reflecting reduced travel resulting from fears about terrorism. Patterns of importation re-flect travel destinations; for England and Wales the commonest source of imported falciparum malaria is West Africa, followed by East and Central Africa.

Clinical features

Malaria may present with almost any clini-cal pattern. The most classical symptom is the malarial rigor, the periodic nature of the at-tacks of fever may give a clue as to the diagno-sis. The disease must be considered in anyone who has been exposed to the parasite, by travel, blood transfusion or the rare airport malaria. It may follow a progressive course with high mortality in non-immune subjects. The rise in chloroquine resistance means that there are few areas in the world where chloroquine can be relied on for treatment.

Complications are associated with high par-asitaemia and are therefore more common in non-immunes and children. The course may

be rapid: delay in diagnosis of *P. falciparum* malaria is associated with increased mortality.

Laboratory confirmation

Diagnosis is by demonstrating parasites in the peripheral blood. A minimum of three speci-mens should be taken at the height of fever. Thick films are of particular value when the parasitaemia is low; the technique requires ex-perience. A thin film enables a parasite count (number of parasites per 100 RBC) to be per-formed and the parasite species to be more clearly identified.

Slides should be reviewed by an expert so that a species diagnosis, essential to guide chemotherapy, can be made. Serology has no part to play in diagnosis of acute malaria. Anti-gen detection methods for malaria antigen are under development, but none yet com-pare with the sensitivity and specificity of microscopy.

Transmission

Malaria is transmitted by the bite of the fe-male anopheline mosquito. Absence of the in-sect vector in Europe means that there is no risk of secondary cases. Rare cases of 'airport malaria' happen when an infected mosquito introduced to Europe bites a host before dy-ing. There are also rare transmissions through blood donation, needlestick or poor hospital infection control.

Acquisition

The incubation period (time from infection to appearance of parasites in blood) varies with infecting species:

P. falciparum: 5–7 days
P. vivax: 6–8 days
P. malariae: 12–16 days
P. ovale: 8–9 days

In transfusion-associated malaria the incuba-tion period is much shorter.

In *P. vivax* and *P. ovale* some parasites remain dormant in the liver (hypnozoites): these can take up to a year before becoming active.

Prevention

- Good advice to those travelling is essential. The risk of those visiting relatives is often underestimated by travellers and those providing advice: pre-existing immunity will probably have waned.
- Prevention of mosquito bites (the mosquitoes bite mainly at night):

  Sleep in fully air-conditioned or screened accommodation and use knockdown insecticide in room each evening.

  If room cannot be made safe, sleep under bed nets; impregnation with pyrethrum enhances the efficacy of nets.

  Electrical pyrethroid vapouriser in room may also be useful.

  Wear long-sleeved garments and long trousers between dusk and dawn. Use mosquito repellents.
- Suppression of the malaria parasite with chemoprophylaxis. Regular antimalarial prophylaxis should be taken for 1 week before travel to an endemic area and 4 weeks after return. Changing patterns of resistance mean that specialist advice should be consulted.
- Control of malaria in populations depends on diminishing or eradication of the vector, the *Anopheles* mosquito. Methods include spraying of houses with insecticides and the destruction of larval sites by removing standing water.

Surveillance

- Malaria is notifiable in many countries, including the UK.
- Cases should be reported to national authorities so that advice on prophylaxis can be based upon observed patterns of risk.

Response to a case

- A travel history should be taken.
- If there is no travel history, information about transfusions or injections (including drug misuse) and proximity to airports should be sought.

- Patients should be reviewed 28 days after treatment to confirm parasitological and clinical cure. Patients who have splenic enlargement should avoid body contact sports and strenuous exercise due to a risk of splenic rupture.

Investigation of a cluster and control of an outbreak

- If clusters arise from areas where malaria has not previously been recognised, the national authorities should be informed. Travel advice should be reviewed.
- If cases occur in people who have not been abroad, consider blood, nosocomial and airport exposures.

Case definitions

Clinical: fever and/or compatible illness in person who has travelled to an area in which malaria is endemic.

WHO categories:
- Autochthonous

  indigenous: malaria acquired by mosquito transmission in an area where malaria is a regular occurrence;

  introduced: malaria acquired by mosquito transmission from an imported case in an area where malaria is not a regular occurrence.
- Imported: malaria acquired outside a specific area.
- Induced: malaria acquired through artificial means (e.g. blood transfusion, common syringes or malariotherapy).
- Relapsing: renewed manifestation (i.e. of clinical symptoms and/or parasitaemia) of malarial infection that is separated from previous manifestations of the same infection by an interval greater than any interval resulting from the normal periodicity of the paroxysms.
- Cryptic: an isolated case of malaria that cannot be epidemiologically linked to additional cases.

3.47 Measles

Measles is a systemic viral infection caused by a paramyxovirus. Its main features are fever, rash and respiratory disease. The public health significance of measles is that it is highly infectious and can be prevented by vaccination.

Suggested on-call action
None usually necessary.

Epidemiology

In the pre-vaccination era, most people were infected in childhood; the average age at infection was 4 years. Large epidemics occurred every 2 years in the UK until 1968, the year that routine childhood immunisation was introduced. The epidemiology of measles in the post-vaccination era varies across Europe, depending on the evolution of vaccine strategies and vaccine coverage (see Table 3.47.1). In countries where coverage has been high for many years, the disease has been virtually eliminated. These include all the Scandinavian countries, the Baltic States and most of Eastern Europe. In contrast Germany, France, Belgium and Italy all have low coverage, below 90%; here outbreaks are still common. An outbreak has been ongoing in Ireland since 2003. In the UK, despite declining vaccine coverage (currently 81% for the first dose by 2 years of age), there were only 442 confirmed cases in 2003, although clusters were reported among

Table 3.47.1 Measles incidence and vaccine policy in Europe

Country	Incidence per 100,000	1st dose MMR (months)	2nd dose MMR (years)
Austria	n/a	14	7
Belgium	32.6	15	11–12
Cyprus	n/a	n/a	n/a
Denmark	0.5	15	12
Czech Republic	0.1	15	2
Estonia	0.8	12	13
Finland	0.0	14–18	6
France	66.6	12	5
Germany	7.3	11–14	2
Greece	0.6	15	4–6
Hungary	0.1	15	11
Ireland	12.6	15	4–5
Italy	17.5	15	5–12
Latvia	0.1	15	7
Lithuania	0.5	15	12
Luxembourg	0.4	15–18	5–7
Malta	0.7	15	5–7
Netherlands	4.3	14	9
Poland	1.5	13–14	7
Portugal	0.7	15	5–6
Slovakia	4.3	14	11
Slovenia	0.2	12–18	7
Spain	1.5	15	3–6
Sweden	0.4	18	12
UK	0.2	12–15	3–5

Source: World Health Organization. Strategic plan for measles and congenital rubella infection in the European Region of WHO (www.who.dk/document/e81567.pdf).
Figures given are for most recent year reported to WHO. n/a = data not reported to WHO.

travelling communities, and schools and nurseries in London. The WHO has set a target of measles elimination in Europe by 2010.

Clinical features

In an unvaccinated child, there is a prodromal illness with a high fever and a coryzal respiratory infection. There is cough, conjunctivitis and runny nose. Koplik's spots appear during the early stage of the illness – these look like grains of salt on a red inflamed background and are found on the mucosa of the cheek next to the upper premolars and molars. The rash of measles starts on day 3 or 4, initially in the hairline, but spreads rapidly to cover the face, trunk and limbs. It is maculopapular but not itchy. Koplik's spots fade as the rash appears. The rash fades over a week to 10 days.

In a vaccinated child, the illness is usually mild with a low-grade fever, transient rash and absent respiratory features.

Complications of measles include pneumonitis, secondary bacterial infection, especially acute otitis media and pneumonia, and encephalitis. Complication rates are higher in malnourished or immunosuppressed children. Subacute sclerosing panencephalitis is a late, slow-onset, progressive complication that occurs in about 1 per million cases. It is always fatal.

Laboratory confirmation

The diagnosis can be confirmed by culture (in blood, nasopharyngeal and conjunctival secretions and urine) or serology (single raised IgM or rise in IgG). Measles IgM can now reliably be detected in saliva if the specimen is collected between 1 and 6 weeks after the onset of symptoms.

Transmission

Man is the only reservoir. Carriers are unknown. Spread is from person to person by direct contact with nose and throat secretions or respiratory droplets; less commonly indirectly by articles freshly soiled with nose and throat secretions.

Acquisition

The incubation period (to onset of fever) is 8–13 days, usually about 10 days. The period of communicability starts just before the onset of the prodrome and lasts until 4 days after the rash appears. Measles is highly infectious, with a reproduction rate of 15–17, i.e. between 15 and 17 secondary cases in a susceptible population for every index case. Natural infection provides lifelong immunity. Vaccine-induced immunity is lower, but is also usually lifelong and can be boosted by exposure to circulating wild virus. In developed countries, maternal antibody persists for up to 12 months; this period may be shorter when the maternal immunity is vaccine-induced.

Prevention

• Vaccinate with a combined measles/mumps/rubella (MMR) vaccine. Two doses are given in Europe. The first dose is at 12–18 months of age; the timing of the second dose varies from 2 to 13 years of age (see Table 3.47.1). In the UK the second dose is given at entry to primary school at age 3–5 years. The main purpose of this second dose is to protect children who failed to respond to the first dose; it also boosts waning vaccine-induced immunity in children who did respond to the first dose.

• The only contraindications to measles vaccine are immunosuppression, allergy to neomycin or kanamycin and a severe reaction to a previous dose. There is increasing evidence that measles vaccine can be safely given to children with egg anaphylaxis.

• Vaccination should not be given within 3 weeks of another live vaccine (except OPV) or within 3 months of an injection of immunoglobulin.

Surveillance

Measles is notifiable in nearly all countries in Europe, including the UK. The clinical diagnosis is unreliable in a highly vaccinated population, so laboratory confirmation (e.g. salivary IgM) should be sought in all notified suspected cases.

Response to a case

- Obtain laboratory confirmation (e.g. saliva test).
- Check vaccination status of contacts.
- Immunise previously unimmunised contacts.
- Determine source of infection (including travel history).
- Exclude from school until 5 days from the onset of rash.
- Give HNIG to immunosuppressed close contacts and those under 12 months of age.

Response to a cluster and investigation of an outbreak

As per case investigation, but also check vaccination coverage in the population where the cluster is occurring, and arrange for vaccination of all children in that population without a documented history of vaccination. In a larger outbreak it may be necessary to conduct a mass campaign to interrupt transmission.

Suggested case definition

Suspected case:
- Fever (>38°C if measured) *plus*
- rash plus one of
- conjunctivitis, cough, coryza.

Confirmed case:
- measles virus in blood, urine, conjunctival or nasopharyngeal secretions; *or*
- measles IgM in blood or saliva; *or*
- fourfold or greater rise in measles IgG in blood.

3.48 Meningococcal infection

Meningococcal infection is the spectrum of disease caused by the bacterium *Neisseria meningitidis*. The infection may present as meningitis, septicaemia or a combination of both. The public health significance of meningococcal infection lies in the severity of the disease, the absence of effective vaccines, the ability of the infection to cause unpredictable clusters and the intense public anxiety that inevitably accompanies a case or cluster.

Suggested on-call action

- Ensure rapid admission to hospital and administration of pre-admission benzyl penicillin.
- Initiate lab investigations to confirm diagnosis.
- Arrange chemoprophylaxis for close contacts of confirmed or probable cases.

Epidemiology

The incidence of meningococcal infection in Europe varies from 1 to 10 per 100,000 population. In most countries the incidence is relatively stable, although the UK saw an increase during the 1990s from 4 to 6 per 100,000. Much of this increase was due to an epidemic of serogroup C cases among older children. Spain, Ireland, Holland and the Czech Republic also experienced outbreaks of serogroup C disease during the 1990s.

Since 2000 the incidence has generally declined across Europe, partly due to the impact of meningococcal C vaccines in some countries, but also due to a general decline in serogroup B disease.

There are 13 serogroups of *N. meningitidis*. In Europe, serogroups B and C account for over 95% of cases. Serogroup B is commoner than C.

Children under the age of 5 years are most frequently affected, with a peak incidence at about 6 months of age, which coincides with the loss of maternally derived immunity. There is a second, smaller peak in teenagers.

Most cases arise sporadically, although clusters occur from time to time. These are unpredictable, although they often occur in educational establishments or in the military. Serogroup C disease tends to cause clusters more than serogroup B.

The infection is seasonal, with a higher incidence in the winter months. There are geographical variations in the disease, although these are not consistent over time. Local increases are often associated with the arrival of a strain not previously seen in that community.

There are a number of factors that predispose to meningococcal infection. These include passive smoking, crowding, recent influenza type A infection, absence of a spleen and complement deficiency. Travellers to the meningitis belt of Africa (where outbreaks of serogroup A disease are common) may be at risk of disease. Cases (serogroup A, but more recently serogroup W135) among pilgrims to the Hajj in Mecca have prompted the government of Saudi Arabia to require a certificate of meningococcal vaccination from visitors.

Clinical features

The early symptoms are non-specific and are often mistaken for a viral infection. In infants there is fever, floppiness, high-pitched crying and sometimes vomiting. Older children and adults have a fever, malaise, increasing headache, nausea and often vomiting. The illness usually progresses rapidly, with the clinical picture changing hourly, although sometimes there is a slower onset, which causes diagnostic difficulty. In infants there is progressive irritability, altered consciousness and sometimes convulsions. Older children and adults develop photophobia and neck stiffness with a positive Kernig's sign, although these features are sometimes absent.

An important feature is the appearance of a petechial rash (see Plate 1a *facing p. 20*), which indicates that there is septicaemia. The rash is not always present, or there may be only a few petechiae, so a careful search for petechiae is important in suspected cases. The 'glass test' can be used to distinguish a haemorrhagic rash from other types of rash (see Plate 1b *facing p. 20*).

Patients with rapidly advancing disease may develop hypotension, circulatory collapse, pulmonary oedema, confusion and coma. The overall case fatality rate is about 10%, although for patients without septicaemia the outlook is better. Approximately 15% of survivors have permanent sequelae, including deafness, convulsions, mental impairment and limb loss.

Laboratory confirmation

Obtaining laboratory confirmation in suspected cases is essential for public health management. This requires close co-operation between clinicians, microbiologists and the public health team. Specimens should be taken as soon as a suspected case is seen in hospital (see Box 3.48.1). The single most important specimen is blood for culture and PCR diagnosis (a 2.5-mL EDTA or citrated specimen is needed for PCR). There is often reluctance to do a lumbar puncture because of the risk of coning; however, where CSF sample has been obtained, this should be submitted for microscopy, culture and PCR. A throat swab should also be obtained for culture (the yield from cases is about 50% and is unaffected by prior administration of antibiotic).

Box 3.48.1 Suggested laboratory specimens in suspected meningococcal infection

- Blood for PCR and culture.
- Throat swab for culture.
- CSF for microscopy, antigen detection, culture and PCR.
- Paired serum samples for serology.

A rash aspirate for microscopy is a further useful specimen. A throat swab from family members before chemoprophylaxis may also help to identify the causative organism, although counselling is advised before swabbing to prevent feelings of guilt should a household member be found to be the source of infection. Acute and convalescent serology can also provide a diagnosis, although the result is often obtained too late to affect either clinical or public health management; it may however be useful in the investigation of a potential cluster as it provides serogroup information.

It is important determine the serogroup of the infecting organism, to inform decisions about vaccination. PCR diagnosis is serogroup-specific and a result is available within a few hours. Latex agglutination tests are also available as a rapid screening method when there is a positive culture, although the national reference laboratory should ideally confirm the result. Genotyping methods such as *porA* sequencing are becoming increasingly available and provide a much more precise typing than phenotype-based methods.

Transmission

The infection is spread from person to person through respiratory droplets and direct contact with nose and throat secretions. Infectivity is relatively low and transmission usually requires prolonged close contact such as that occurs in the household setting or through 'wet' mouth kissing.

Man is the only reservoir and the organism dies quickly outside the host. Approximately 10% of the population carries the organism harmlessly in the nasopharynx. Carriage confers natural immunity. Carriage rates are lowest in children under 5 years, and then rise to peak at 20–25% in teenagers and young adults. During outbreaks, carriage rates of the outbreak strain may rise sharply, to high as high as 50%. There is, however, no consistent relationship between carriage rates and disease, and some outbreaks occur in the absence of normal carriage. Increased rates of carriage have been observed in smokers, in crowded conditions and among military recruits.

The most common setting for transmission to occur is within households, where a member of the household (usually an adult) has recently become a carrier and infects a susceptible household member (usually a child). The absolute risk, in the absence of chemoprophylaxis, of a second case in the same household in the month following an index case is about 1 in 300. In comparison, transmission in other settings is rare; the estimated risks of a second case in the month following an index case in a pre-school group, primary and secondary school are respectively 1 in 1500, 1 in 18,000 and 1 in 33,000. Transmission from patients to healthcare workers has been documented, but is also rare; occurring where there has been direct exposure to nasopharyngeal secretions.

Acquisition

The incubation period is usually 3–5 days, although it may occasionally be up to 10 days. For public health purposes, an upper limit of 7 days is generally accepted. Patients are usually no longer infectious within 24 hours of starting antibiotic treatment, although it should be noted that some antibiotics used in treatment (e.g. penicillin) will only temporarily suppress carriage. For this reason a chemoprophylactic antibiotic should be given before hospital discharge.

Maternal immunity to meningococcal infection is passed across the placenta to the neonate, but only lasts for a few months. Subsequent carriage of pathogenic and non-pathogenic meningococci confers serogroup-specific natural immunity, which usually develops within 7 days of acquisition. Carriage of pathogenic meningococci is unusual in infancy and early childhood, rises progressively to peak at 25% in 15- to 19-year-olds and then slowly declines through adult life. Conversely, carriage of *N. lactamica* (which induces some cross-immunity to *N. meningitidis*) is predominantly in infants and young children, with carriage rates low in teenagers and young adults. It has been speculated that a variety of factors may affect susceptibility. This could, e.g. account for the increased risk of invasive disease that follows influenza type A infection.

Prevention

• Vaccines offer the only prospect for prevention. Polysaccharide vaccines against serogroups A, C, W135 and Y are available; however, they offer only short-lived (2–3 years) protection and are ineffective in young children, in whom the disease incidence is greatest. They are only of value where short-term protection is required, e.g. during outbreaks or for travellers to the meningitis belt or the Hajj.

• Serogroup B vaccines have to date performed poorly in clinical trials (particularly in children) and are not yet generally available (with the exception of some Latin American countries). Genetically engineered serogroup B vaccines are now undergoing clinical trials and appear promising.

• Improved polysaccharide-protein conjugate vaccines against serogroup A, C, W135 and Y strains are in development. They induce immunological memory, which is likely to be lifelong. Conjugate serogroup C vaccines have now been introduced into the childhood immunisation schedules in a number of countries in Europe. In the UK, the first country to introduce the vaccine, three doses are given at 2, 3 and 4 months of age; children over 12 months require only a single dose. The impact of the programme has been dramatic with a reduction in disease incidence of over 90%.

Surveillance

• Both meningococcal infection and meningococcal disease are notifiable in most European countries, including the UK.

• Laboratory reports are another important source of data in most countries, although increasing use of pre-admission antibiotics means that there is now greater reliance on non-culture diagnoses for surveillance.

Response to a case

• Public health action is indicated for confirmed or probable cases; it is not indicated for possible cases or infection in non-sterile sites (except for meningococcal conjunctivitis, which is as an indication for public health action because of the high immediate risk of invasive disease).

• There are four key actions for the public health practitioner:

1 Ensure rapid admission to hospital and that pre-admission benzyl penicillin has been given (see Box 3.48.2). Prompt action may reduce the case fatality rate by up to 50%.

2 Ensure that appropriate laboratory investigations are undertaken (see Box 3.48.1).

Box 3.48.2 Immediate dose of benzyl penicillin for suspected meningococcal infection

Adults and children aged 10 years or over	1200 mg
Children aged 1–9 years	600 mg
Children aged 1 year	300 mg

The dose should be given intravenously (or intramuscularly if there is peripheral shutdown). If there is a history of penicillin anaphylaxis (which is very rare), chloramphenicol by injection (1.2 g for adults, 25 mg/kg for children under 12 years) is a suitable alternative.

Box 3.48.3 Doses for chemoprophylaxis

Rifampicin: 600 mg twice daily for 2 days (adults and children over 12 years); 10 mg/kg twice daily for 2 days (children aged 1–12 years); 5 mg/kg twice daily for 2 days (infants under 12 months).
Or
Ciprofoxacin (unlicensed for this use): 500 mg single oral dose (adults only).
Or
Ceftriaxone: 250 mg single i.m. dose (adults); 125 mg in children under 12 years.

---

3 Arrange for chemoprophylaxis for close contacts, and vaccine if the infection is due to a vaccine-preventable strain (see Box 3.48.3).

The aim of chemoprophylaxis is to eradicate the infecting strain from the network of close contacts, and thus prevent further cases among susceptible close contacts. Chemoprophylaxis should be given as soon as possible. Close contacts are defined as people who have had close prolonged contact with the case in the week before onset. This usually includes household members, girlfriends/boyfriends, regular childminders and sometimes students in a hall of residence. Classroom, nursery and other social contacts do not need chemoprophylaxis.

The aim of vaccination is to prevent late secondary cases. There is less urgency for vaccination, as chemoprophylaxis aims to prevent the early secondary cases. Vaccine should be offered to all close contacts as defined above; unvaccinated contacts of serogroup C disease should be given conjugate and not polysaccharide vaccine.

4 Provide information about meningococcal disease to parents, GPs and educational establishments. The aim here is to improve the outcome of any secondary cases that may occur and to prevent rumours and anxiety.

Investigation of a cluster

• Obtain serotyping or genotyping to see if cases are potentially linked.
• Look for links to educational or other institutions.

Response to an outbreak

• Seek expert advice and establish an outbreak control team.
• Information dissemination is essential.
• Where clusters occur in an educational establishment, the following action is recommended:

1 Two or more possible cases (see case definition): prophylaxis to household or institutional contacts is not recommended.
2 Two confirmed cases caused by different serogroups: only give prophylaxis to household contacts.
3 Two or more confirmed or probable cases which are, or could be, caused by the same strain within a 4-week period: prophylaxis to household contacts and to a defined close contact group within the establishment. This may include, e.g. classroom contacts, children who share a common social activity or a group of close friends.
4 Two or more confirmed or probable cases which are, or could be, caused by the same strain separated by an interval of more than 4 weeks: consider wider prophylaxis, but seek expert advice.

• Where clusters occur in the wider community, age-specific attack rates should be calculated: the numerator is the number of confirmed cases and the denominator is the population within which all the cases reside. This may be difficult to define.
• Vaccination and chemoprophylaxis for the community may be indicated for clusters of serogroup C disease where attack rates are high (e.g. above 40 per 100,000).

• Establish an outbreak control team and seek expert advice.

Suggested case definitions

Confirmed case: invasive disease (meningitis, septicaemia or infection of other normally sterile tissue) confirmed as caused by *Neisseria meningitidis*.

Probable case: clinical diagnosis of invasive meningococcal disease without laboratory confirmation, in which the CCDC, in consultation with the clinician managing the case, considers that meningococcal disease is the likeliest diagnosis. In the absence of an alternative diagnosis a feverish, ill patient with a petechial/purpuric rash should be regarded as a probable case of meningococcal septicaemia.

Possible case: as probable case, but the CCDC, in consultation with the clinician managing the case, considers that diagnoses other than meningococcal disease are at least as likely. This includes cases treated with antibiotics whose probable diagnosis is viral meningitis.

3.49 Molluscum contagiosum

Molluscum contagiosum is a skin infection caused by a poxvirus that replicates in epidermal cells to produce characteristic smooth-surfaced white or translucent papules 2–5 mm in diameter.

Epidemiology

Molluscum contagiosum is more common in boys than in girls. Incidence peaks at 10–12 years of age and again in young adults, due to sexual transmission. It is more common in people who are immunocompromised and prevalence rates of 5–18% have been reported in persons with HIV infection. UK General Practitioners reported a mean weekly incidence in 2003 of 4.5 per 100,000 population, similar to previous years.

Diagnosis

Molluscum contagiosum may occur on any part of the body but in adults often affects the anogenital area. There are usually about 20 lesions, but they may be more extensive in HIV infection and atopic eczema. The lesions resolve spontaneously after 6–24 months and treatment is only justified on cosmetic grounds or if there is discomfort. If necessary, diagnosis can be confirmed by the typical appearance of the contents of the lesions on light microscopy or by electron microscopy.

Transmission and acquisition

Transmission is by direct contact, both sexual and nonsexual, from human cases. Indirect spread can occur as a result of contaminated objects and environmental surfaces. Autoinoculation also occurs as a result of scratching. The incubation period is between 2 and 12 weeks and a person will remain infectious as long as the lesions persist. Transmission is thought to be higher in families than in other community settings such as schools.

Control

Normal personal and environmental hygiene should be observed. There is no need for an affected person to stay away from work or school. A child with molluscum contagiosum can take part in most school activities, including swimming.

3.50 MRSA (methicillin-resistant *Staphylococcus aureus*)

Staphylococcus aureus is a common cause of infection, ranging from minor skin sepsis to life-threatening septicaemia. There are many subtypes of *S. aureus*, which may be distinguished by phage typing. Over 80% of *S. aureus* produce penicillinases and are resistant to benzyl penicillin. Cloxacillin and flucloxacillin are not inactivated by this enzyme and were generally the antibiotics of choice before resistance to these antibiotics became common in the mid-1980s, particularly in hospitals. Laboratory identification of these resistant strains uses methicillin, an antibiotic no longer used therapeutically, and they are referred to as methicillin-resistant *Staphylococcus aureus* (MRSA). The mechanism of methicillin resistance is usually the production of a low-affinity penicillin-binding protein rather than the production of a β-lactamase. Most MRSA are sensitive to vancomycin but isolates with intermediate-level resistance to vancomycin (VISA) have been reported. Staphylococcal food poisoning is an intoxication rather than an infection (see Chapter 3.72).

Suggested on-call action

• The local health protection team should be prepared to assist the infection control doctor to investigate and control nosocomial outbreaks of MRSA.
• The public health team may be asked to advise on the management of a cluster of cases of methicillin-sensitive *S. aureus* (MSSA) or MRSA infection in the community.

Epidemiology

In the UK, levels of MRSA in hospitals have risen over the last decade and it has emerged as a major public health problem and source of public and political concern. This rise has been attributed to the appearance of new strains with epidemic potential, hospital patients who are increasingly vulnerable to infections like MRSA, failure to maintain good hospital hygiene including hand washing, more intensive bed usage, greater throughput of patients, more transfer of patients between wards and hospitals and reductions in staffing levels.

In England and Wales, MRSA as a proportion of total *S. aureus* bacteraemias increased from 2% in 1990 to 42% in 2000 but has now stabilised at this level. A mandatory MRSA bacteraemia surveillance scheme for all acute hospitals in England was introduced in April 2001. *S. aureus* bacteraemias totalled 19,311 in 2003 of which 40% were MRSA. MRSA rates per 1000 bed days ranged from 0.04 to 0.33 for general hospitals, they were higher in specialist hospitals and lower in single specialty hospitals. However these data do not distinguish between hospital-acquired and community-acquired infections or indeed whether they were acquired in the UK. The incidence of *S. aureus* bacteraemia in England is 10 per 100,000 population per year. About one-third of these are community-acquired, although most of those acquired in the community will have healthcare-related risk factors. Methicillin sensitive *S. aureus* (MSSA) colonisation rates in the community are around 30%, while MRSA rates in the community are 1%. Independent risk factors for MRSA colonisation in one study were recent hospital admission and diabetes. The prevalence of MRSA among persons without risk factors is 0.24% or lower.

The European Antimicrobial Resistance Surveillance System (EARSS) indicates that the proportion of MRSA bacteraemias in UK is 44% compared to 44% in Greece, 33% in France, 23% in Spain, 38% in Italy, 18% in Germany and less than 3% in Scandinavia and the Netherlands. The reason for these large variations in MRSA levels in European countries is the historical differences in their approaches to MRSA control. Those with low levels have pursued strict case finding, isolation and eradication programmes. Those with high levels initially followed a similar path but in the face of rising incidence as the epidemic strains emerged they adopted a targeted approach, concentrating on controlling MRSA in

Table 3.50.1 Clinical syndromes associated with *S. aureus*

Infection	Comments
Acute osteomyelitis	Infection is usually haematogenous but may spread from adjacent structures or arise in association with peripheral vascular disease.
Bacteraemia and septicaemia	Often associated with infection in other sites such as pneumonia, cellulitis or wound infection.
Skin infection	Folliculitis, carbuncle, furunculosis (boils), impetigo.
Cellulitis	May follow trauma.
Conjunctivitis	
Septic arthritis	May be due to haematogenous spread from distant site or direct inoculation from a penetrating wound or bite, from adjacent osteomyelitis, prosthetic joint surgery or when intra-articular injections are given. Risk factors include trauma, joint diseases such as rheumatoid arthritis or osteoarthritis, debility, immunosuppressive therapy and intravenous drug abuse.
Staphylococcal pneumonia	Rare but may follow influenza, measles, chronic bronchitis or surgery. May occur in children in the first 8 weeks of life and may be complicated by pleural effusion, empyema or lung abscess.
Staphylococcal scalded skin syndrome (SSSS)	Fever, tender erythematous rash, large bullae and exfoliation of sheets of skin due to certain *S. aureus* phage groups that produce an exotoxin.
Toxic shock syndrome (TSS)	Due to exotoxins produced by *S. aureus* and comprises fever, hypotension, thrombocytopenia, vomiting and diarrhoea, skin rash with later desquamation, renal, hepatic and CNS dysfunction. Associated with tampon use but can occur with infection at other sites.

high-risk areas, such as surgical units, and generally accepting its presence in other areas.

Clinical features

The clinical syndromes associated with *S. aureus* infection are summarised in Table 3.50.1. MRSA causes infection or colonisation in the same way as MSSA. However, because there are fewer antibiotic treatment options MRSA infections are more difficult to treat and morbidity, length of hospital stay and treatment costs may all be increased.

Laboratory confirmation

The laboratory diagnosis of *S. aureus* infection requires microbiological examination of appropriate clinical specimens. As a minimum a gram stain, culture and antibiotic sensitivities should be requested. Biochemical tests, phage typing and genome analysis are available. Sixteen different strains of MRSA have been

characterised in the UK. These differ in their ability to spread in hospital and to colonise and cause infection. Currently EMRSA-15 and EMRSA-16 are the dominant strains in the UK. The polymorphic X-region of the protein A gene (spa) can be used to type MRSA strains. This spa typing is more sensitive than phage typing and allows the spread of MRSA strains within and between hospitals to be tracked.

Transmission

The reservoir of *S. aureus* is colonised or infected humans and, rarely, animals. The main sites of colonisation are the anterior nares and skin, whilst purulent discharges from wounds and other lesions are the main sources in infected persons. Infection is spread directly on hands and indirectly via skin scales, fomites, equipment and the environment. In about a third of cases infection is endogenous. Some carriers are more efficient at spreading infection than others. MRSA rarely invades intact skin but can invade pressure sores, surgical wounds and intravascular catheter sites and may then lead to severe infections.

Acquisition

The incubation period is 4–10 days and a person will remain infectious to others as long as the infection or carrier state persists. Risk factors for nosocomial acquisition of MRSA include prolonged hospital stay, intensive care, prolonged antimicrobial therapy and surgical procedures.

Prevention

• Guidelines are available for the control of MRSA in both hospitals and the community (see Appendix 2).
• In UK hospitals a targeted approach is usually adopted in which the control measures are determined by the type of ward (non-acute, acute, intensive care or high risk), the presence of susceptible patients and the background level of MRSA.
• In addition to basic infection control measures such as handwashing and PPE, interventions may include isolation, case finding by microbiological screening of patients and staff and clearance of MRSA using topical or systemic antibiotics and antiseptic detergents and dusting powder.
• Movement of patients within and between hospitals should be minimised and appropriate antibiotic prophylaxis should be used during surgery.
• Attention to hospital hygiene, an antibiotic policy, support from senior management and a properly resourced infection control team are further important requirements.

Surveillance

• In the community, specimens for microbiological examination should be collected from cases of suspected staphylococcal infection.
• It is not usually necessary to report individual cases of MRSA in the community but

clusters of cases should be reported to the local health protection team.
• In hospitals the infection control team should agree testing protocols. As a minimum all patients with clinical lesions should be sampled. In many hospitals nasal and skin swabs are collected routinely on patients who are admitted to high-risk areas of the hospital such as ITU. Cases of MRSA will then be readily detected by alert organism surveillance.

Response to a case or carrier

• Treatment guidelines for cases and carriers in hospitals and the community should be used. Antibiotic treatment should be guided by the results of antibiotic sensitivity testing.
• Discharging lesions should be covered with impermeable dressings if practicable.
• Contact with infants and other susceptible groups should be avoided and school-age children and cases in high-risk occupations should stay at home until no longer infectious.
• Colonisation with MRSA should not prevent a patient being discharged from hospital to their own home or to a nursing home if their general clinical condition allows it. There should be good communication between the hospital infection control team and the nursing home staff.

Investigation of a cluster and control of an outbreak

• Despite the implementation of infection control measures, outbreaks of MRSA (and less commonly of MSSA) are reported from hospitals, community nursing homes, military barracks, day-care settings and amongst groups of people participating in contact sports such as wrestling or rugby.
• An MRSA outbreak may be defined as an increase in cases of MRSA infection or colonisation or a clustering of new cases due to the transmission of a single strain in a particular setting.
• Outbreaks are investigated in a systematic fashion including search for infected cases and carriers; requesting appropriate laboratory tests; typing to confirm that cases are caused by

the same strain; screening staff to detect carriers who may be the source of infection; environmental investigation and microbiological sampling; reviewing clinical practice such as wound closure and antibiotic use; and reviewing infection control practice, including handwashing, cleaning of equipment and care of catheter sites.

• In an MRSA outbreak additional control measures may be required including restricting or suspending admissions, restricting the movement of staff and patients, limiting the use of temporary staff and ward closure.

Suggested case definitions

• A patient or staff member who has MRSA isolated for the first time from a clinical sample or screening swab.
   OR
• A patient or staff member who is positive for a second or subsequent time having been successfully treated and shown to be microbiologically clear of MRSA.

Cases are classified as infected if any of the signs and symptoms of infection are present, otherwise they are classified as colonised.

3.51 Mumps

Mumps is a systemic viral infection characterised by parotitis. It is caused by a paramyxovirus. The public health significance of mumps is that complications are common and it is preventable by vaccination.

Suggested on-call action

None usually required.

Epidemiology

Before vaccination was introduced in 1988, mumps caused epidemics every 3 years, with highest attack rates in children aged 5–9 years. Following the introduction of MMR, a rapid fall in the incidence was observed and by the mid-1990s there were fewer than 2000 cases notified a year (although only about 30% of these were confirmed on laboratory testing). Since 1998, the incidence in the UK has increased, mostly in unvaccinated older children and young adults. Outbreaks have been reported in secondary schools, universities and military settings.

Deaths from mumps are rare, although meningitis is a relatively common complication: in the pre-vaccine era, mumps was the commonest viral cause of meningitis.

Clinical features

Tenderness and swelling of the parotid occur in about 70% of cases. It can be confused with swelling of the cervical lymph nodes. Other common features of mumps include meningitis (which is mild), orchitis (in adult males) and pancreatitis. Rare features are oophoritis, arthritis, mastitis and myocarditis.

Laboratory confirmation

Saliva, CSF or urine may be collected for viral culture. Serological diagnosis is best achieved either by demonstrating S antibody by complement fixation or IgM antibody by ELISA: blood or saliva (gingival fluid) may be used.

Transmission

Man is the only reservoir. Carriage does not occur. Mumps is moderately infectious, with transmission occurring through droplet spread and direct contact with saliva of a case.

Acquisition

The incubation period is 2–3 weeks (average 18 days). Cases are infectious for up to a week (normally 2 days) before parotid swelling until 9 days after.

Prevention

Routine MMR vaccination; two doses required (in the UK these are given at 12–15 months and 3–5 years).

Surveillance

- Notifiable disease in the majority of EU countries, including the UK, Ireland, Germany and Scandinavian countries.
- Seek laboratory confirmation in all cases, e.g. by salivary testing of clinical notifications.

Response to a case

- Exclusion from school for 5 days from onset of parotid swelling.
- Check vaccination status.
- Arrange for laboratory confirmation (e.g. saliva test).

Response to a cluster and control of an outbreak

As for a case, but also consider school, institution or community-wide vaccination if coverage is low or during outbreaks.

Suggested case definition for an outbreak

Clinical: acute onset of parotid swelling, in the absence of other obvious cause.
Confirmed: positive by culture, IgM or fourfold rise in IgG. Does not need to meet clinical case definition.

3.52 *Mycoplasma*

Mycoplasma pneumoniae causes acute respiratory infection and is an important cause of community-acquired pneumonia during its' 4 yearly epidemics.

Suggested on-call action

None, unless outbreak suspected in institution containing frail individuals (treat symptomatic contacts if so).

Epidemiology

Most *M. pneumoniae* infection is never diagnosed. Epidemics occur approximately every 3–5 years and last 12–18 months, peaking in winter(s). *M. pneumoniae* may be responsible for up to a third of community-acquired pneumonia during these epidemics. The next epidemic in the UK is most likely to occur from late 2005 to early 2007. Outside of epidemic periods, as little as 1% of pneumonias may be due to this organism. Incidence rates are highest in school-aged children with a secondary peak in adults aged 30–39 years. Outbreaks particularly occur in military recruits.

Clinical features

Mycoplasma classically presents with fever, malaise and headache with upper respiratory tract symptoms such as coryza, sore throat or unproductive cough. Up to 10% will then progress to tracheobronchitis or 'atypical' pneumonia with a more severe cough, although mucopurulent sputum, obvious dyspnoea and true pleuritic pain are rare. Onset is usually insidious, with presentation often delayed 10–14 days. Asymptomatic infection may also occur. Those with sickle-cell anaemia or Down's syndrome may be more severely affected.

Laboratory confirmation

The mainstay of diagnosis is demonstration of a fourfold rise in serum-specific IgG antibodies. However, it may take several weeks for such a rise to become apparent. Quicker but less-sensitive alternatives may be available including culture on special media, detection of serum specific IgA or IgM (positive after 8–14 days of illness), and antigen detection or PCR testing of sputum or nasopharyngeal aspirates (or less optimally throat swabs).

Transmission

Humans are the sole reservoir. Transmission requires relatively close contact: although school-age children appear to be the main vectors of transmission, they usually only infect family members and close playmates and rarely start school outbreaks. Air-borne spread by inhalation of droplets produced by coughing, direct contact with an infected person (perhaps including asymptomatics) and indirect contact with items contaminated by nasal or throat discharges from cases probably all contribute to transmission.

Acquisition

The incubation period is reported as ranging from 6 to 32 days. Two weeks is a reasonable estimate of the median. The infectious period probably does not start until coryza or cough is evident (the case-to-case interval is usually about 3 weeks). The length of infectiousness is unclear: 3 weeks from onset of illness can be used as a rule of thumb if coughing has ceased, although excretion may be prolonged despite antibiotics. Immunity does occur postinfection, but later re-infection is recognised. Patients with functional asplenism may be more prone to overwhelming infection.

Prevention

• Avoid overcrowding in closed communities.
• Safe disposal of items likely to be contaminated by respiratory secretions.

Surveillance

• Notifiable in a few countries, including the Netherlands, Finland and Switzerland, but not the UK.

• Report to local public health authorities if associated with institution.
• Report laboratory confirmed cases to national surveillance systems.

Response to case

• Hygiene advice and care with respiratory secretions.
• Not to attend work or school whilst unwell.
• Avoid contact with those with sickle-cell anaemia, Down's syndrome or asplenism, where possible.

Investigation of a cluster

• Look for links to institutions; however, more likely to be links between families via school-aged children.
• Although clustering of onset dates may indicate a common exposure, opportunities for active intervention are likely to be limited.

Control of an outbreak

• Re-inforce hygiene and infection control practices, especially relating to respiratory secretions and handwashing.
• Avoid introduction of new susceptibles into affected institutions with frail individuals (e.g. nursing home).
• Warn local clinicians and remind them of appropriate antibiotics for cases with lower respiratory infection (macrolides, tetracyclines or quinolones, i.e. not the usual first choice for pneumonia).
• Consider feasibility of separating coughing residents from asymptomatic ones.
• There is some evidence of the effectiveness of prophylactic antibiotics (e.g. azithromycin 500 mg on day 1 followed by 4 days on 250 mg) to reduce the secondary attack rate for symptomatic infection in vulnerable populations.

Suggested case definition

Confirmed: serological confirmation of illness (IgM, IgA or fourfold rise in IgG) or demonstration of antigen or PCR in respiratory secretions.
Clinical: pneumonia, bronchitis or pharyngitis without other identified cause in member of affected institution.

3.53 Norovirus

Noroviruses (also known as small round structured viruses (SRSV) or Norwalk-like viruses) are the most common cause of gastroenteritis in Europe. Although generally causing mild illness, spread may be rapid, particularly in institutions. Other causes of viral gastroenteritis include other caliciviruses, rotavirus (see Chapter 3.65), adenovirus and astrovirus.

Suggested on-call action

• If in group at risk for further transmission (Box 2.2.1), exclude from work or nursery.
• If you or reporting clinician/microbiologist is aware of related cases, consult local outbreak plan.

Epidemiology

Approximately 3500 laboratory-confirmed cases of norovirus infection are now reported annually in the UK. However, true incidence of disease is likely to be at least 1% of the population per year. All age groups are affected: incidence is highest in young children, but severe infection is most frequent in the elderly. Infection occurs throughout the year, but reported cases and hospital outbreaks in the UK are more common during the cooler months. Recorded outbreaks in the UK, the Netherlands and Spain occur mainly in hospitals or residential institutions (e.g. nursing homes) but are occasionally reported from day-care centres, food outlets, hotels, schools and cruise ships. Norovirus has a worldwide distribution.

Clinical features

Norovirus infection is relatively mild, lasting 12–60 hours. Abdominal cramps and nausea are usually the first symptoms, followed by vomiting and/or diarrhoea. Forceful vomiting is particularly characteristic. Diarrhoea is usually mild, with no blood, mucus or white blood cells in the stool. Other symptoms may include anorexia, lethargy, myalgia, headache and fever. Illness may be severe in elderly or debilitated patients. Asymptomatic infection may also occur.

Laboratory confirmation

Diagnosis is traditionally by electron microscopy (EM) of faecal specimens, which should be collected within the first day or two of illness and preferably be unformed. However many laboratories do not routinely test all stools by EM. Samples of vomit may also be examined by EM. ELISA testing for the 15 most common strains is now widely available and is replacing EM. PCR tests, which are much more sensitive than EM, are available from some reference laboratories and genotyping of isolates may also be available. Serology (paired samples 3–4 weeks apart) may also be available.

If laboratory confirmation is lacking or awaited, epidemiological criteria can be used to assess the likelihood of an outbreak being due to norovirus (Box 3.53.1).

Transmission

Humans are the only known reservoir of norovirus. Spread between humans may occur via the following:
• Infected food handlers may contaminate food that is eaten raw (e.g. salads) or post-cooking, via hands contaminated by faeces.
• Contaminated foods: the most commonly contaminated food is shellfish that have concentrated the virus from sewage-contaminated waters. If eaten raw (e.g. oysters) or insufficiently cooked, such shellfish can cause disease.

> **Box 3.53.1 Epidemiological criteria for suspecting that an outbreak is due to norovirus**
>
> - Stool cultures negative for bacterial pathogens*. (N.B.: check that all relevant pathogens have actually been tested for).
> - Incubation period, if known, of 15–50 hours*.
> - Vomiting in over 50% of cases*.
> - Diarrhoea generally mild without blood or mucus.
> - Over half have nausea and abdominal cramps, and over a third have malaise, low-grade fever, myalgia and headache.
> - Mean duration of illness is 12–60 hours*.
> - High secondary attack rate. Even if originally food-borne, likely to be signs of ongoing person-to-person spread (see Box 2.2.3).
> - Staff are also affected.
>
> *'Kaplan criteria'.

Outbreaks have also been linked to imported fruits such as raspberries and strawberries.

- Person-to-person spread: norovirus is easily spread via the faeco–oral route, either directly or indirectly due to contamination of environmental surfaces and other items and consequently there is a high secondary attack rate. Norovirus may remain viable for many days on carpets or curtains. Norovirus may also be spread by vomiting leading to a contaminated environment or to aerosol transmission. This may explain spread in some outbreaks in hospitals and residential institutions.
- Water-borne: drinking water that is inadequately chlorinated or contaminated posttreatment may transmit norovirus, as may swimming in contaminated water.

Acquisition

The incubation period is usually 15–50 hours but ranges of 4–77 hours have been reported from outbreaks. The infectious period lasts until 48 hours after the resolution of symptoms, but is highest in the first 48 hours of illness. The infective dose is extremely low and the attack rate high (often around 50%). Immunity occurs postinfection, but may only last a few months (sufficient to remove recovered cases from the pool of susceptibles in an outbreak). This, plus the existence of several antigenic types, means later re-infection is possible.

Prevention

- Good standards of personal and food hygiene.
- Good standards of infection control in hospitals and residential homes, including adequate cleaning arrangements.
- Hospital patients admitted with history consistent with norovirus should go into side-rooms.
- Cook raw shellfish before consumption and wash fruit if to be eaten raw.

Surveillance

- Cases should be reported to local public health authorities and national surveillance systems.
- Not formally notifiable in the UK except as 'suspected food poisoning' (although gastroenteritis in children under 2 years is notifiable in Northern Ireland).

Response to case

- Exclude cases in groups with risk of further transmission (Box 2.2.1) until 48 hours after resolution of diarrhoea and vomiting.
- Enteric precautions with particular attention to environmental contamination related to vomitus.
- Cases in institutions should be isolated where practicable.

- Treat symptomatic contacts in high-risk groups (Box 2.2.1) as cases.
- Hygiene advice to cases and contacts.
- Collect basic risk factor data.

Investigation of a cluster

- Most recognised clusters are associated with an institution or a social function.
- If an institution, use Box 2.2.3 to help assess likelihood of person-to-person spread or food-borne source.
- If a social function, consider infected food handler, contaminated premises and contaminated food, especially shellfish.
- If a community outbreak, describe by person, place and time and obtain full food details (especially seafood, fruit, salad, sandwiches), occupational, family and social histories including links to hospitals, residential institutions, hotels and restaurants 10–50 hours before onset as a hypothesis generating exercise. Organise further case finding, e.g. requesting faecal samples from cases of gastroenteritis presenting to GPs.

Control of an outbreak

- For outbreaks in institutions, form an outbreak team, which includes a senior manager who has authority to commit the institution to agreed action.
- Reinforce good infection control (especially handwashing) and food hygiene practices. Ensure toilet facilities are adequate.
- Increase cleaning, particularly of toilet areas and 'contact points' (e.g. taps and doorhandles). Wear disposable gloves and aprons for cleaning potentially contaminated areas.
- Disinfect contaminated areas with 1000 ppm hypochlorite. Immediate cleaning of areas contaminated by vomiting.
- Isolate cases where practicable in residential institutions. Cohorting of cases otherwise.
- Exclude cases in non-residential institutions until symptom-free for 48 hours.
- Staff to wear gloves and aprons and to observe enteric precautions when dealing with infected patients.
- Exclude staff with gastrointestinal symptoms until 48 hours after resolution. Nausea and cramps may precede vomiting and diarrhoea; do not wait until they vomit on the premises!
- Do not admit more susceptible individuals into an outbreak area, preferably until 72 hours since last episode of diarrhoea or vomiting. Outbreaks in institutions will normally terminate in 1–2 weeks if new susceptibles are not introduced. There is evidence that the earlier that hospital units or nursing homes are closed, the sooner the outbreak terminates.
- Do not discharge potentially incubating patients into another institution.
- Restrict unnecessary patient and staff movements between wards: the main aim is to prevent transmission to other wards, whilst outbreak 'burns-out' in affected ward.
- Staff working in affected wards should not then work in unaffected wards until remaining asymptomatic for 48 hours from last exposure.
- Exclude non-essential personnel from the ward.
- Give advice on norovirus and hand hygiene to adult visitors. Restrict visiting by children if possible.
- Thoroughly clean before re-opening to admissions. Change curtains in hospital.
- The Infection Control Nurse or Environmental Health Officer will need to maintain constant supervision to ensure that the agreed actions are fully implemented and maintained.

3.54 Ophthalmia neonatorum

Ophthalmia neonatorum (ON) is an acute infection of the eye or conjunctiva occurring in the first 3 weeks of life, caused by bacteria present in the birth canal. Infection due to *Neisseria gonorrhoea* is the most serious and that due to *Chlamydia trachomatis* the most common. ON may also be caused by staphylococci.

Suggested on-call action
Usually none required.

Epidemiology

The incidence of ON depends on the prevalence of maternal infection in the population. Following exposure the attack rate is 30% giving an estimated incidence of 1–2% of births. Historically ON has been notifiable in England and Wales because of the serious nature of gonococcal ON and the need for prompt treatment; recently there have only been 100–200 reports per year, but this underestimates the true incidence.

Diagnosis

In gonococcal ON there is swelling and redness of the eye, with purulent discharge, within 1–5 days of birth. Without prompt treatment the cornea may be damaged. Chlamydial ON starts between 5 and 12 days after birth. There is an acute purulent phase, which may be followed by chronic inflammation with corneal scarring. Diagnosis should be confirmed by microscopy using appropriate staining or culture.

Transmission and Acquisition

Spread is by direct contact with an infected birth passage. Secondary spread may take place by direct or indirect contact with eye discharges. The infant will remain infectious until treated.

Control

Infection may be prevented by identification and treatment of infection in pregnancy. Routine use of appropriate prophylactic eyedrops for newborn infants prevents gonococcal but not chlamydial ON. ON is notifiable in some countries, including England and Wales. Obtain microbiological diagnosis and treat with appropriate antibiotics. Contact precautions should be observed. If the infection is chlamydial or gonococcal, the mother and her sexual partners should be investigated and treated for genital infection, even if they are symptom-free.

Suggested case definition
Purulent conjunctivitis within 3 weeks of birth.

3.55 Paratyphoid fever

Paratyphoid fever is caused by *S. paratyphi* A, B or occasionally C. *S. paratyphi* is now often referred to as *S. enterica* serovar Paratyphi. It produces an illness similar to typhoid (see Chapter 3.81), though usually less severe.

Suggested on call action
• Exclude cases and contacts who are food handlers or in other risk groups (see below).

Epidemiology

Infection results from the ingestion of water or food contaminated by human faeces. Infection occurs worldwide and is associated with poor sanitation. About 200 laboratory reports of paratyphoid are made annually in the UK, 80–90% of which are imported, most commonly from the Indian subcontinent. A large cluster of cases across eight European countries in 1999 was associated with travel to Turkey.

Clinical features

S. paratyphi may cause gastroenteritis or enteric fever (EF). EF begins with fever and possibly rigors. Patients complain of headache, cough, malaise, myalgia and may be constipated. Later in the course diarrhoea, abdominal tenderness, vomiting, delirium and confusion may occur. In paratyphoid fever cases, spots are more frequent and brighter red than in typhoid. Complications are less common than for typhoid and typically arise in the third week. Up to 5% cases may relapse.

Laboratory confirmation

Blood, urine, faeces and bone marrow aspirate can be cultured. Definitive diagnosis is by culture of the organism from a normally sterile site (e.g. blood). Around 90% of UK cases are serogroup A, with the remainder group B. Phage typing and, possibly, molecular typing of isolates may be available. Sero-diagnosis may also be available. Organisms initially reported as *S. paratyphi* B may actually be *Salmonella java*, which does not usually cause enteric fever. *S. java* is common in poultry in the Netherlands and Germany.

Transmission

Transmission is predominantly food-borne from the consumption of foods contaminated by a human case or occasionally by an asymptomatic carrier, including fruit or vegetables washed in water contaminated by sewage. Water-borne outbreaks and milk-borne infection are recorded. Person-to-person spread is possible in poor hygienic conditions. Serogroup B is occasionally associated with cattle.

Acquisition

The incubation period for enteric fever is usually between 1 and 2 weeks and for paratyphoid gastroenteritis 1–10 days. Commonly bacteria are excreted up to 2 weeks after convalescence. A small number of persons infected with *S. paratyphi* become chronic carriers. Partial immunity results from infection.

Prevention

• Control depends on sanitation, clean water and personal hygiene.
• There is no effective vaccine against paratyphoid.

Surveillance

• Paratyphoid is a notifiable disease in most countries, including the UK.

• Report to local public health departments on clinical suspicion.
• Laboratory confirmed cases should be reported to local and national public health agencies.

Response to a case

• Check antibiotic resistance of isolate.
• Enteric precautions and hygiene advice for cases; isolation if hospitalised.
• Obtain food and travel history for the 3 weeks prior to onset of illness.
• Cases who have not visited an endemic country in the 3 weeks before onset should be investigated to determine the source of infection.
• Exclude cases who are
   food handlers (Box 2.2.1: risk group 1) until 6 consecutive negative stool specimens taken at 1-week intervals and commencing 3 weeks after completion of antibiotic therapy.
   health/social care workers, children aged under 5 years and cases with poor personal hygiene (risk groups 2, 3 and 4) until three consecutive negative faecal samples taken at weekly intervals, commencing 3 weeks after completion of treatment.
• Exclude all other cases until clinically well for 48 hours with formed stools and hygiene advice given.
• Exclude contacts in risk groups 1–4 until two negative faecal specimens taken 48 hours apart and hygiene advice given. If any other contacts unwell, exclude from work/school until well for 48 hours.
• Quinolones may reduce the period of carriage in those for whom exclusion is producing social difficulties.

Investigation of a cluster

• Clusters should be investigated to ensure that secondary transmission has not occurred within Europe.
• Check each case (and their household contacts) for travel abroad.
• Interview cases to identify the source of infection. This could be contact with a chronic

carrier, with faecal material, or with contaminated food, milk, water or shellfish. Obtain and compare food histories. Explore family and social links between cases.

Control of an outbreak

• Exclude cases and contacts as above.
• Exclude and test food handlers in any associated institution or food premises. Ensure adequate personal and food hygiene.
• Organise testing and withdrawal of any implicated food. Ensure that only pasteurised milk, treated water and cooked shellfish are used.

Suggested case definition

Clinical illness compatible with paratyphoid and isolate from blood or stool.

3.56 Parvovirus B19 (fifth disease)

Parvovirus B19 is the cause of a common childhood infection, erythema infectiosum, also known as fifth disease or slapped cheek syndrome. It is important because of the risk of complications in pregnancy, in those with haemoglobinopathies and the immunocompromised.

Suggested on-call action

If the case is a healthcare worker in contact with high-risk patients, consider either exclusion from work or avoiding contact with high-risk patients.

Epidemiology

Infection occurs at all ages, although children aged 5–14 years are at greatest risk. School outbreaks usually occur in early spring. Fifth disease is now more common than rubella in children in the UK.

Clinical features

The first symptom is fever, which lasts for 2–3 days until the rash appears. The rash is maculopapular and is found on the limbs, less commonly the trunk. The cheeks often have a bright red ('slapped cheek') appearance. In a healthy person, the illness is usually mild and short-lived, although persistent joint pain, with or without swelling sometimes occurs, especially in young women, most commonly in knees, fingers, ankles, wrists and elbows.

Parvovirus infection in the first 20 weeks of pregnancy can cause foetal loss (9%) and hydrops foetalis (3%); it is, however, not teratogenic. In patients with haemoglobinopathies it can cause transient aplastic crises, and in immunodeficient patients red cell aplasia and chronic anaemia can occur.

Laboratory confirmation

This is important to distinguish from rubella, especially in pregnant women or their contacts. The diagnosis can be confirmed by testing serum for B19 IgM.

Transmission

Man is the only reservoir; cat and dog parvoviruses do not infect humans. Transmission is from person to person by droplet infection from the respiratory tract; rarely by contaminated blood products. Long-term carriage does not occur.

Acquisition

Parvovirus is highly infectious. The incubation period is often quoted as 4–20 days, but is usually between 13 and 18 days. The infectious period is from 7 days before the rash appears until the onset of the rash. In aplastic crises infectivity lasts for up to a week after the rash appears, and immunosuppressed people with severe anaemia may be infectious for several months or even years.

Prevention

Consider avoiding exposure of patients at risk of complications (see above) to potential cases in outbreak situations.

Surveillance

- Not notifiable in most other European countries, including the UK.
- May only come to the attention of the public health department as a result of investigation of a case of suspected rubella, or when there is an outbreak of a rash illness in a school.

Response to a case

- Arrange for laboratory confirmation.
- Isolation or school exclusion of cases is of no value as any transmission occurs before the onset of symptoms.
- Consider exclusion of a nonimmune healthcare worker who has been exposed to a case, if a fever develops, until either the rash appears or for 15 days from the last contact with the case. Alternatively advise the healthcare worker to avoid contact with high-risk patients (women in the first 20 weeks of pregnancy, those with haemoglobinopathies and the immunocompromised), or to take respiratory precautions until a rash appears or for 15 days. Screening of healthcare workers may be justified for those who have frequent contact with high-risk patients, or for laboratory workers who work with infectious material known to contain B19 virus.
- If infection confirmed in a healthcare worker, test high-risk contacts (as above) for immunity and monitor for evidence of infection, as they need specialist care if infected. Consider human normal immunoglobulin 400 mg/kg intravenously for 5–10

days for immunosuppressed contacts (efficacy uncertain).

Investigation and control of an outbreak

In addition to measures described above for a case, it may be worth excluding susceptible teachers who are in the first 20 weeks of pregnancy from a school in which an outbreak is occurring, until they are more than 20 weeks pregnant.

Suggested case definition
IgM or em positive in presence of clinically compatible illness.

3.57 Plague

Plague is a serious and potentially highly infectious disease caused by *Yersinia pestis*.

Suggested on-call action
• Ensure that cases are isolated.
• Ensure staff monitoring is instituted.
• Ensure samples are handled appropriately.
• Identify contacts and others at risk.
• Liaise with rodent and flea control experts if possibility of local acquisition.

Epidemiology

Y. pestis is a pathogen of rodents in many parts of the New and Old World. Man comes into contact with infected fleas by disturbing the natural hosts (ground squirrels, gerbils, etc.) or if domestic rats acquire them. Northern Europe is free of plague, but cases occur in the former Soviet Union.

Clinical features

Bubonic plague, acquired cutaneously, is an illness with rapid onset of high fever, malaise and delirium. Regional adenopathy and tender buboes draining the site of infection develop. Petechial or purpuric haemorrhages are common. The disease progresses to septic shock, with an untreated mortality of 60–90%.

Pneumonic plague, acquired by respiratory spread, is a severe illness with high fever, tachypnoea, restlessness and shortness of breath. Respiratory signs are often absent. Frothy blood-tinged sputum is usually produced as a pre-terminal event. The untreated mortality is 100%.

Laboratory confirmation

The organism can be isolated from the blood, sputum and buboes. Organisms in smears can be Gram-stained. Serology and antigen detection may also be available. The definitive tests for *Y. pestis* are

• culture from a clinical specimen with confirmation by phage lysis and
• a significant ($\geq$ fourfold) change in antibody titre to F1 antigen in paired serum samples.

Transmission

Bubonic plague is transmitted by the bite of infected rat fleas. Spread is from the bite site to lymph nodes, rapidly followed by septicaemia and pneumonia. Pneumonic plague is acquired directly by the respiratory route from another case of pneumonic plague.

Acquisition

The incubation period for bubonic plague is 1–6 days and for pneumonic plague is 10–15 hours. Patients are infectious until at least 48 hours of appropriate chemotherapy received and a favourable clinical response seen. Partial immunity results from infection.

Prevention

• Control of rats and fleas is essential.
• Laboratory staff likely to come into contact with the organism should be vaccinated. The organism should be handled only in Class 4 laboratory facilities.

Surveillance

• Notifiable: cases should be reported to national authorities and to WHO.
• Any suspected case should be reported to local public health departments as a matter of urgency.

Response to a case

• Streptomycin and tetracyclines or chloramphenicol are the drugs of choice. Treatment after 15 hours probably does not influence the course of pneumonic plague.
• Patients should be considered highly infectious and should be strictly isolated.
• All care should be taken with specimens.
• Staff should be monitored carefully for fever and treated promptly.
• Household contacts should be offered tetracycline prophylaxis.
• Patients and possessions must be disinfected of fleas.
• If pneumonic plague in someone who has not been to an endemic area, consider deliberate release.

Investigation of a cluster and control of an outbreak

• The source should be identified as a matter of urgency and rodent and flea control instituted as necessary.
• Contacts should be offered prophylaxis.
• Consider deliberate release if two or more suspected cases linked in time and place, or if

any confirmed case has not been to endemic area.

Response to a deliberate release

• Report to local and national public health authorities.
• Define exposed zone and identify individuals exposed within it (some may have left scene).
• Cordon off exposed zone.
• Decontaminate those exposed: remove clothing and possessions, and then shower with soap and water.
• Chemoprophylaxis (currently ciprofloxacin for 7 days) as soon as possible for those exposed.
• Record contact details for all those exposed.
• Some health and emergency workers may also need prophylaxis.
• Police may take environmental samples.
• More general information in Chapter 4.14 and specific information on HPA website.

Suggested case definitions

Suspected case
  The diagnosis should be considered if the following clinical presentations occur in previously healthy patients, especially if two or more cases arise that are linked in time and place:
  • Sudden onset of severe, unexplained febrile respiratory illness.
  • Unexplained death following a short febrile illness.
  • Sepsis with Gram-negative coccobacilli identified from clinical specimens.
  In the event of a known or suspected deliberate release, or among contacts of plague cases, the threshold for making a diagnosis of plague should be lower.
Confirmed case
  A case that clinically fits the criteria for suspected plague and, in addition, positive results are obtained on one or more specimens by the Reference Laboratory.

3.58 Pneumococcal infection

Streptococcus pneumoniae ('pneumococcus') is the commonest cause of community-acquired pneumonia and a common cause of bacteraemia and meningitis.

Suggested on-call action

• If case of meningitis, reassure contacts that no prophylaxis is needed.
• If outbreak in institution suspected, consult local outbreak control plan.

Epidemiology

Around 5000 invasive pneumococcal infections are reported annually in the UK, but true incidence is much higher, e.g. pneumococcal pneumonia is estimated to affect 0.1% of adults per annum. All ages are affected, but the distribution is bimodal: half of cases occur in the over 65-year-olds but rates are also high in infants. Pneumococcal pneumonia and meningitis are both more common in the winter. Pneumococcal infection is more common in smokers, heavy drinkers and those who live in overcrowded sleeping quarters. Incidence increases during influenza epidemics.

Although the incidence of pneumococcal meningitis is highest in young children, its relative importance is highest in middle-aged and elderly adults, in which it is the most common cause of bacterial meningitis. Reported national rates in Europe in 1996 varied from 0.04/100,000 in Greece to 2.6/100,000 in Iceland.

Resistance to antibiotics such as erythromycin (15% in England in 2000), penicillin (7%) and cephalosporins has been increasing in most European countries and is particularly high in Spain and Malta, but generally lower in Germany and the Netherlands.

Pneumococcus is the most important bacterial cause of otitis media, which is particularly common in children under 3 years of age. Overall, one recent study estimated that pneumococcal infection causes 2 million GP consultations (93% due to otitis media, mostly children), 75,000 hospitalisations (72% due to pneumonia) and 17,000 deaths (93% from pneumonia, mostly elderly) a year in England and Wales.

Clinical features

Approximately a third of pneumococcal infections affect the respiratory tract, a third are focal infections (mostly otitis media) and a third are fever or bacteraemia without obvious focus. The most common symptoms of pneumococcal pneumonia are cough, sputum and fever. Factors that may suggest pneumococcal rather than 'atypical' pneumonia in an outbreak include mucopurulent or bloodstained sputum, pleuritic chest pain and prominent physical signs. Respiratory symptoms may be less obvious in the elderly. Many cases have predisposing illnesses such as chronic respiratory, cardiac, renal or liver disease, immunosuppression or diabetes. Bacteraemia may occasionally lead to meningitis. Case fatality for bacteraemia or meningitis is 20% and for pneumonia is about 10% (higher in the elderly).

Laboratory confirmation

Gram staining and culture of good quality sputum specimens are the mainstay of diagnosis of pneumococcal pneumonia, although they are only 60% sensitive and 90% specific. Twenty-five per cent of cases of pneumonia will also have a positive blood culture, which can be useful confirmation that the pneumococcus is a pathogen rather than a co-incidental commensal. Antigen detection in sputum or urine may be available in some laboratories. Gram positive diplococci in CSF suggest pneumococcal meningitis. Serotyping of strains is available: there are over 90 serotypes of varying pathogenicity. The most common pathogenic

serotypes in Europe in 1999 were 14, 9, 19, 6, 23, 3, 1, 8, 4 and 7 (six of which are in the conjugate vaccine), but serotype distribution showed variation by age-group and country. Serology may be available for retrospective clinical diagnosis.

Transmission

Pneumococci find their ecological niche by colonising the human nasopharynx. Carriage is common, ranging from about 10% in adults to 50% in children in day-care centres, and is higher in winter. However, not all serotypes are pathogenic. Transmission requires extensive close contact with cases or carriers and is usually by droplet spread, but may also be via direct oral contact or articles soiled by respiratory discharges. Pneumococci remain viable in dried secretions for many months and may be cultured from the air or dust in hospitals, although the importance of this for transmission is unclear. In hospitals, spread is usually to patients in the next one or two beds. Staff may also become colonised.

Cases of pneumococcal meningitis are viewed as sporadic; indeed many cases are autoinfections.

Acquisition

The incubation period for exogenous infection is probably about 1–3 days. However, endogenously acquired invasive disease in asymptomatic carriers also occurs, giving an 'incubation period' of weeks.

The infectious period probably lasts as long as there are viable bacteria in nasal, oral or respiratory secretions. However, penicillin renders patients with susceptible organisms noninfectious in 48 hours.

Type-specific immunity follows infection and is long lasting. Colonisation may also lead to immunity: one study estimated that two-thirds of those who became colonised developed antibody within 30 days. Risk of infection is higher in those with splenic dysfunction, (including sickle-cell and coeliac disease) and immunodeficiency, e.g. due to chemotherapy, diabetes and HIV.

Prevention

• A single-dose polysaccharide vaccine with 50–70% efficacy for bacteraemia in those over 2 years of age is available (effectiveness for pneumonia, otitis media and exacerbations of bronchitis remains unproven). Current UK recommendations (and those of most other European countries) are that vaccine should be given to all those in whom pneumococcal infection is likely to be more common and/or dangerous. This includes all those aged over 65 years of age and those with chronic renal, heart, lung or liver disease, splenic dysfunction, immunosuppression, diabetes, cochlear implants or CSF Shunts. The present vaccine covers 23 serotypes that are responsible for 96% of serious infections, including all common antibiotic resistant strains.
• A multidose conjugate vaccine covering seven common serotypes (responsible for 82% of serious infections in children and 66% in adults) is also available and is recommended in the UK for at-risk children aged between 2 months and 5 years. Conjugate vaccine reduces the risk of pneumococcal meningitis, bacteraemia, pneumonia and otitis media. Polysaccharide vaccine should also be given when the child reaches 2 years of age. The conjugate vaccine may be introduced into routine childhood immunisation schedules in the future.
• Avoid overcrowding in institutions such as hospitals, day-care centres, military camps, prisons and homeless shelters.
• Safe disposal of discharges from nose and throat.

Surveillance

• Single cases of meningitis are notifiable in many European countries, including England, Wales, Northern Ireland, Republic of Ireland, Denmark and Norway.

• Possible outbreaks of pneumococcal infection should be reported to local public health authorities.
• Isolates from blood, CSF or other normally sterile sites should be reported to national surveillance systems. Isolates from sputum are not usually reported because of their uncertain clinical significance. Antibiotic sensitivity (especially penicillin) should be given for all reported cases.

Response to a case

• Safe disposal of discharges from nose and throat.
• Antibiotic therapy as appropriate to clinical condition and sensitivity will reduce infectivity.
• There may be some value in separating patients from others with an increased risk of serious disease until 48 hours of appropriate antibiotics received.
• Immunisation of children under 5 years of age who have suffered pneumococcal meningitis or bacteraemia.

Investigation of a cluster

• Organise serotyping of strains.
• Check for links via institutions. Otherwise no action usually necessary.

Control of an outbreak

• Immunise all contacts that are at higher risk of serious infection: polysaccharide vaccine usually protects more quickly than conjugate.
• Check antibiotic sensitivity and serotype of isolates.
• If outbreak in institution/ward, vaccinate all residents (unless known to be strain not in vaccine). Institute case finding and early treatment of symptomatics for at least 7–10 days.
• Ensure adequate environmental decontamination.

**Suggested case definition
for an outbreak**

Confirmed: clinically compatible illness
with isolate from normally sterile site
(e.g. blood or CSF).
Probable: clinically compatible illness with
either:
  (i) isolate of outbreak serotype from non-
sterile site (e.g. sputum), or
  (ii) antigen positive from normally sterile site (e.g. urine).

3.59 Poliomyelitis

Poliomyelitis is an acute viral infection of the
nervous system caused by poliovirus types 1,
2 and 3. Its public health importance lies in
the ability of polioviruses to cause permanent
paralysis and sometimes death. It is readily
transmitted, causing both endemic and epidemic disease.

Suggested on-call action

- Arrange for urgent laboratory confirma-
tion.
- Obtain vaccination and travel history.
- Notify national surveillance unit.

Epidemiology

Poliomyelitis has been eliminated from most
developed countries by vaccination. The last
indigenous case of polio in the UK (an unvaccinated gypsy boy) was in 1983, and the
WHO declared the UK polio-free in 1997. Imported cases occur occasionally, mainly from
the Indian subcontinent. Vaccine-associated
polio, a complication of live oral polio vaccine
(OPV), occurs at a rate of two cases per million doses. There are on average two cases of
vaccine-associated polio a year in the UK, half
of which are in vaccine recipients (usually an

infant following the first dose of OPV) and half
are in unvaccinated contacts of recently vaccinated individuals (usually a parent of a recently
vaccinated infant).

The epidemiology in other EU countries is
similar, although there was an outbreak in the
Netherlands during the 1990s among unvaccinated members of a religious community.
Many countries have switched to using inactivated polio vaccine (IPV), which carries no risk
of vaccine-associated polio. Global eradication
of polio is now in sight. The disease remains
endemic in only seven countries and 98% of
cases occur in India, Nigeria and Pakistan.
Europe was declared polio-free in 2002.

Clinical features

Most cases of polio are asymptomatic or
present with a sore throat or diarrhoea. A few
cases develop meningitis that is indistinguishable from other causes of viral meningitis.
Paralysis is relatively rare: the proportion of
paralytic cases increases with age from about
1 in 1000 in infants to 1 in 10 in adults. Post-
polio syndrome may develop 10–40 years after
recovery from an initial paralytic attack and is
characterised by further weakening of previously affected muscles.

Poliomyelitis should be considered in any
patient with acute flaccid paralysis with a
history of recent travel to an endemic area.
Vaccine-associated polio should be considered
in a recently vaccinated individual with acute
flaccid paralysis (particularly after the first
dose) or in a close contact of a recently vaccinated individual. The main differential diagnosis is Guillain–Barré syndrome. The paralysis in polio is usually asymmetric, whereas in
Guillain–Barré syndrome it is usually symmetrical. There is always residual paralysis in polio, whereas patients with Guillain–Barré syndrome usually recover completely.

Laboratory confirmation

The most important diagnostic specimen is a
stool sample, which should be sent for viral

culture. Poliovirus can be recovered from faeces for up to 6 weeks and in nasopharyngeal secretions for up to 1 week from onset of paralysis. At least two stool samples, 24 hours apart, should be obtained within 7 days of the onset of paralysis. All cases of acute flaccid paralysis should be investigated to exclude polio. The diagnosis can also be made serologically or by CSF examination.

Transmission

Polio is spread by the faeco–oral route. Man is the only reservoir. Long-term carriage does not occur. Poor hygiene favours spread.

Acquisition

The usual incubation period is 7–14 days for wild cases and vaccine-associated (recipient) cases, although it may be as long as 35 days. For vaccine-associated (contact) cases the incubation period may be up to 60 days. Immunodeficiency is a risk factor for vaccine-associated paralysis, and immunodeficient patients with either vaccine-associated or wild polio may excrete virus for many months.

Prevention

• Vaccination – most countries in Europe (including the UK) now use IPV. Three doses are given at 2, 3 and 4 months of age with boosters at 3–5 years and 15–19 years (see Box 4.7.1).
• Boosters are required at 10-year intervals for travel to endemic areas. No individual should remain unvaccinated against polio.

Surveillance

• Notifiable in most countries, including the UK. Report on clinical suspicion.
• Many countries have specific systems for the surveillance and investigation of acute flaccid paralysis (AFP).

Response to a case or cluster

• Immediate notification, by telephone, to the CCDC and to the regional and national epidemiologist.
• Request urgent stool virology.
• Treat a single case of indigenous wild polio as a national public health emergency.
• If confirmed, mass vaccination with OPV would be required, possibly at the national or subnational level.
• In the event of an outbreak, involve international agencies such as WHO.
• For an imported case, notify WHO or relevant national surveillance unit.
• For vaccine-associated cases, no specific action is required, although it may be an opportunity to review vaccine coverage locally.

Suggested case definition

Possible: acute flaccid paralysis without other apparent cause.
Probable: acute onset of flaccid paralysis with decreased/absent tendon reflexes, without other identified cause, and without sensory or cognitive loss.
Confirmed: serological evidence or isolation of virus, together with clinically compatible illness.

3.60 Q fever

Q fever is a zoonotic disease caused by the rickettsia *Coxiella burnetii*. It causes an acute febrile illness, which may occur as outbreaks or, more rarely, a serious chronic infection.

Suggested oncall action

None required unless outbreak suspected.

Epidemiology

Around 70 cases of Q fever are reported in the UK per annum but because much infection with *C. burnetii* is mild or asymptomatic, the true incidence of infection is not known. Reported cases in children are rare, probably because of an increased likelihood of infection being asymptomatic, and males are more than twice as likely to be reported with Q fever than females, mainly due to occupational exposure. In Europe, human infection increases in the spring, particularly in April and May. Reported incidence has not increased over the last decade in the UK, but, reports have trebled in Germany, mainly due to outbreak associated cases. Historically, Germany shows a cyclical pattern, with peaks occurring every 5–10 years. Most UK cases are sporadic or associated with occupational exposure to animals, but occasionally large outbreaks occur, including in urban areas. *C. burnetii* infection occurs in most countries, although New Zealand is an exception.

Clinical features

Infection may be asymptomatic, an acute febrile or pneumonic illness or chronic infection, particularly endocarditis or hepatitis. Almost all acute clinical cases have fever and fatigue, and most have chills, headaches, myalgia and sweats. Other features may be cough, weight loss and neurological symptoms (particularly in the UK) or acute hepatitis (particularly in France and southern Spain). Tiredness and malaise may persist for months after infection.

Laboratory confirmation

The diagnosis of Q fever is usually confirmed by the demonstration of a fourfold rise in serum antibodies: this usually takes 14–20 days to become apparent (range: 7 days to 6 weeks). IgM may be detected earlier than IgG (7–10 days) and usually persists for 6 months, although occasional persistence up to 2 years makes a single high titre non-diagnostic of an acute event. 'Phase II' antibody generally occurs in acute infection and 'Phase I' in chronic. Culture of this organism is potentially hazardous. Strain typing is not routinely available.

Transmission

The natural reservoir for *C. burnetii* is a number of animal species, particularly sheep, cattle, goats, cats, dogs, wild rodents, birds and ticks. Most infected animals are asymptomatic, although abortions may occur. In mammals such as sheep and cats, the infection localises to the endometrium and mammary glands and is reactivated during pregnancy to be aerosolised during parturition. These aerosols may be inhaled directly or may contaminate the environment for many months, leading to the creation of secondary aerosols. Animal excreta or carcasses may also contaminate the environment with *C. burnetii*. Human infection is usually via inhalation from close exposure to animals, wind-borne aerosols (possibly over many miles) or contaminated fomites such as wool, straw and fertilizer. Infection via raw milk is described but its importance is unclear. Blood and marrow transfusion, necropsy and laboratory animals (especially pregnant sheep) have all been sources of infection.

Acquisition

The incubation period varies from 14 to 39 days (average 20 days) and is generally shorter the larger the infecting dose. Although person-to-person spread has been reported it is rare and, in practice, human cases can be viewed as non-infectious under normal circumstances. The infective dose is low, perhaps only 1–5 organisms: 1 g of placenta from an infected sheep may contain 10^9 infective doses. Immunity from previous illness is probably lifelong. Children may be less susceptible to clinical disease than adults, females possibly less susceptible than males, and the immunocompromised and cigarette smokers more susceptible than the general population.

Prevention

• Vaccination of high-risk occupations not generally recommended in Europe.
• Adequate disposal of animal products of conception.
• Pasteurisation of milk.
• Good infection control in microbiology and animal research laboratories.

Surveillance

• Q fever is statutorily notifiable in some countries (e.g. Belgium, Germany, Italy, Netherlands, Portugal and Switzerland), but not in others, including the UK.
• However, all laboratory-confirmed cases should be reported to the relevant surveillance centre. Potential clusters or linked cases should be reported to local public health authorities.

Response to a case

• Check for exposure to animals.
• No exclusion/isolation necessary, although avoid blood/tissue donation.

Investigations of a cluster

Undertake hypothesis generating study to cover 6 weeks before onset, including
• full occupational history.
• full travel history.
• exposure to sheep, cattle, goats and other farm animals or farm equipment, clothing, etc?
• exposure to pets, especially cats, or pet owners/household after parturition? Visit to petshop?
• exposure to potentially contaminated fomites including straw, hay, peat, manure and wool?
• general outdoor exposure. Check local veterinary and meteorological data for clues (e.g. sheep abortions, wind conditions).
• Consider possibility of bioterrorism incident.

Control of an outbreak

• Plot dates of onset as an epidemic curve: is there ongoing exposure?
• Remove any continuing source.
• Treat human cases.

Suggested case definition for an outbreak

1 Fourfold rise in serum antibodies to *C. burnetii*. No need to demonstrate symptoms.
Or
2 Acute febrile or pneumatic illness with single high convalescent IgM and no other cause identified.

3.61 Rabies

Rabies is an infection of the CNS caused by a lyssavirus (a genus of rhabdovirus). The public health significance of rabies is that there are many animal hosts, the disease is always fatal and both human and animal vaccines are available.

Suggested on-call action

Possible exposure:
• Advise cleansing of wound if recent.
• Assess need for post-exposure prophylaxis. If in doubt, seek expert advice.
Possible case:
• Seek history of animal bite, travel and vaccination status.
• Contact virus reference laboratory to arrange lab confirmation.
• Arrange admission to specialist unit.
• Prepare list of close contacts.
• Inform CDSC (or equivalent).
• Inform state veterinary service (or equivalent).

Table 3.61.1 Rabies risk in EU and EFTA countries

No risk (no vaccine required post-exposure, except for bat exposures – seek specialist advice)
  Cyprus, Finland, Gibraltar, Greece, Iceland, Ireland, Italy (except Northern and Eastern borders), Spain (including the Canary and Balearic islands), Malta, Norway, Portugal (including Madeira), Sweden, the UK (incl. Jersey and the Isle of Man).

Low risk (only vaccine required post-exposure)
  Austria (except Hungarian border – high risk), Belgium, Denmark, France, Germany (except Northrhine-Westphalia, Hessen, Bavaria and Saxonia – high risk), Luxembourg, Netherlands, Switzerland.

High risk (immunoglobulin and vaccine required post-exposure)
  Czech Republic, Estonia, Hungary, Lithuania, Latvia, Poland, Slovakia, Slovenia.

Adapted from Health Protection Agency guidelines for rabies post-exposure prophylaxis.

Epidemiology

Rabies exists in animal populations in many countries of Europe, although human cases are extremely rare; most occur in Russia. The risk of rabies from an animals bite varies in different countries; a number of EU countries (including the UK) are rabies-free (Table 3.61.1); however, bats are a potential source of infection in the UK and other rabies-free countries such as Spain.

Clinical features

The early features of human rabies are often mistaken for hysteria, with altered personality and agitation. Pain or numbness at the site of an animal bite is a useful early clue. Painful spasms of the face induced by attempts to drink ('hydrophobia') are the classical feature. The case fatality is 100%.

Laboratory diagnosis

This is only possible after the onset of symptoms. The national virus reference laboratory must be involved. Serum antibodies appear after 6 days. Rabies virus can be isolated from saliva, brain, CSF and urine, or demonstrated by immunofluorescent antibody staining of impression smears of skin, cornea or other material.

Transmission

Animal reservoirs include dogs, cats, foxes, wolves, bats, squirrels, skunks and occasionally horses. Transmission is from the bite or scratch of an infected animal, or a lick on a mucosal surface such a conjunctiva. Air-borne spread has been demonstrated in bat caves, but this is unusual. Rare cases have occurred in recipients of corneal grafts from patients who died of undiagnosed rabies.

Acquisition

The incubation period is usually 3–8 weeks, but may be as short as 9 days or as long as 7 years, depending on the amount of virus introduced, the severity of the wound and its proximity to the brain.

Prevention

• Control rabies in domestic animals by vaccination before travel to infected countries and implantation of a microchip device.
• Oral vaccination of foxes (using baits), the principal reservoir in Europe.
• Vaccinate high-risk travellers to endemic areas and those at occupational risk such as some laboratory workers and animal handlers (including bat handlers, although immunisation may not protect against some bat lyssaviruses). The primary course is three doses at days 0, 7

Table 3.61.2 Rabies post exposure prophylaxis

Rabies risk in country of incident	Unimmunised/incompletely immunised individual	Fully immunised individual
No risk	None	None
Low risk	5 doses of vaccine at days 0, 3, 7, 14 and 30	2 doses of vaccine at days 0 and 3–7
High risk	5 doses of vaccine plus human rabies-specific immunoglobulin	2 doses of vaccine

Adapted from *Immunisation Against Infectious Disease,* UK health departments, HMSO, 1996.

and 28, given in the deltoid (N.B.: the response may be reduced if vaccine is given in the buttock) with a booster at 6–12 months.

• Give post-exposure prophylaxis following a bite (or cat-scratch) in an endemic area according to nature of exposure (Table 3.61.2). Cleanse the wound thoroughly as soon after injury as possible: as a minimum with soap or detergent under running water for at least 5 minutes; antiseptics should also be used if available. Obtain as much information on the exposure as possible (place, species, bite/scratch, behaviour, owned/stray), including name and address of owner of the animal so it can be observed for the next 10 days for abnormal behaviour. All bat bites (some of which are not immediately obvious), including those in 'no-risk' countries such as the UK should be given post-exposure prophylaxis with vaccine; expert advice should be sought as to whether immunoglobulin is also indicated.

Surveillance

Rabies is notifiable. Local and national public health authorities should be informed immediately.

Response to a case

• Isolation in a specialist unit for the duration of the illness.
• Healthcare workers attending the case should wear masks, gloves and gowns.
• Vaccination and immunoglobulin for contacts who have open wound or mucous membrane exposure to the patient's saliva (according to the schedule above).
• Investigate source of infection.
• Disinfect articles soiled with patients' saliva.

Investigation of a cluster and control of an outbreak

A cluster of human cases from an indigenous source is unlikely in the UK. Local authorities should have plans to eradicate rabies in the animal population should it occur.

Suggested case definitions

Clinical: acute encephalomyelitis in an exposed individual.
Confirmed: clinically compatible case confirmed by vial antigen, isolate or rabies neutralising antibody (prevaccination).

3.62 Relapsing fever

Louse-borne relapsing fever is a systemic disease due to *Borrelia recurrentis*. Tick-borne disease may be caused by a number of different *Borrelia* species.

Suggested on-call action

None required unless ongoing transmission suspected because of the presence of lice. In which case institute delousing procedures.

Epidemiology

Louse-borne fever is found in Africa, especially highland areas of East Africa and South America. Endemic (tick-borne) disease is widespread, including foci in Spain.

Clinical features

The illness is characterised by periods of high fever lasting up to 9 days, which are interspersed with afebrile periods of 2–4 days.

Laboratory confirmation

Definitive diagnosis is by visualising spirochetes in peripheral blood smear. Multiple smears may need to be examined (thick and thin, Wright and Giemsa stains).

Transmission

Relapsing fever is vector borne; there is no person-to-person spread. The disease is classically epidemic where spread by lice and endemic when spread by ticks.

Acquisition

The incubation period is 5–11 days.

Prevention

Maintenance of personal hygiene and by impregnation of clothes with repellents and permethrin in endemic areas.

Surveillance

• Relapsing fever is a notifiable disease in many EU countries, including the UK, Germany, the Netherlands, Norway and Sweden.
• Cases should also be reported to WHO.

Response to a case

• The case does not need isolation once deloused.
• The immediate environment should also be deloused.

Response to a cluster/control of an outbreak

Vector control.

3.63 Respiratory syncytial virus

Respiratory syncytial virus (RSV) causes bronchiolitis in infants and upper and lower respiratory tract infection at all ages. It may cause serious nosocomial outbreaks in children, the elderly and the immunocompromised.

Suggested on-call action

• Suggest case limits contact with infants, frail elderly and immunocompromised.
• If linked cases in an institution suspected, activate Outbreak Control Plan.

Epidemiology

RSV epidemics occur every winter in December and January with lower activity between October and April. Almost all children who have lived through 2 epidemics in urban areas will have become infected, causing 20,000 hospital admissions a year in the UK. Most cases are not specifically diagnosed as RSV, but 80% of cases of bronchiolitis and 20% of pneumonia in young children are caused by RSV. Reinfections occur throughout life. About 5% of elderly people suffer RSV infection each year, and it is a significant cause of infection and outbreaks in nursing homes, day units and hospitals, particularly neonatal units. Male gender, age under 6 months, birth during first half of RSV season, crowding and/or siblings, and day-care exposure are recognised risk factors for severe RSV infection.

Clinical features

The most common presentation is upper respiratory tract infection with rhinitis, cough and often fever. Children may also get otitis media or pharyngitis. Bronchiolitis (wheeze, dyspnoea, poor feeding), pneumonia or croup may develop after a few days. Infants with congenital heart disease or chronic lung disease risk severe disease as do those under 6 weeks of age and premature infants. In adults, RSV infection is usually confined to the upper respiratory tract but it may cause exacerbations of asthma or chronic bronchitis, or, particularly in the elderly, acute bronchitis or pneumonia. Few infections are asymptomatic. Case fatality is particularly high in the immunocompromised.

Laboratory confirmation

Nasopharyngeal aspirates (NPAs) taken early in the illness may be positive for RSV by antigen detection, which can provide immediate results, or viral culture, which takes 3–7 days but is slightly more sensitive. NPAs may not be obtainable from elderly patients: nose or throat swabs are less sensitive and, as the elderly do not shed the organism for as long as infants and often present later in the illness, the diagnosis rate is low in this group. PCR is available from some specialist laboratories and is more sensitive for these patients. Serology is also available for retrospective diagnosis.

Transmission

Humans are the only known reservoir of RSV. Spread occurs from respiratory secretions either directly, through large droplet spread,

or indirectly via contaminated hands, handkerchiefs, eating utensils or other objects or surfaces. RSV may survive for 24 hours on contaminated surfaces and 1 hour on hospital gowns, paper towels and skin. Infection results from contact of the virus with mucous membranes of the eye, mouth or nose. Hospital staff and visitors are thought to be important vectors in hospital outbreaks and in the relatively common transmission of sporadic nosocomial infection.

Acquisition

The incubation period is 2–8 days with an average of 5 days. The infectious period starts shortly before to (usually) 1 week after commencement of symptoms. Some infants may shed RSV for many weeks. Immunity is incomplete and short-lived, although re-infections are usually milder. Those with defective cellular immunity are at increased risk of more severe disease.

Prevention

• Personal hygiene, particularly handwashing and sanitary disposal of nasal and oral discharges.
• Good infection control in hospitals, nursing homes and day units. Avoid overcrowding.
• Avoid young infants, frail elderly and immunocompromised coming into contact with individuals with respiratory infection.
• RSV vaccines are under development.
• Consider use of RSV specific immunoglobulin prophylaxis for certain high risk groups during RSV season, e.g.:
  children under 2 years of age who have received treatment for bronchopulmonary dysplasia in the last 6 months.
  infants born at 35 weeks gestation or less and who are aged under 6 months at the onset of the RSV season.

Surveillance

• RSV infection is not notifiable in the UK, but cases associated with institutions should be reported to local public health authorities.
• Laboratory confirmed cases should be reported to the relevant national surveillance system.
• Hospitals should include RSV in nosocomial surveillance programmes.

Response to a case

• Contact isolation for hospital patients.
• Avoid contact with infants, frail elderly and immunocompromised until well.
• Exclude from nursery, work, school or non-residential institution until well.
• Sanitary disposal of nasal and oral discharges.

Investigation of a cluster

• Rarely investigated unless link to institution thought likely. Undertake case finding at any institution containing infants, elderly or immunosuppressed, if linked to a case.
• Antigenic and genomic fingerprinting may be useful in investigating hospital clusters, but beware that more than one strain may be involved, i.e. there may be more than one source.

Control of an outbreak

• Contact isolation and cohorting of suspected cases in hospitals. Closest feasible equivalent in nursing and residential homes.
• Reinforce hygiene and infection control measures, particularly handwashing and sanitary disposal of nasal and oral discharges.
• Exclude staff and day attenders at institutions with respiratory infection until well. Restrict visiting.

• Active surveillance of new and existing patients in hospital for respiratory infection with rapid testing for RSV.
• Cancel non-urgent admissions.
• Consider other measures to limit transfer of RSV by hospital staff (e.g. use of eye-nose goggles, gloves and perhaps gowns and masks).
• Maintaining adequate compliance with the above recommendations will require constant monitoring and reinforcement.
• Consider use of RSV specific immunoglobulins in high-risk individuals.

Suggested case definition for use in an outbreak
Upper or lower respiratory tract infection and antigen or culture positive for RSV.

3.64 Ringworm

The dermatophytoses, tinea and ringworm are synonymous terms that refer to fungal infections of the skin and other keratinised tissues such as hair and nails. These infections are common throughout the world. They are caused by various species of the genera *Trichophyton*, *Epidermophyton* and *Microsporum*, and are classified according to the area of the body that is affected, namely corporis (body), faciei (face), cruris (groin), pedis (foot), manuum (hand), capitis (scalp), barbae (beard area) and unguium (nail).

Suggested public health on-call action
Advise on laboratory diagnosis and treatment.

Epidemiology

Tinea capitis
Zoophilic: *Microsporum canis* (cat, dog),
  Trichophyton verrucosum (cattle)
Anthropophilic: *T. tonsurans, T. violaceum,*
  T. soudanense, M. audouinii, T. schoenleinii
	Mainly affects children.
	In UK and North America prevalence has increased recently
	  due to anthropophilic *Trichophyton tonsurans,* which
	  particularly affects children of African Caribbean ethnic
	  origin.
	Spread occurs in families and at school and asymptomatic
	  infection is common. Hairdressing practices may be risk
	  factors.
	In other countries *M. canis* is the commonest cause.

Tinea corporis, Tinea cruris, Tinea barbae,
  Tinea pedis
M. canis, T. tonsurans, T. rubrum,
T. mentagrophytes, Epidermophyton
floccosum
	In Northern Europe since the 1950s *T. rubrum* has replaced
	  M. audouinii and *E. floccosum* as the most frequently
	  isolated dermatophytes.
	In Southern Europe and the Middle East zoophilic
	  dermatophytes, such as *M. canis* and *T. verrucosum,* are
	  the most frequent.

Tinea unguium (Onychomycosis)
T. rubrum, T. mentagrophytes
	T. rubrum and T. mentagrophytes account for 90% of
	  onychomycoses.
	Increasing age, diabetes, acquired immunodeficiency
	  syndrome and peripheral arterial disease are risk factors
	  and there is a familial pattern.

Clinical features

Tinea capitis	The clinical presentation is variable comprising generalised diffuse scaling
	  of the scalp, patchy hair loss, broken-off hair stubs, scattered pustules,
	  lymphadenopathy, boggy tumour (kerion), favus (hair loss caused by
	  T. schoenleinii, largely confined to Eastern Europe and Asia). Infection
	  with *T. tonsurans* may cause lightly flaky areas, indistinguishable from
	  dandruff or small patches of hair loss.

Tinea corporis Tinea cruris	Lesions are found on the trunk or legs and have a prominent red margin with a central scaly area.
Tinea barbae, barber's itch	Infection of the beard area of the face and neck with both superficial lesions and deeper lesions involving the hair follicles.
Tinea pedis, athlete's foot	Affects the feet particularly the toes, toe webs and soles

Tinea unguium
  (Onychomycosis)
	Infection of the nails, usually associated with infection of the adjacent skin.
	  There is thickening and discolouration of the nail.

Confirmation

Hair infected with *Microsporum* species fluoresce green under filtered ultraviolet (Wood's) light. Hairs infected with most *Trichophyton* species do not fluoresce. Fungal spores and hyphae can be detected by microscopic examination of the hair after preparation in potassium hydroxide. Definitive diagnosis requires culture of the infecting fungus. Specimens for culture are collected by scraping the affected area with a scalpel or glass slide.

Specimens can also be obtained using a scalp massage brush. The scalp is brushed 10 times, and the contaminated brush pressed into the surface of an agar-coated Petri dish, which is then incubated for up to 3 weeks. A culture taken from an infected child will usually produce a fungal colony from each of the 130 inoculation points, whereas one taken from a carrier often produces only 1–10 colonies. Identification of the fungus helps determine the source of infection (either an animal or another child) and allows appropriate treatment and control measures.

Transmission

The reservoir of some dermatophyte species such as *T. rubrum* and *T. tonsurans* is exclusively human (anthropophilic). Others species have animal reservoirs (zoophilic) including cats, dogs and cattle. Soil (geophilic) species are less common causes of human infection. Transmission is by direct skin-to-skin contact with an infected person or animal or by indirect contact with fomites (seat backs, combs and brushes) or environmental surfaces (showers, changing rooms) contaminated with hair or skin scales. The risk of spread is low in schools but higher with prolonged exposure in families and particularly where there is broken skin.

Acquisition

The incubation period varies with the site of infection but is typically 2–6 weeks. The infectious period lasts for as long as infection is present, which may be from months to years if untreated. Persons who are immunosuppressed, including those with HIV infection, are at increased risk of dermatophyte infection. Certain occupations, such as veterinary surgeons, are at risk of infections of animal origin.

Prevention

• Early recognition of animal and human cases and carriers and prompt effective treatment.
• Maintain high levels of personal and environmental hygiene with attention to handwashing, care of pets, regular cleaning and maintenance of floors and surfaces at home, in schools and in swimming pools and communal changing rooms.

Surveillance

• Cases of scalp and body ringworm in school-aged children should be reported to the school nurse.
• Clusters of cases should be discussed with the local health protection team.

Response to a case

• Anthrophilic dermatophytes can spread between children at school, but exclusion of an infected pupil from school is unnecessary once treatment has started. However, activities involving physical contact or undressing, which may lead to exposure of others, should be restricted.
• Confirm diagnosis and identity of infecting fungus with skin, nail or hair samples for microscopy and culture.
• Start effective treatment. Most cases of dermatophyte infections respond readily to topical agents used for 2–4 weeks, but oral treatment is required for nail and scalp infection. Treatment guidelines have been published. Topical treatment may reduce the risk of transmission to others before oral treatment is established. Selenium sulphide shampoo, used twice weekly, reduces the carriage of viable spores and may also reduce infectivity. It is not recommended for use in children aged less than 5 years, for whom an alternative antifungal lotion may be used.
• If cultures show that the infecting fungus is of human rather than animal or soil origin, a search should be made for other cases. Signs of infection in others may be minimal and so

samples should be requested for culture. Those with mycological evidence of carriage may be offered treatment.
• If the source is an animal, family pets should be screened by a veterinary surgeon.

Investigation of a cluster

• Clusters of cases of scalp or body ringworm may be reported from schools or nurseries.
• Spread is well recognised amongst members of wrestling teams (Tinea corporis gladiatorum).
• Nosocomial spread has also been documented from patients to nursing staff.

Control of an outbreak

• Confirmation of the diagnosis is important and all contacts should be examined to identify cases and carriers. Samples should be requested for culture.
• The local health protection team should be available to give advice and practical assistance.
• Prompt effective treatment should be offered to cases and carriers (see above).
• Exclusion from school is not normally necessary once treatment has started, but may be considered if control proves difficult.
• An environmental investigation should be carried out to ensure a high standard of hygiene, particularly in communal changing rooms. Additional cleaning may be recommended. Possible animal sources should be investigated.
• In hospitals and nursing homes, cases should be nursed with source isolation precautions, and gloves and aprons should be used.

Suggested case definition for cluster investigation

Characteristic lesions reported amongst household or other close contacts, with or without laboratory confirmation by microscopy or culture.

3.65 Rotavirus

Rotaviruses are the commonest cause of childhood diarrhoea. The public health significance of rotavirus diarrhoea is the high level of morbidity and the imminent availability of vaccines.

Suggested on-call action

• Exclude cases in risk groups (Box 2.2.1) until 48 hours after the diarrhoea and vomiting have settled.
• If linked to other cases in an institution, consult outbreak control plan.

Epidemiology

Over 10,000 laboratory-confirmed cases are reported in the UK every year, although this only represents a small fraction of the total. It has been estimated that a third of hospital admissions for childhood diarrhoea are due to rotavirus. A similar pattern been reported in other European countries.

The peak incidence is between 6 months and 2 years of age; clinical infection is unusual above 5 years, although subclinical infection is probably common. Most cases occur in winter. Mortality is low in developed countries, although there are an estimated one million deaths each year in developing countries. Many outbreaks are reported every year, mostly associated with residential institutions, nurseries or hospitals.

Clinical features

There is sudden onset of diarrhoea and vomiting, often with a mild fever. Occasionally there is blood in the stools. The illness usually lasts for a few days only.

Laboratory confirmation

This is needed to differentiate rotavirus infection from other viral infections of the gastrointestinal tract. Rotavirus particles can usually be demonstrated in diarrhoea stools by EM. Serology is also available. There are three serogroups, of which group A is by far the commonest.

Transmission

There are both animal and human rotaviruses, although animal-to-human transmission does not occur. Person-to-person transmission is mainly by the faeco–oral route, although there may also be spread from respiratory secretions and sometimes via contaminated water. Long-term carriage does not occur. Outbreaks may occur in nurseries, and nosocomial spread may occur in paediatric, and occasionally geriatric units, where the virus may contaminate the environment. It is resistant to many disinfectants, but is inactivated by chlorine.

Acquisition

The incubation period is 1–3 days. Cases are infectious during the acute stage of the illness and for a short time afterwards; this is usually for less than a week in a healthy child, but may be as long as a month in an immunocompromised patient. Re-infection may occur after some months.

Prevention

• No specific preventive measures.
• General enteric precautions may help limit spread in households, nurseries and hospitals. In nurseries, children should have clothing to cover their nappies.
• A vaccine, which does not appear to cause intussusception, has recently been licensed in Mexico; it is not yet available in Europe.

Surveillance

• Must be based on laboratory reports. This significantly underestimates the true incidence, as only hospitalised cases are likely to be investigated.
• Gastroenteritis in children under 2 years of age is formally notifiable in Northern Ireland.

Response to a case

• Isolate hospitalised cases with enteric precautions.
• Give hygiene advice to the family in the community.
• Exclude from nursery or school (or risk occupation, see Table 2.2.1) until 48 hours after the diarrhoea and vomiting have settled.

Investigation of a cluster

• Not often reported, unless linked to an institution.
• Consider also the possibility of a common source, e.g. contaminated water supply.

Control of an outbreak

• Remind the local population of the importance of good hygiene (although this will probably not play an important role in controlling the outbreak).
• In institutions with cases, ensure adequacy of hygiene and toilet facilities.

Suggested case definition

Confirmed: diarrhoea or vomiting with laboratory confirmation.
Clinical: diarrhoea or vomiting in a person linked to a confirmed case.

3.66 Rubella

Rubella (German measles) is a systemic virus infection characterised by a rash and fever. Rubella virus is a member of the togaviridae. The public health importance of rubella is the consequences of infection in pregnancy and the availability of a vaccine.

Suggested on-call action

• Exclude from school until 5 days from onset of rash.
• Advise limiting contact with those known to be pregnant.

Epidemiology

Rubella is now rare in most of Europe, including the UK, where immunisation programmes have been in place for many years. Before immunisation, epidemics occurred at 6-year intervals, affecting mainly children in primary school but also adolescents and some adults. During epidemics, up to 5% of susceptible pregnant women caught the disease, leading to congenital rubella syndrome and rubella-associated terminations of pregnancy.

In the post-immunisation era, rubella outbreaks still occur among susceptible young adult males who are too old to have been immunised. There are now fewer than 10 cases a year of congenital rubella syndrome in the UK.

Clinical features

The main differential diagnosis is parvovirus, which is now common than rubella. In rubella, there is sore throat, conjunctivitis and mild fever for 2 or 3 days before the macular rash appears. The lymph nodes of the neck are often swollen. Recovery is usually rapid and complete, although, as in parvovirus infection, persistent joint infection sometimes occurs, especially in adults.

The features of congenital rubella syndrome range from mild sensorineural deafness to multiple defects of several organ systems.

Laboratory confirmation

This is particularly important in pregnancy. The simplest method is by IgM detection in serum or saliva. Other methods are viral culture from serum or urine, or a rising IgG antibody titre.

Transmission

Man is the only reservoir. Transmission is by direct person-to-person contact by respiratory droplets. There are no carriers.

Acquisition

Rubella is moderately infectious, although not as infectious as parvovirus or measles. The incubation period is 2–3 weeks. Infectivity is from 1 week before the onset of rash to about 4 days after onset.

The risk of congenital rubella syndrome in a susceptible pregnant woman infected in the first trimester is greater than 90%. This risk declines to about 50% in the second trimester and is zero near term.

Prevention

• Immunise all children with combined MMR vaccine. Two doses are required to ensure seroconversion and maintain herd immunity. The only contraindications are immunosuppression and pregnancy, although women accidentally immunised in pregnancy can be reassured that the risk of foetal damage is minimal.
• Screen all women in early pregnancy and immunised post-partum if found to be susceptible.

Surveillance

Notifiable in the UK, although clinical diagnosis is unreliable and surveillance should be based on obtaining laboratory confirmation (e.g. by salivary IgM).

Response to a case

• Seek laboratory confirmation (saliva test in the UK), especially in pregnancy or if the case has been in contact with a pregnant woman.
• Check immunisation status of the case and arrange for immunisation if un-immunised.
• Exclude children from school for 5 days from the onset of rash.
• Test pregnant women who have been in contact with a case, particularly during the first trimester, for susceptibility or evidence of early infection (IgM antibody) (Fig 2.4.2). Immunise susceptible women post-partum; offer infected women termination. In later pregnancy there is a balance between the risk of foetal damage and the desirability of termination.

Investigation of a cluster and control of an outbreak

Laboratory confirmation essential. In addition to the measures described above for all cases, consider a community-wide immunisation programme if coverage is low.

Suggested case definitions

Confirmed:
• presence of IgM in blood, urine or saliva; *or*
• fourfold or greater rise in haemagglutination inhibition antibody in serum; *or*
• positive viral culture in blood, urine or nasopharyngeal secretions.
Suspected (for investigation):
• generalised maculopapular rash, fever and one of cervical lymphadenopathy or arthralgia or conjunctivitis.

3.67 Salmonellosis

Salmonella infection is a common cause of gastroenteritis that can result in large outbreaks, particularly due to food-borne transmission, and severe infection in the elderly, immunosuppressed and pregnant women. One outbreak of salmonellosis in a hospital in England in 1984 led to 19 deaths.

Many Agencies now use a new system of nomenclature for *Salmonella* organisms, based on DNA relatedness, which suggests that all salmonellae probably belong to a single species, *enterica*, which has seven subgroups. Most human pathogens belong to a subgroup also called *enterica*, so that *S. enteritidis* would now be termed *S. enterica*, subgroup *enterica* serotype Enteritidis, or *S.* Enteritidis for short. This chapter continues to use the familiar system. (For *S. paratyphi* and *S. typhi*, see Chapters 3.55 and 3.81 respectively.)

Suggested on-call action

• Exclude cases in risk groups for onward transmission (Box 2.2.1) until formed stools for 48 hours.
• If you or reporting laboratory/clinician is aware of other potentially linked cases, consult local outbreak plan.

Epidemiology

Salmonellosis is one of the most commonly reported causes of gastrointestinal infection in Europe, except in the Nordic countries. It is the second most commonly reported bacterial cause of infectious intestinal disease in the UK, although it is only responsible for about 3% of community cases of gastroenteritis: this discrepancy is due to the relative severity of salmonellosis. Incidence in the UK, as measured by reports of laboratory confirmed cases, has nearly halved from 33,000 (1992–1997) to 17,000 per annum. This decrease has affected most serotypes and is reflected across Europe, with the notable exception of Spain. A major reason for this decrease in the UK is the vaccination of poultry flocks, which had been the source for the huge increase in human infection with *S. enteritidis* PT4 in the years from 1988 to 1997; as a result, PT4 infections in humans have fallen by 73%, although non-PT4 infections have increased during the same period. In Denmark compulsory slaughter of infected poultry flocks is thought to be a major contributor to the decrease in human infection with *S. enteritidis*. In recent years there has been an increase in *S. typhimurium* DT104 and 204b resistant to a number of antibiotics.

Salmonellosis occurs at all ages, although incidence rates of confirmed infection are highest in young children, partially due to testing bias. Laboratory isolates of *Salmonella* show a consistent seasonal pattern, peaking in late summer (Fig 2.2.1); this is thought to be related to more rapid multiplication at higher ambient temperatures and perhaps seasonal variation in raw food consumption. *Salmonella* is recorded as the cause of death in an average of 40 people per year in the UK. Although most cases are sporadic or part of family outbreaks, outbreaks associated with institutions or social functions are not uncommon. Travel abroad is also a risk factor in low prevalence countries.

Clinical features

It is difficult to differentiate salmonellosis from other causes of gastroenteritis on clinical grounds for individual cases. The severity of the illness is variable but in most cases stools are loose, of moderate volume, and do not contain blood or mucus. Diarrhoea usually lasts 3–7 days and may be accompanied by fever, abdominal pain, myalgia and headache. Other symptoms, particularly nausea, may precede diarrhoea, and malaise and weakness may continue after resolution of the gastroenteritis. Rare complications include septicaemia and abscess formation. Factors that may suggest salmonellosis as the cause of a cluster of cases of gastroenteritis include fever in most cases, headache and myalgia in a significant minority, and severe disease in a few. With some

serotypes, e.g. *S. dublin, S. choleraesuis* and, to a lesser extent *S. virchow*, septicaemia and extraintestinal infection are more common.

Laboratory confirmation

Diagnosis is usually confirmed by culture of a stool specimen, rectal swab or blood culture. Using a stool sample rather than a rectal swab, collecting at least 5 g of faecal material and, especially when looking for asymptomatic excretors, collecting two or more specimens over several days all increase sensitivity. Excretion usually persists for several days or weeks beyond the acute phase of the illness. Refrigeration and/or a suitable transport medium may be necessary if there will be a delay in processing specimens, especially in warm weather.

The laboratory may be able to issue a provisional report within 48 hours of receiving the specimen (further confirmatory tests will be necessary), although a further day is often required. Serotyping (e.g. 'typhimurium') is available for all salmonellae and phage typing ('PT' or 'DT') is available for *S. agona, S. enteritidis, S. hadar, S. java, S. newport, S. pullorum, S. thompson* and *S. virchow,* usually via reference laboratories. These tests are often useful in detecting and controlling outbreaks of rarer salmonellae. However, for *S. enteritidis* PT4 or *S. typhimurium* DT104,further more discriminatory tests may be required; pulsed field gel electrophoresis (PFGE) 'fingerprinting' has already been shown to be useful and antibiograms may be a useful marker for case finding in an outbreak.

Transmission

Salmonella infection is acquired by ingestion of the organisms. In most cases this is through the consumption of a contaminated food.
• *Salmonella* infection or carriage affects many animals (Table 3.67.1) leading to contamination of foodstuffs before their arrival in the kitchen. If such foods are eaten raw or undercooked then illness can result. Such food sources include undercooked poultry or meat,

Table 3.67.1 Frequency and some possible sources of common *Salmonella* serotypes

Serotype	No. of human cases pa, (England & Wales, 2001–03)	Animal reservoirs (DT/PT)	Some additional vehicles found in outbreaks
S enteritidis	10,474	Chickens, other poultry, cattle (PT8)	Egg (PT14b in Spanish eggs), dairy produce, Chinese meals
S. typhimurium	2,131	Cattle (104, U302, RDNC) Pigs (193, 104, U308a, U302, 170) Poultry (104), Sheep (104)	Halva (from Turkey), manure, salad
S. virchow	297	Chickens	Eggs
S. hadar	208	Chickens, other poultry	Turkey (PT10), roast beef (PT2)
S. braenderup	163	Poultry, cattle	Curry powder
S. infantis	154	Calves, pigs	Chicken drumsticks
S. newport	149	Poultry, cattle	Peanuts (from China), lettuce, horsemeat, mango
S. agona	145	Turkeys, chickens	Kosher snack
S. java	124	Poultry (Netherlands, Germany), tropical fish, terrapins	Desiccated coconut
S. stanley	106		Peanuts (from China), alfalfa sprouts

Rarer serotypes associated with particular animals include *S. arizonae* (sheep), *S. binza* (gamebirds), *S. derby* (pigs, sheep), *S. dublin* (cattle), *S. indiana* (ducks), *S. livingstone* (chicken, ducks), *S. mbandaka* (chicken) and *S. seftenberg* (chicken).

raw or undercooked eggs (often used in mayonnaise, sweets such as mousse or tiramisu, and 'egg nog' drinks) and raw or inadequately pasteurised milk. Such foodstuffs, particularly raw poultry or meat, may be the source of cross-contamination to other foods that may not be cooked before eating (e.g. salad). This cross-contamination may also occur via food surfaces or utensils. Contamination of food by an infected food handler may occur, but is thought to be uncommon in the absence of diarrhoea. Salmonellae can multiply at temperatures ranging from 7 to 46°C, and thus inadequate temperature control will allow a small number of contaminating organisms to develop into an infective dose. Heating to at least 70°C for at least 2 minutes is required to kill the organism.

• Imported foods (e.g. salad, halva, peanuts) may be contaminated before their arrival in Europe. *Salmonella* is also a risk to travellers abroad.

• Person-to-person spread via the faeco–oral route may occur without food as an intermediary. The risk is highest during the acute diarrhoeal phase of the illness. Person-to-person spread due to inadequate infection control practices may prolong food-borne outbreaks in institutions. Children and faecally incontinent adults pose a particular risk of person-to-person spread.

• Other, rarer, causes of salmonellosis include direct contact with animals, including exotic pets; contamination of non-chlorinated water; nosocomially via endoscopes, breast milk, blood transfusion and soiled bedclothes; and contamination of bedding, toys and clothing by excreta.

Acquisition

The incubation period may range from 6 hours to 3 days or occasionally longer and is affected by the number of organisms ingested. Most cases occur within 12–36 hours of ingestion. The infectious period varies enormously: most cases excrete the organism for a few days to a few months with a median duration of 5 weeks. Approximately 1% of adults and 5% of children under 5 years of age will excrete the organism for at least a year.

In most cases the infective dose for salmonellae is 10^3–10^5 organisms but certain food vehicles are thought to protect the organism against gastric acid, reducing the infective dose to only a few organisms. High-fat foods such as chocolate and cheese may be examples. Immunity to *Salmonella* infections is partial, with re-infection possible, if milder. Those at increased risk include patients with low gastric acidity (including antacid therapy), immunosuppression, debilitation or on broad spectrum antibiotics.

Prevention

Prevention of food-borne salmonellosis is a classic case of the need for a 'farm to fork' strategy:
• At the farm, action is required to reduce infection and carriage in food animals, particularly poultry to reduce contaminated meat and eggs. Vaccination of poultry flocks is recommended. Slaughter and processing practices for poultry require attention to reduce cross-contamination. The Scandinavian experience suggests that *Salmonella*-free poultry can be achieved.
• Commercial food processing should be subject to the HACCP (Hazard Analysis Critical Control Point) system to identify, control and monitor potential hazards to food safety. Specific measures for *Salmonella* include use of only pasteurised eggs and milk; adequate cooking of meat and poultry; practices to avoid cross-contamination; exclusion of food handlers with diarrhoea; and adequate temperature control. This is particularly important in establishments serving food to vulnerable groups (the very young, the very old and the immunocompromised).

• In the home, routine food and personal hygiene measures need to be supplemented by particular care with raw poultry and eggs. The public need to be made aware that all poultry should be viewed as contaminated and how to prevent cross-contamination from it. Consumption of raw or undercooked eggs should be avoided, and date stamped eggs from vaccinated flocks are preferable. In the UK, Lion-marked eggs are recommended, and at the time of writing, there is evidence that eggs imported from Spain are more likely to be contaminated.

Surveillance

• Salmonellosis is notifiable in the majority of EU countries including Ireland, Germany, Sweden and Norway (in the UK notify as suspected 'Food Poisoning').
• Laboratory isolates of *Salmonella* should be reported to local and national surveillance systems. Isolates should be sent for further typing to aid epidemiological investigation.
• On a European level, salmonellosis is monitored via the EnterNet System (Chapter 5.1).

Response to a case

• Hygiene advice, particularly on handwashing, should be given to all cases. Ideally, the case should not attend work or school until he/she has normal stools (preferably for 48 hours).
• Occupational details should be sought: cases in risk groups 1–4 (Box 2.2.1) should be excluded until 48 hours after the first normal stool.
• Enquiry for symptoms in household contacts (or others exposed to the same putative source) should be made; those with symptoms, particularly diarrhoea, should be treated as cases.
• Enteric precautions for those admitted to hospital (especially for handling faeces or soiled bedding or clothing) should be followed.
• Asymptomatic excretors rarely require exclusion, provided adequate personal hygiene precautions are followed. This requires

adequate knowledge and co-operation of the individual (or a responsible adult) and adequate facilities.

• If illness acquired in hospital, inform hospital control of infection team.

Investigation of a cluster

• Arrange with local and reference laboratories for serotyping and phage typing of strains to check if similar organisms.

• Some salmonellae are particularly associated with specific animal hosts (Table 3.67.1); the national reference laboratory can advise on this.

• Although some clues may be obtained by analysis of person/place/time variables, administration of a hypothesis-generating questionnaire is usually necessary (see Chapter 4.3). A general semi-structured questionnaire for investigating clusters of food-borne illness should be routinely available; this can be modified in light of the epidemiology of the specific pathogen (e.g. known animal reservoirs or vehicles associated with previous outbreaks) and outbreak specific factors (e.g. most cases in children).

Control of an outbreak

• In food-borne outbreaks, microbiological examination of faeces from infected patients and food can reveal the organism responsible and a cohort or case-control study may reveal the vehicle of infection. However, in order to prevent recurrence the question 'how did the food consumed come to contain an infective dose of the organism?' needs to be answered. Particular factors to bear in mind in a food-borne outbreak of salmonellosis are as follows:

(i) Were any potentially contaminated foods consumed raw or inadequately cooked? In the case of *S. enteritidis* PT4, was poultry inadequately cooked or were raw eggs used in any recipes? Can the raw food be checked for the organisms?

(ii) Are food preparation procedures and hygiene practices adequate to prevent cross

contamination, particularly from raw meat or poultry?

(iii) Did any food handlers have symptoms of gastrointestinal infection? All food handlers should provide faecal samples for analysis, but remember that they may also have eaten the vehicle of infection and so be victims of the outbreak rather than the cause.

(iv) What happened to the food after cooking? Was there scope for contamination? Was it refrigerated until just before eating? Was it adequately reheated?

• Many outbreaks require more than one problem to occur in food preparation. An example is a sandwich tea made for a sports match that used raw egg mayonnaise and then was stored in the boot of a car on a hot summer day until consumed.

• Secondary spread is common in outbreaks of *Salmonella* infection. Outbreak cases should receive intervention as outlined earlier for sporadic cases. Plotting of an epidemic curve may help identify the contribution of person-to-person spread (see Box 2.2.3 for other clues).

• Outbreaks in hospitals or nursery homes require particular care because of the vulnerable nature of the residents.

Case definition for analytical study of a *Salmonella* outbreak

Clinical: diarrhoea or any two from abdominal pain/fever/nausea with onset 6–72 hours after exposure.

Confirmed: clinical case with isolate of outbreak strain.

3.68 SARS (Severe acute respiratory syndrome)

Severe acute respiratory syndrome (SARS) is a recently discovered severe viral respiratory illness caused by SARS-associated coronavirus (SARS-CoV).

Suggested on-call action

• Assess whether case fits current case definition. If so, inform National Surveillance Centre.
• The response to the following groups should be considered: cases, potential cases, contacts of cases, the worried well.
• Patient(s) should be immediately isolated and respiratory transmission-based precautions instituted.
• Samples should be taken urgently for laboratory diagnosis.
• Contacts of persons under investigation for SARS should be traced and quarantined until SARS has been ruled out as the cause of the illness. Contacts are those who have cared for, lived with, or having had direct contact with the respiratory secretions, body fluids and/or excretions (e.g. faeces) of cases of SARS.
• Individuals with risky exposures to a person or persons in a SARS alert cluster should be managed as contacts until SARS has been ruled out as the cause of the illness.
• Contacts within the health care setting should be managed as follows:
  (i) Inpatients should be isolated or cohorted and transmission-based (respiratory, body fluids and faecal) precautions instituted. They should be placed on fever surveillance.
  (ii) Exposed staff should be placed on active fever surveillance, and either cohorted to care for exposed patients (as above) or placed on home quarantine.
• Community contacts should be
  (i) given information on the clinical picture, transmission, etc. of SARS.
  (ii) placed under active surveillance for 10 days and voluntary home quarantine recommended.
  (iii) visited or telephoned daily by a member of the public health care team.
• Temperature recorded daily.
• If the contact develops disease symptoms, they should be investigated locally at an appropriate healthcare facility.

Epidemiology

An unusual respiratory illness emerged in southern China in November 2002; the outbreak developed outside China in February 2003 and ended in July 2003. For cases of SARS to reappear, the virus has to re-emerge (from a possible animal source, a laboratory accident or undetected transmission in humans). Since 5 July there have been confirmed SARS-CoV infections resulting from laboratory accidents (Singapore and Taiwan) and from exposure to animal sources or environmental contamination (China); none of these cases has been fatal nor resulted in secondary transmission. According to the WHO, a total of 8098 people worldwide became sick with SARS during the 2003 outbreak. Of these, 774 died. Healthcare workers and close (e.g. household or face-to-face) contacts of cases are at particular risk. The case fatality rate is about 10% and increases with age.

Clinical features

In general, SARS begins with a high fever (temperature greater than 38°C [100.4°F]). Other symptoms may include headache, an overall feeling of discomfort and body aches. Some people also have mild respiratory symptoms at the outset. About 10–20% of patients have diarrhoea. After 2–7 days, SARS patients may develop a dry cough. Most patients develop pneumonia and the majority of cases have an abnormal chest radiograph at some stage.

Laboratory confirmation

The most effective diagnostic tests are RT-PCR or real-time PCR of genomic fragments or cultured virus. RT-PCR can be used to make a relatively early diagnosis. A positive RT-PCR test should be repeated by the national reference laboratory using a second, unopened aliquot. Respiratory, serum, stool and urine specimens should be taken for virus isolation and for acute phase serology. Respiratory samples should include nasopharyngeal aspirates, provided full infection control procedures are in place to protect staff and other patients. Respiratory and stool specimens should be routinely collected for virus isolation or detection of viral genome utilising RT-PCR during the first and second weeks. Serum specimens should also be collected for serology in the second and third weeks to detect a rising titre by testing acute and convalescent sera in parallel.

Clinical samples should be separated into three aliquots at the time of collection, or in a secure laboratory, which is clean and in which there is no ongoing work on SARS-CoV strains. One aliquot should be used by the local diagnostic laboratory, the second aliquot should only be used, unopened, by the national reference laboratory, and the third aliquot should be retained for use by the WHO SARS Reference and Verification Laboratory, should verification be necessary.

Transmission

SARS is mainly spread by respiratory droplets, and SARS-CoV is also shed in faeces; faecal shedding is more prolonged than respiratory. The number of new cases(R_0) arising from each case of SARS in the absence of interventions is about 3, public health interventions can reduce R_0 to below 1 and control the disease. Risk of transmission is greatest around the tenth day of illness. Transmission is reduced if the case is isolated within 3 days of onset. Mild cases are infectious; more severely ill patients seem to be more infectious. Super spreading events occur but are not understood or predictable. Asymptomatic patients are not infectious and cases are no longer infectious 10 days after fever resolution. Children are very rarely affected and are not known to transmit SARS.

Acquisition

The mean incubation period is 5 days (range 2–10 days), although incubation periods of up to 14 days have been reported.

Available information suggests that persons with SARS are most likely to be infectious when symptomatic. Patients are most contagious during the second week of illness. Current advice is that recovering patients limit their interactions outside the home for 10 days after they are afebrile and respiratory symptom free.

Prevention

Control of SARS is by identifying and isolating all cases as early in the illness as possible, rigorous infection control at all stages with monitoring the health of close contacts, so that any infected are identified and isolated before they become infectious. This includes
• isolation and contact tracing to break chains of transmission.
• care in laboratory handling of specimens (containment level 3).
• good hospital infection control
• WHO recommendations that patients with probable SARS should be isolated and accommodated as follows in descending order of preference:
(i) negative pressure rooms with the door closed.
(ii) single rooms with their own bathroom facilities.
(iii) cohort placement in an area with an independent air supply and exhaust system. Turning off air conditioning and opening windows for good ventilation is recommended if an independent air supply is unfeasible. Wherever possible, patients under investigation for SARS should be separated from those diagnosed with the syndrome.

Surveillance

• Report urgently to local and national public health authorities.
• National public health authorities should report every laboratory confirmed case of SARS to WHO (see below).

Response to a case

See on-call box

Investigation of a cluster

• Look for a history of travel abroad, contact with a case or recent exposure to a healthcare setting.
• If none of the above explains cases, undertake full hypothesis-generating study.

Control of an outbreak

• Deal with individual case as above.
• Set up dedicated triage area, and patients under investigation for SARS should be separated from the probable cases.
• Provide suspected patients with a face mask to wear, preferably one that provides filtration of their expired air.
• Provide triage staff with a face mask and eye protection.
• Ensure good infection control/handwashing procedures in place.
• Disinfectants, such as fresh bleach solutions, should be widely available at appropriate concentrations.
• Guidance for clinical and laboratory management, and case definitions available on WHO and Health Protection Agency websites.

Suggested case definition

Clinical: The following clinical case definition has been developed for public health purposes.
• A person with a history of fever (≥38°C) *and*
• One or more symptoms of lower respiratory tract illness (cough, difficulty breathing, shortness of breath) *and*
• Radiographic evidence of lung infiltrates consistent with pneumonia or Respiratory Distress Syndrome (RDS) OR autopsy findings consistent with the pathology of pneumonia or RDS without an identifiable cause *and*
• No alternative diagnosis can fully explain the illness *and*

Continued

• In Europe, a history of travel to an area with reported cases or exposure to a case would normally be required for the case-definition.
Laboratory: A person with symptoms and signs that are clinically suggestive of SARS *and* with positive laboratory findings for SARS-CoV based on one or more of the following diagnostic criteria:
• PCR positive for SARS-CoV – PCR positive using a validated method from
  (i) at least two different clinical specimens (e.g. nasopharyngeal and stool) *or*
  (ii) the same clinical specimen collected on two or more occasions during the course of the illness (e.g. sequential nasopharyngeal aspirates) *or*
  (iii) two different assays or repeat PCR using a new RNA extract from the original clinical sample on each occasion of testing.
• Seroconversion by ELISA or IFA:
  (i) Negative antibody test on acute serum followed by positive antibody test on convalescent phase serum tested in parallel *or*
  (ii) Fourfold or greater rise in antibody titre between acute and convalescent phase sera tested in parallel.
• Virus isolation:
  (i) Isolation in cell culture of SARS-CoV from any specimen *and*
  (ii) PCR confirmation using a validated method.

3.69 Scabies

Scabies is an inflammatory disease of the skin caused by the mite *Sarcoptes scabiei* var. *hominis*.

On-call action

Advise on treatment and recommend immediate control measures.

Epidemiology

Scabies is associated with overcrowding and poor personal hygiene. It is more prevalent in children and young adults, in urban areas and in winter. Scabies infection shows a cyclical pattern with a periodicity of 10–30 years. In UK scabies has increased since 1991 and there have been reports of outbreaks in hospitals and in nursing and residential homes where both patients and staff may be affected. UK General Practitioners reported a mean weekly incidence of scabies in 2003 of 4.5 per 100,000 population, similar to previous years. This probably underestimates the true incidence.

Diagnosis

There may be no sign of infection for 2–4 weeks after exposure, when an allergy develops to mite saliva and faeces and an itchy symmetrical rash appears. The rash comprises small, red papules and is seen anywhere on the body. If the person has had scabies before, the rash may appear within a few days of re-exposure. The itching is intense, particularly at night. Burrows are the only lesions caused directly by the mite and may be seen in the webs of the fingers and on wrists and elbows. In infants, young children, the elderly and the immunocompromised, mites can also infect the face, neck, scalp and ears. Usually only about 12 mites are present on an affected person at any one time but if there is impaired immunity or altered skin sensation large numbers of mites may be present and the skin is thickened and scaly. This condition is known as atypical, crusted or Norwegian scabies. Scabies is often misdiagnosed, but skin scrapings can be examined under the microscope for mites, eggs or faeces.

Transmission and acquisition

The pregnant female, which is about 0.3 mm long, burrows in the epidermis and lays 2–3 eggs each day before dying after 4–5 weeks. The eggs hatch after 3–4 days into larvae that move to hair follicles where they develop into adults after a further 7–10 days. Mating takes place and the female embeds in a new burrow within 1 hour.

Classical scabies is transmitted via direct skin-to-skin contact so that the risk of transmission is higher in families than, e.g. in schools. In crusted scabies transmission can also occur via skin scales on bedding, clothes and upholstery. It is therefore more infectious. Scabies remains infectious until treated. Animal scabies is called mange or scab. It can be passed to humans but only causes a temporary problem since the mites cannot multiply and soon die out.

Prevention

Prevention of scabies depends on early recognition of cases and prompt effective treatment. This in turn depends on public and professional education and a high level of awareness and diagnostic suspicion.

Surveillance

Scabies is not notifiable; however, clusters of cases of scabies in residential and day-care settings should be reported to the local public health team.

Response to a case

• Aqueous malathion lotion or permethrin dermal cream should be applied to the whole body, including the scalp, neck, face, ears, between the fingers and toes and under the nails. Earlier guidance only recommended application from the neck down for most healthy adults. A hot bath prior to application should be discouraged as it increases systemic absorption. Ideally the scabicide should be left on for 24 hours and should be reapplied if the hands are washed during that time. The patient should then have a bath or shower, dress in clean clothes and change bed sheets. A second

Table 3.69.1 Responsibilities in control of scabies

Local health protection team (CCDC and CICN in England)	Receive reports of scabies in community settings. Advise on management. Involve district nurses, health visitors, school health nurses, GPs, managers and owners of residential and nursing homes. Make available information on scabies for the public and professionals.
General practitioners	Maintain a high level of diagnostic suspicion. Diagnose, treat and follow up cases of scabies amongst their patients and contacts. Make referrals and request second opinions as appropriate. Discuss with local health protection team (LHPT) whenever an outbreak of scabies is suspected in a residential or nursing home. Co-operate with the LHPT in dealing with such an outbreak.
Residential and nursing home managers, owners and staff	Remain vigilant to the possible diagnosis of scabies. Involve the GP in diagnosing, treating, referral and follow-up Recognise outbreaks and alert the LHPT. Co-operate with the LHPT in dealing with such an outbreak.
Families of those with scabies	Ensure treatment is carried out correctly. Inform all close contacts, particularly those in a day-care or nursing setting if scabies is suspected. Follow advice from their GP or the LHPT, particularly relating to treatment and exclusion from work or school.

application after 7 days will kill any larvae that hatch from eggs that survived the first application. Itching may continue for 2–3 weeks after successful treatment and may require treatment with anti-pruritics.

• All household, close and sexual contacts should receive simultaneous treatment, even if symptom free.

• Clothing and bedding should be laundered on a hot washing machine cycle. Any items that cannot be washed in this way should be set aside and not used for 7 days. Under these conditions mites will become dehydrated and die. Normal hygiene and vacuuming of chairs, beds and soft furnishings will minimise environmental contamination with skin scales.

• In crusted scabies more intensive treatment is necessary, which may be continued for some time. Oral ivermectin (as a single oral dose of 200 μg/kg or two doses 1 week apart) has been shown to be effective in difficult cases and in those with HIV infection. Cases can return to school or work after the first application of scabicide.

Control of an outbreak

• Clusters of cases of scabies may be reported from hospitals, nursing homes or other residential health or social-care settings. Confirmation of the diagnosis is important in these settings. All patients and residents may need to be examined in an attempt to identify the index case, who is often someone with an unrecognised case of crusted scabies. The GP of the patient, client or service user should be asked to advise. He/she may ask for a second opinion from a consultant dermatologist. A high level of diagnostic suspicion should be maintained. Atypical scabies can spread from patients to nurses and others who provide close care. Use of standard precautions including gloves and aprons will minimise this.

• Outbreaks of scabies in a community setting should be referred to the local public health team.

• The cases, whether members of staff or residents, should be promptly treated (see above).

• Staff can return to work once treatment has been completed.

• If practicable, while affected residents are undergoing treatment they should be separated from other residents.

• If the case is a member of staff, treatment is recommended for his/her close household contacts.

• If the case is a client it may not be practicable to treat everyone else in the residential setting, but if there are several cases and the situation appears to be out of control then it may be necessary to treat all residents, staff and their families simultaneously on an agreed treatment date.

• A skin monitoring record form should be used for each person following treatment so that apparent treatment failures and recurrences can be assessed.

• If itching persists for 2–3 weeks after treatment and close monitoring of skin condition shows no improvement then misdiagnosis, treatment failure or re-infection should be suspected. The patient should be re-examined to confirm the diagnosis, further coordinated applications of scabicide correctly applied may be advised and a search should be made for an unrecognised source case of crusted scabies.

Case definition for outbreak

A rash of typical appearance and itching particularly at night. Often with other similar cases reported amongst household and other close contacts.

3.70 *Shigella*

Shigellae cause intestinal infection including 'bacillary dysentery'. *Shigella sonnei* is the most common species in Western Europe and causes relatively mild illness. Most *S. flexneri* and all *S. boydii* and *S. dysenteriae* are imported and are more severe. *S. dysenteriae* type 1 may cause very severe illness due to production of an exotoxin.

Suggested on-call action

• If the case is in risk group for further transmission, advise exclusion.

• If you or reporting clinician/microbiologist is aware of other linked cases, activate Local Outbreak Plan.

• If infection with *S. dysenteriae*, obtain details of household and ensure symptomatic contacts are excluded.

• If *S. dysenteriae*, ensure symptomatic contacts receive medical assessment.

Epidemiology

Shigella infection has decreased dramatically since the peak incidence period of 1950–1969, when 20–40,000 cases per annum were reported in the UK. Most years since 1980 have seen less than 5000 reports, with the exception of a small epidemic in the mid-1980s and a larger one in the early 1990s, both due primarily to *S. sonnei*. There were only 1294 laboratory reported cases in the UK in 2003, of which 74% were *S. sonnei*, 19% *S. flexneri*, 4% *S. boydii* and 3% *S. dysenteriae*.

Shigellosis is primarily a disease of children, with the highest rates reported in those less than 5 years of age followed by those aged 5–14 years. The mean age of infection is lower in epidemic years than non-epidemic. Boys have higher rates than girls, but the reverse is seen in those aged 15–44 years. There is no longer a winter excess of cases in the UK. The most common settings for *S. sonnei* outbreaks are schools and nurseries, but may also occur in men who have sex with men and in residential institutions. Large outbreaks of non-sonnei infection are uncommon in the UK, but family outbreaks appear to be more frequent in those of south Asian ethnicity. Travel abroad is a risk factor for non-sonnei shigellosis in the UK and for all shigellae in Scandinavia and the Netherlands.

Clinical diagnosis

S. sonnei infection often causes only mild and transient diarrhoea and rarely causes dysentery. Other species are more likely to follow the classic picture of an initial illness of abdominal pain and diarrhoea (often watery), which may be accompanied by malaise, fever, nausea, vomiting, tenesmus and toxaemia. Approximately 40–50% then develop mucus and/or frank blood in the stool (dysentery). In developed countries illness is usually self-limiting, lasting an average of 7 days. *S. dysenteriae* 1 may cause toxic megacolon and haemolytic uraemic disease and has a case-fatality rate of 10–20%. Asymptomatic *Shigella* infection and excretion may also occur.

Laboratory confirmation

Diagnosis is usually confirmed by isolation of the organism from faeces; testing is routine in most laboratories. Provisional results are usually available within 48 hours. Speciation should always be carried out as control measures vary between species. Serotyping based on 'O' antigens is also available if epidemiologically indicated, e.g. any case of *S. dysenteriae* or possible clusters of *S. boydii* (18 serotypes) or *S. flexneri* (six serotypes and two variants, e.g. 'type 2a'). *S. sonnei* is antigenically homogeneous; phage typing or colicin typing may be available from reference laboratories.

Transmission

Man is the only significant reservoir of infection. Transmission to other humans is via the faeco–oral route either directly or by contamination of food, water or the environment. Direct person-to-person spread is extremely common in households and institutions, particularly those with young children: 30–50% of contacts of cases became infected. Cases with diarrhoea are a much greater risk than asymptomatic excretors, with inadequate handwashing after defaecation the main cause. Such individuals may also contaminate food. Young children may act as a transmission link between households.

Shigellae, particularly *S. sonnei* may also survive for up to 20 days in favourable environmental conditions (i.e. cool, damp and dark). This may lead to transmission via lavatory seats, towels and any other vehicle that could become contaminated by faeces, either directly or via unclean hands. Flies may also transfer the organism from faeces to food.

Food- and water-borne outbreaks are relatively uncommon but do occur. Recent outbreaks in Europe have been due to imported iceberg lettuce (several countries), imported baby maize (Denmark), a food handler contaminating cheese (Spain) and contaminated drinking water (Greece and Germany).

Acquisition

The incubation period is between 12 and 96 hours, but may be up to 1 week for *S. dysenteriae* type 1. The infectious period is primarily during the diarrhoeal illness; however, cases maintain a low level of infectivity for as long as the organism is excreted in the stool, which is 2–4 weeks on average. The infective dose is very low: infection may follow ingestion of as few as 10 organisms of *S. dysenteriae* type 1. The average infective dose for *S. sonnei* is about 500 organisms. Immunity post-infection does occur and lasts for several years, at least for the same serotype. Longer-term immunity does not appear to be important.

Prevention

• Adequate personal hygiene, particularly handwashing after defaecation.
• Adequate toilet facilities in schools. Supervised handwashing in nursery and infant schools. Regular and frequent cleaning of nurseries and schools, particularly for toilet areas.
• Safe disposal of faeces and treatment of drinking and swimming water.

- Care with food and water for travellers to developing countries.
- Routine cooking kills shigellae.

Surveillance

All clinical cases of diarrhoea or dysentery should be reported to local public health authorities. Dysentery is formally notifiable in the UK. Laboratory isolates of *Shigella* species from symptomatic patients should be reported to the relevant national surveillance system.

Response to a case

- Hygiene advice to case and contacts.
- Enteric precautions for case and symptomatic contacts. In institutions, isolate if possible.
- If case or symptomatic contact, exclude from work or school until well (preferably until no diarrhoea for 48 hours).
- For higher risk groups (see Box 2.2.1) with *S. sonnei*, exclude until 48 hours after first normal stool and give hygiene advice.
- For higher risk groups with non-sonnei shigellae, exclude until 2 consecutive negative faecal specimens taken at least 24 hours apart.
- Contacts of cases with non-sonnei shigellae should be screened microbiologically if in a higher risk group. If positive or symptomatic, treat as case.
- Obtain details of any nursery or infant school attended. Check to see if other cases and reinforce hygiene measures. Check that adequate toilet facilities and supervision available.
- For species other than *S. sonnei* , check that case has been abroad in the 4 days before onset (7 days for *S. dysenteriae* type 1) or has been in contact with another case who was ill abroad or on return. If no link abroad, obtain details of contacts and full food history for 4 days before onset (7 for *S. dysenteriae*).
- Mild cases will recover without antibiotics and multiple drug resistance is increasing. Antimotility drugs should be avoided.

Investigation of a cluster

- Liaise with microbiologist to organise typing of isolates (may be more than one type in an outbreak).
- Does epidemic curve suggest point source (plus secondary cases) or continuing exposure? Does age/sex/ethnic/geographic analysis of cases suggest common factor?
- Look for links via institutions such as nurseries, schools, social clubs, care facilities and links between affected families via child networks. Administer hypothesis generating food questionnaire for 12–96 hours before onset. Ask about water consumption, hobbies, swimming, social functions and occupation. For non-sonnei species, look for social networks that include travellers to developing countries.

Control of an outbreak

- Re-inforce hygiene measures, particularly handwashing. Supervised handwashing for children aged under 8 years.
- Check toilet and handwashing facilities are adequate. Increase cleaning of risk areas in toilets (e.g. seats and 'touch points') to at least twice a day.
- Ensure regular and frequent cleaning of all other areas and objects that could become contaminated. Ensure facilities for disinfection after faecal accidents.
- Exclusion of cases.
- Provide hygiene advice to families of those in affected institutions.

Suggested case definition for outbreak

Confirmed: diarrhoea and/or abdominal pain with *Shigella* species of outbreak strain identified in faeces.

Clinical: diarrhoea in member of population of affected institution, without alternative explanation

3.71 Smallpox

Smallpox is an acute contagious disease caused by the variola virus – a DNA virus member of the orthopox genus. Naturally occurring infection has been eradicated worldwide, so its public health importance now lies in the potential of a deliberate release in a bioterrorist attack and the consequent need to re-consider vaccination and other control strategies.

Suggested on-call action

If diagnosis is likely, isolate at the point of contact and notify national surveillance unit.

Epidemiology

The WHO confirmed the global eradication of smallpox in 1980. The virus still officially exists in two WHO designated laboratories in the USA and Russia; however, there is concern that stocks may exist in other laboratories.

Clinical features

There are two clinical forms of the disease: variola major (severe) and variola minor (mild). In variola major there is typically a rapid onset of flu-like symptoms – fever, headache, malaise and aching head and back. The distinctive vesicular rash then appears over the next 1–2 days, eventually covering the whole body. Vesicles are most concentrated peripherally – on the face, arms and leg, also the mouth and throat (unlike chickenpox, which is commonest on the trunk). The vesicles develop into pustules over the next week; these crust and fall off over the next 3–4 weeks, leaving permanent pitted scars. The case fatality rate in a nonimmune person is 30%. There is no specific effective treatment, although vaccination early in the incubation period can modify the course of the disease and reduce mortality. In malignant smallpox, the most severe form, the rash is haemorrhagic and the case fatality rate is over 90%. Variola minor has a much less severe course and most patients recover.

Smallpox may be confused with chickenpox: diagnostic clues are given in Table 3.71.1 and photographs of the different rashes are shown in Plate 3 (*facing p. 212*). Other differential diagnoses include disseminated herpes simplex infection, and (rarely) cowpox and monkeypox. Other diseases involving a rash (measles,

Table 3.71.1 Distinguishing smallpox from chickenpox in a well, nonimmune person

	Smallpox	Chickenpox
Overall illness	Almost always severe	Usually mild
Initial signs	Headache, back pain	Mild malaise
First spots	Forehead, face, scalp, neck, hands and wrist	Trunk
'Cropping'	Pocks in one area, e.g. face appear all at once	Generalised
Limb distribution of spots	More on hands and wrists than upper arms; similarly more on feet and ankles than the thighs	More on upper arms than hands and wrists, more on thighs than feet and ankles
Hands and feet	Circular flattened grey Vesicles are characteristic	Such vesicles never seen in chickenpox
Itchiness	Not in first few days of rash	Common in the first few days of the rash and then continuing

enterovirus, parvovirus B19 and HHV-6) are much less likely to be confused with smallpox.

Laboratory confirmation

This is by EM identification of orthopox virus from vesicular fluid, scrapings from the base of lesions, scabs or vesicle crusts. This must be confirmed by PCR and viral isolation from culture. Confirmation can only be done in a specialised containment level 4 laboratory. EM takes 2 hours and PCR takes 6 hours.

Varicella and herpes simplex viruses are easily distinguished from parvovirus on EM. Parapox particles (e.g. from Orf) should also be distinguishable from orthopox viruses (such as smallpox). If an orthopox virus is found on routine EM, a clinical history will be required. Molluscum is the only orthopox infection in the UK for which EM is routinely performed.

Transmission

There is no known animal reservoir or vector. The virus spread from person to person by droplet nuclei or aerosols expelled from the orophayrynx of an infectious case. Close contact (e.g. household, hospital ward) is normally required; however, air-borne transmission via drafts and air conditioning can occur, also from contaminated clothing and bedding. Under normal conditions, the virus is unlikely to survive more than 48 hours in the environment, although prolonged survival is possible in dry scabs.

Acquisition

The incubation period is usually 12–16 days (range 7–17 days). Patients are infectious from the onset of fever until the last scabs fall off. The infectious dose is assumed to be very low (<100 virus particles). Immunity following natural infection is lifelong. Past vaccination offers some degree of protection.

Prevention

• Smallpox vaccine is a live vaccine produced from vaccinia virus. It is delivered by multiple skin puncture with a bifurcated needle; a 'take' is successful when a pustule develops, which progressively crusts. Serious vaccine complications occasionally occur (encephalitis, eczema vaccinatum). Revaccination is recommended after 3 years for those at continuing risk; after revaccination protection lasts for about 10 years.
• Vaccination should be considered for laboratory workers working with closely related viruses and for frontline workers who might have to care for cases in the event of a deliberate release.
• Individuals such as archaeologists who have direct contact with corpses that may have died from smallpox are not at risk.

Surveillance

• Any suspected case must be reported immediately to the national surveillance unit.
• Smallpox is statutorily notifiable in many countries including the UK and Ireland.
• All suspected cases are investigated by WHO; a number are investigated every year and usually turn out to be another poxvirus infection such as monkeypox.

Response to a case

• Isolate any probable or confirmed case at point of diagnosis, pending transfer to a high-security unit with negative-pressure isolation. Patients should be isolated until all crusts have fallen off.
• Confirm the diagnosis (with appropriate precautions).
• Decontaminate all waste before disposal by autoclaving.
• Vaccination of contacts in the first 4 days of the incubation period reduces mortality by 50%. Anti-viral drugs may also be considered.

• Any confirmed case should be assumed to be a deliberate release.

Investigation and management of a cluster

• Assume deliberate release and implement control plan. Many health and emergency planning agencies would be involved with Central Government co-ordination.
• A national plan exists in the UK and is available on the Department of Health website. Actions include isolation of cases, verification and management of contacts, vaccination and enhanced surveillance.

Response to an overt deliberate release

• Activate local and national plans and take expert advice.
• Define exposed zone and identify exposed people.
• Decontaminate exposed people: remove clothing, shower and wash hair.
• Vaccinate all exposed.
• Trace those who have left the scene for decontamination and vaccination.
• Isolate exposed zone to allow natural decontamination: formal decontamination unnecessary.
• Full biological protective equipment for those who enter exposed zone.
• Vaccination of frontline workers.

Suggested case definition

Clinical: acute onset of fever >38°C, which is persistent, followed by a vesicular or pustular rash with lesions all at the same stage of development without obvious cause and with a centrifugal distribution
Confirmed: identification of orthopox particles by EM and PCR; in an outbreak EM alone is adequate for cases with epidemiological links with others.

3.72 Staphylococcal food poisoning

Staphylococcal food poisoning is an uncommon food-borne disease (FBD) caused by heat-stable enterotoxins produced when certain strains of *Staphylococcus aureus* multiply in food.

Suggested on-call action

If you or reporting clinician/microbiologist know of associated cases, consult outbreak control plan.

Epidemiology

Staphylococcal food poisoning occurs throughout the world, but is now rarely reported in the UK. However, many people with FBD do not seek medical advice.

Clinical features

There is sudden onset of nausea, cramps, vomiting, diarrhoea, hypotension and prostration. The illness lasts 1–2 days; serious sequelae are uncommon, but admission to hospital may occur because of the intensity of symptoms.

Laboratory confirmation

Gram-positive cocci may be seen on Gram staining of food vehicles. *S. aureus* may be cultured from unheated food at levels of 10^5–10^6 organisms per gram or from the vomit or faeces of cases. Enterotoxin may be detected in food samples. *S. aureus* of the same phage type may be found in the implicated food vehicle and on the skin or lesions of food handlers.

Transmission

Food handlers colonised with *S. aureus* or with infected skin lesions contaminate foods such as cooked meats, sandwiches and pastries. These are stored with inadequate refrigeration, allowing the organism to multiply and produce toxin before being eaten. Two hours at room temperature may be long enough to produce a significant amount of toxin. Even with further cooking or heating the toxin may not be destroyed. Outbreaks have followed contamination of dairy products as a result of staphylococcal mastitis in cattle.

Acquisition

The incubation period is 1–7 hours (usually 2–4 hours). Staphylococcal food poisoning is not communicable from person to person.

Prevention

Staphylococcal food poisoning can be prevented by
• strict food hygiene including kitchen cleaning and handwashing.
• minimising food-handling.
• safe food storage in particular temperature control above 60°C or below 10°C.
• excluding food handlers with purulent lesions. Nasal carriers do not need to be excluded.

Surveillance

Cases and outbreaks of staphylococcal food poisoning should be reported to local public health departments (formally notifiable in UK). Outbreaks should be reported to national surveillance centres.

Response to a case

• Enquire about food consumed in the 24 hours before onset of symptoms.
• Exclude risk groups (Box 2.2.1) with diarrhoea or vomiting.

Investigation of a cluster

• Discuss further microbiological investigation (e.g. phage typing) with microbiologist.
• Undertake hypothesis-generating study covering food histories particularly restaurants, social functions and other mass catering arrangements.
• Investigate the origin and preparation methods of any food items implicated in the outbreak. Submit any leftover food for laboratory analysis.
• Search for food handlers with purulent lesions.

Control of an outbreak

• Identify and rectify faults with temperature control in food preparation processes.
• Exclude any implicated food handler.

Suggested case definition

Vomiting occurring 1–7 hours after exposure to potential source with appropriate laboratory confirmation.

3.73 Streptococcal infections

Streptococci are part of the normal flora and colonise the respiratory, gastrointestinal and genitourinary tracts. Several species cause disease, including the following:
• Group A streptococci (beta-haemolytic streptococci, BHS, *Streptococcus pyogenes*) cause sore throat and skin infection (impetigo, cellulitis, pyoderma), scarlet fever, necrotising fasciitis, streptococcal toxic shock syndrome, wound infections, pneumonia and puerperal fever.
• Group A organisms may also cause postinfectious syndromes, such as rheumatic fever, glomerulonephritis; and Sydenham's chorea.

• Group B streptococci cause neonatal meningitis and septicaemia.
• Group C and G streptococci can cause upper respiratory infections such as tonsillitis.
• Viridans streptococci are a common cause of bacterial endocarditis.

Suggested on-call action

Not usually necessary unless outbreak suspected.

Epidemiology

Streptococcal sore throat and scarlet fever are found worldwide, though less commonly in the tropics. Up to 20% of individuals may have asymptomatic pharyngeal colonisation with group A streptococci. Particular 'M types' are associated with various sequelae (e.g. 1, 3, 4, 12 with glomerulonephritis). The incidence of sequelae depends upon the circulating M types. Acute rheumatic fever has become rare in most developed countries, though occasional cases and outbreaks are seen. It is associated with poor living conditions and is most common in those aged 3–15 years.

Impetigo is most commonly seen in younger children. The M types associated with nephritis following skin infection are different from those associated with nephritis following upper respiratory infection.

Asymptomatic carriage of group B streptococci (GBS) is common in pregnant women.

Clinical features

• *Sore throat*: it can be difficult to differentiate streptococcal from viral sore throat; various scoring systems have been proposed but they lack predictive power.
• *Skin infection*: streptococcal skin infection commonly presents as acute cellulitis or impetigo.
• *Scarlet fever*: this may accompany pharyngeal or skin infection and is characterised by a skin rash, classically a fine punctate erythema,

sparing the face, but with facial flushing and circumoral pallor. During convalescence, desquamation of the finger and toe tips may occur.
• *Puerperal infection*: puerperal fever occurs in the post-partum or post-abortion patient and is usually accompanied by signs of septicaemia.
• *Necrotising fasciitis*: this involves the superficial and/or deep fascia; group A streptococci are implicated in about 60% of cases.

Laboratory confirmation

Streptococci are classified by a number of systems including haemolytic type, Lancefield group and species name.

Group A streptococcal antigen can be identified in pharyngeal secretions using rapid antigen detection; negative tests require confirmation. Detection of antibody to streptococcal extracellular toxins may be useful in the diagnosis of necrotising fasciitis.

Confirmation is by culture on blood agar, the production of a zone of haemolysis and showing inhibition with bacitracin.

A rise in antistreptolysin O, anti-DNA-ase or antihyaluronidase antibodies between acute and convalescent sera may be helpful in retrospective diagnosis.

Transmission

Streptococcal infection is commonly acquired by contact with patients or carriers, particularly nasal carriers. Transmission via contaminated foodstuffs, particularly unpasteurised milk and milk products is recognised.

Group B disease is acquired by the newborn as (s)he passes through the genital tract of the mother.

Acquisition

Group A streptococcal pharyngitis

The incubation period is 1–4 days for acute infection. The mean time for appearance of immunological sequelae is 10 days for acute glomerulonephritis, 19 days (1–5 weeks) for acute rheumatic fever and several months for Sydenham's chorea. The infectious period is commonly 2–3 weeks for untreated sore throat. Purulent discharges are infectious. Penicillin treatment usually terminates transmissibility within 48 hours.

Group B infection in infants

Early-onset infection occurs at a mean age of 20 hours. Late-onset infection occurs in infants with a mean age of 3–4 weeks, range 1 week to 3 months.

Immunity develops to specific M types and appears to be long-lasting. Repeated episodes due to other M types occur.

Prevention

Primary

- Personal hygiene.
- Avoid unpasteurised milk.
- Reduce need for illegal abortions.

Secondary

- Prevention of immune-mediated sequelae.
- Prompt recognition, confirmation and treatment of streptococcal infection.
- Those with a history of rheumatic fever should be offered antibiotic prophylaxis to prevent cumulative heart valve damage. Prophylaxis should be for at least 10 years; for patients with established heart disease it should be at least until 40 years of age.

Prevention of group B streptococcal infection

- Intrapartum antibiotic treatment of women colonised with group B streptococcus appears to reduce neonatal infection.
- Screening strategies to detect maternal colonisation are under development and should be considered.

Surveillance

Scarlet fever and/or puerperal fever are notifiable in some countries including England, Wales and Northern Ireland (SF) and Scotland (PF).

Response to a case

- Report acute cases of scarlet fever, puerperal fever and post-streptococcal syndromes to local health authorities.
- Careful handling of secretions and drainage fluids until after 24 hours penicillin treatment.
- Personal hygiene advice to case and contacts.
- UK advice is currently to exclude child with scarlet fever until after 5 days of antibiotics.
- Antibiotic chemoprophylaxis is not routinely indicated for close contacts of a case of group A disease. Only administer antibiotics to mother and baby if either develops invasive disease in the neonatal period or to close contacts if they develop symptoms of localised group A disease. Oral penicillin V is the first line drug; azithromycin is a suitable alternative for those allergic to penicillin.

Investigation of a cluster

- Does epidemic curve suggest point source, ongoing transmission (or both) or continuing source?
- Determine mode of transmission, exclude food-borne source, particularly milk, urgently.
- Search for and treat carriers if considered a potential source of infection.

Control of an outbreak

- Activate outbreak plan.
- Identify and treat carriers.
- Antibiotic chemoprophylaxis for household contacts of invasive group A disease is indicated when there are two or more cases within 30 days, or as a control measure in a community clusters or outbreak.
- Identify and remove contaminated food sources.

3.74 Tetanus

Tetanus is an acute illness caused by the toxin of the tetanus bacillus, *Clostridium tetani*. Its public health significance is the severity of the disease and its preventability by vaccination.

Suggested on-call action
None required for public health team.

Epidemiology

There are 10–15 cases notified a year in the UK, although there is probably significant under ascertainment of mild cases. Most cases are in unvaccinated people over 65 years of age, although there has been a recent outbreak in young adult injecting drug users. The case fatality is about 10%. The epidemiology is similar in other western European countries.

Clinical features

In classical tetanus there are painful muscular contractions, especially of the neck and jaw muscles (hence the name 'lockjaw'), muscular rigidity and painful spasms. The symptoms can be mild in a vaccinated person. There is often a history of a tetanus-prone wound, although not always.

Laboratory confirmation

This is infrequently obtained and unnecessary in typical cases. It is sometimes possible to culture the organism from the site of the original wound.

Transmission

The reservoir is the intestine of horses and other animals, including humans. Tetanus spores are found in soil contaminated with animal faeces. Transmission occurs when spores are introduced into the body through a dirty wound, through injecting drug use and occasionally during abdominal surgery. The illness is caused by a toxin. Person-to-person spread does not occur.

Acquisition

The incubation period is 3–21 days, depending on the site of the wound and the extent of contamination; occasionally it may be up to several months. Natural immunity may not follow an attack of tetanus.

Prevention

• Vaccination with tetanus toxoid. The UK schedule is three doses in infancy (in combination with pertussis, diphtheria, polio and Hib) at 2, 3 and 4 months, with boosters at 3–5 years and 13–18 years. Further boosters may be required at the time of injury. In a fully vaccinated individual, routine boosters are not justified, other than at the time of injury.
• Give tetanus vaccine (and tetanus immunoglobulin for tetanus-prone wounds) at the time of injury where more than 10 years have elapsed since the last dose of vaccine. The dose of tetanus immunoglobulin is 250 IU by i.m. injection; 500 IU if more than 24 hours have elapsed since the time of injury.
• Promote safe techniques in injecting drug users (see Chapter 3.4)

Surveillance

Notifiable in most European countries, including the UK.

Response to case

Seek injury history, ascertain vaccination status and arrange for primary course or booster, depending on history.

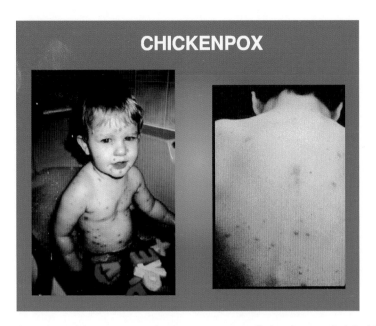

Plate 2 Chickenpox vesicles are sparser and more common centrally (trunk, upper limbs), child is well.

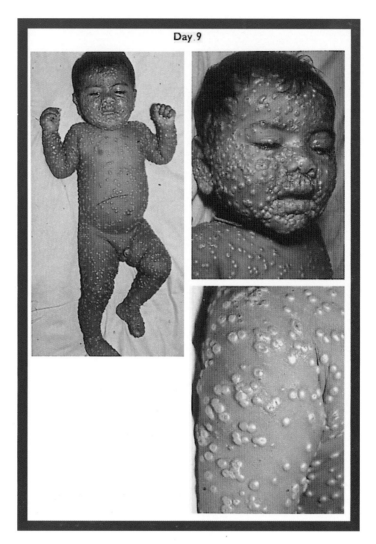

Day 9

Plate 3 Smallpox vesicles are denser and more common peripherally (hands, feet, wrists, ankles). Vesicles are slightly flattened. Child is unwell.

Response to a cluster or outbreak

Outbreaks of tetanus are rare. Look for a common source, e.g. surgery, i.v. drug abuse. Intravenous drug abuser outbreak – liaise with drug services to promote safer drug use and with clinicians to promote early diagnosis and treatment.

Suggested case definition
Physician diagnosis of tetanus.

3.75 Threadworms

Suggested on-call action
None.

Epidemiology

Threadworm (pinworm) infection is an intestinal infection with *Enterobius vermicularis,* a nematode of the family *Oxiuridae.* It is widespread in temperate regions, particularly amongst children. Clusters of cases may occur in household and residential settings. In England in 2003 GPs reported a mean weekly incidence of threadworm infection of 2 per 100,000 population, similar to previous years but undoubtedly this underestimates the true incidence.

Diagnosis

In symptomatic infections there is perianal itching and sleep disturbance. Appendicitis and chronic salpingitis are rare complications of worm migration.

The diagnosis can be confirmed by the presence of eggs on a strip of transparent adhesive tape that has been pressed on to the anal region and then examined under a microscope. Adult worms may be seen in faeces or on pe-

rianal skin. Adult worms live in the caecum. Females are 8–12-mm long but males, which die soon after mating and are rarely seen, are between 2- and 2.5-mm long.

Transmission and acquisition

Mature female worms migrate through the anus and lay thousands of eggs on the perianal skin. Infective embryos develop within 5–6 hours and these are transferred to the mouth on fingers as a result of scratching. Larvae emerge from the eggs in the small intestine and develop into sexually mature worms. Reinfection is common and infectious eggs are also spread to others directly on fingers or indirectly on bedding, clothing and in environmental dust. Adult worms do not live for longer than 6 weeks. Retro-infection may occur as a result of hatched larvae migrating back through the anus from the perianal region.

Prevention

Control is by prompt recognition and treatment of cases and their household contacts, health education and attention to personal and environmental hygiene, particularly handwashing. The perianal area may be washed each morning to remove eggs, and underwear, bedding and nightclothes should be changed regularly.

Response to a case/ cluster/outbreak

• Anti-helminthics such as mebendazole or piperazine are effective against adult worms but must be combined with hygienic measures to break the cycle of auto-infection.
• All household members should be treated.
• Exclude cases in risk groups 1–4 (Box 2.2.1) until treated. No need to exclude from school.
• An initial course of treatment should be followed by a second course 2 weeks later to kill worms that have matured in that time.

3.76 Tick-borne encephalitis

Tick-borne encephalitis (TBE) is a flavivirus infection of the CNS, characterised by a biphasic meningoencephalitis.

Epidemiology

It has a focal distribution throughout forested areas of Central and Eastern Europe and parts of Scandinavia (see Table 3.76.1). Related infections occur in Russia (but more severe) and North America. The disease is most common in early summer and autumn. Cases have not been reported in the UK, although louping ill, a related infection, occurs occasionally in Scotland and Ireland.

Diagnosis

The diagnosis should be considered in a patient with neurological symptoms with a history of a tick bite in an endemic area. Laboratory confirmation is by serology or virus isolation from blood (only in specialist laboratory).

Transmission and acquisition

Ixodes ricinus, the woodland tick, is the principal reservoir in Central and Northern Europe;

in Eastern Europe and Russia it is *Ixodes persculatus*. Sheep and deer are also hosts for louping ill. The incubation period is 7–14 days. Person-to-person transmission does not occur.

Control

Prevention is by wearing of protective clothing against tick bites in endemic areas. Killed vaccines are available and are recommended for at-risk travellers and residents, particularly those in occupations such as forestry and farming. In Austria, routine immunisation of the general population, including infants, has been recommended since the early 1980s. Post-exposure prophylaxis with a specific immunoglobulin is also available in some countries.

3.77 Toxocara

Toxocara canis is an ascarid parasite of dogs. It occasionally causes ocular infection in man.

Suggested on-call action
None required.

Table 3.76.1 Cases and incidence of TBE in European countries

Country	Year	Number of cases	Incidence/100,000
Austria	2003	87	1.09
Czech	2003	n/a	5.9
Finland	2003	107	n/a
Germany	2003	276	n/a
Hungary	2001–2003	63 (average/year)	n/a
Latvia	2003	n/a	15.7
Lithuania	2003	763	22
Norway	2003	1	n/a
Poland	2003	339	0.89
Slovakia	2003	74	1.38
Slovenia	2003	272	13.6

Source: Strauss R *et al.*, *Eurosurveillance Weekly,* 2004, **8**(29).
n/a = not available. No cases have been reported in recent years from Denmark; the only risk area is the island of Bornholm.

Epidemiology

Toxocara canis infection is found worldwide. Infection is more common in young children. Serologic surveys in Europe show seropositivity rates of 19% in the Netherlands, 2.5% in Germany, 5.8–36% in the Czech Republic, 0–37% in Spain and 13% in the Slovak Republic.

Clinical features

Infection may be asymptomatic, and may produce the visceral larva migrans syndrome or ocular disease. Visceral larva migrans mostly occurs in younger children in association with pica. The features include fever, eosinophilia and bronchospasm and an urticarial skin rash. Hepatosplenomegaly may be present. Ocular disease is found in older children; vision may be compromised.

Laboratory confirmation

Diagnosis is based on detecting antibodies to *T. canis* larvae using an ELISA test.

Transmission

The larvae can remain dormant in dogs for long periods, migrate transplacentally and through bitches' milk to infect the pups. Most pups are infected at the time of whelping; the adult worms produce eggs until the majority are expelled when the pups are 6-months old. The eggs, which are the source of human infection, survive in the environment for many years.

Prevention and control

Toxocariasis may be controlled by regular worming of dogs and disposal of dog faeces hygienically. Contact between animal faeces and children should be minimised. No public health response is usually needed in response to cases.

3.78 Toxoplasmosis

Toxoplasma gondii is a protozoan parasite that causes a spectrum of disease from asymptomatic lymphadenopathy to congenital mental retardation, chorioretinitis and encephalitis in the immunocompromised.

Suggested on-call action
None required unless outbreak suspected.

Epidemiology

Human exposure to toxoplasmosis is worldwide and common. Twenty to forty per cent of healthy adults in developed countries are seropositive. It is more common in Mediterranean countries than in Northern Europe.

Clinical features

There are a number of clinical presentations. Acute infection is usually asymptomatic, but may produce a mononucleosis-like illness. Congenital infection may occur following acute infection during pregnancy. Congenital toxoplasmosis is characterised by foetal hepatosplenomegaly, chorioretinitis and mental retardation. In the immunocompromised, cerebral reactivation of toxoplasmosis may occur, with presentation as encephalitis.

Laboratory confirmation

Acute toxoplasmosis may be diagnosed serologically. Specific IgM antibodies appear during the first 2 weeks, peak within 4–8 weeks, and then typically become undetectable within several months. IgG antibodies rise more slowly, peak in 1–2 months, and may remain high for years.

Congenital infection requires the demonstration of IgM in neonatal blood; evidence of acute infection during pregnancy indicates the need for foetal blood sampling at 18 weeks and cord blood at delivery.

Serology is not useful for diagnosis of toxoplasmosis in patients with AIDS. Cerebral toxoplasmosis is usually diagnosed on the basis of clinical features, a positive agglutination test and CT/MRI scan appearance. Specific diagnosis in patients with AIDS and CNS symptoms requires a brain biopsy.

Transmission

The cat is the definitive host and transmits the infection through faecal shedding of oocysts. Children may come into contact with oocysts from pets, soil or sandpits. Adults are usually infected by ingestion of undercooked meat. Congenital infection usually occurs following primary infection in a pregnant woman.

Pathogenesis

The incubation period is 10–25 days. There is no person-to-person spread.

Prevention

• Pregnant women in particular should avoid raw or undercooked meat. Contact with soil or food possibly contaminated with cat faeces should be avoided.
• Chemoprophylaxis has been recommended for AIDS patients with positive IgG serology once CD4 cells are low.
• Protect sandpits and play areas from cats.

Surveillance

• Report to local public health authorities. Notifiable in some countries (Sweden, Baltic states, Hungary, Slovakia, Slovenia and, if congenital, Germany), but not UK.
• Some countries have surveillance of congenital cases.

Response to a case

Investigate likely exposure to cat faeces and raw/undercooked meat.

Investigation/control of a cluster/outbreak

As for response to case.

Suggested case definition for an outbreak

Confirmed: isolate or IgM antibody confirmed.
Clinical: acute fever and lymphadenopathy in person linked epidemiologically to confirmed case.

3.79 Tuberculosis

Tuberculosis (TB) is an infection of the lungs and/or other organs, usually by *Mycobacterium tuberculosis*, but occasionally by *M. bovis*, *M. africanum* or '*M. canettii*'. TB has a long incubation period, produces chronic disease with risk of reactivation and without treatment would often be fatal.

Suggested on-call action

If the case is a healthcare worker, teacher or another individual in contact with particularly susceptible individuals, consult the Outbreak Control Plan. However, action can usually wait until the next working day.

Epidemiology

The incidence of tuberculosis has fallen in western European countries throughout this century. In the UK the rate of decline slowed in the 1960s due to increased immigration from higher prevalence countries. Notifications have increased by about 30% from 1989 to 2003. Current rates vary 15-fold across the EU (Table 3.79.1). Rates are substantially higher in south Asia and are extremely high in much of Sub-Saharan Africa. High rates of

Table 3.79.1 Estimated TB rate in European countries for 2002

Country	Rate per 100,000
Cyprus	5
Sweden	5
Malta	6
Norway	6
Italy	8
Netherlands	8
Switzerland	8
Finland	10
Germany	10
Luxembourg	12
UK	12
Czech Republic	13
Denmark	13
Ireland	13
Belgium	14
France	14
Austria	15
Greece	20
Slovenia	21
Slovakia	24
Spain	30
Hungary	32
Poland	32
Portugal	47
Estonia	55
Lithuania	66
Latvia	78

Source: WHO.

drug-resistant TB are reported from countries of the former Soviet Union.

Within the UK, TB rates are highest in Black Africans (70 times higher than for the indigenous population in 2002), South Asians (35 times higher) and Black Caribbeans (9 times higher). Seventy per cent of cases are now in non-white groups with higher rates in those born abroad. The median time from entry to the UK to development of disease is 4 years. Rates also increase with age and, at least in whites, are higher in deprived communities. Rates are much higher in London, followed by the industrial conurbations of the Midlands, Yorkshire and Lancashire. Other risk factors for TB include HIV infection, other causes of immunosuppression, chronic alcohol misuse and socially marginalised groups such as the homeless, refugees, drug users and prisoners. In the

UK only about 4% of TB patients were thought to be HIV infected in 1998–2000. The overall TB mortality rate is around 0.7 per 100,000 population per year.

TB incidents in institutions are an increasingly recognised problem: passive surveillance in England in 2003 identified 54 incidents in healthcare premises involving potential exposure of patients to infectious staff or other patients, 26 incidents in schools and 5 in custodial settings.

Clinical features

TB is a biphasic disease. Only about 5% of whose who have primary infection develop clinically apparent primary disease, either from local progression in the lungs, or haematogenous or lymphatic spread to other sites. Such spread may lead to serious forms of the disease such as meningitis or milary TB occurring within a few months of the initial infection.

In the remaining 95%, the primary TB lesion heals without intervention, although in at least half of patients, bacilli survive in a latent form, which may then reactivate in later life. Five per cent of those originally infected will develop post-primary disease. The risk of reactivation increases with age, chronic disease and immunosuppression (e.g. HIV/AIDS). Reactivated TB is often pulmonary and, without treatment, carries a high mortality.

Two-thirds of TB in the UK is pulmonary disease, which is initially asymptomatic, although it may be detected on chest X-ray. Early symptoms may be constitutional, such as fatigue, fever, night sweats and weight loss, and often insidious in onset. Chest symptoms often occur in later disease, including cough (usually productive), haemoptysis and chest pain. Hoarseness and difficulty swallowing may occur in laryngeal TB. Symptomatic screening for cases is highly sensitive (most cases have symptoms on enquiry) but not very specific (many other diseases also cause similar symptoms). Chest X-ray has high sensitivity and medium specificity. Specificity is high for sputum smear and very high for sputum culture, but both are of only moderate sensitivity.

Table 3.79.2 Typical action in response to tuberculin testing

Test result		Interpretation and action	
Heaf grade	Mantoux* (100 units/mL)	Scar from previous BCG	No BCG scar
0/1	0–4 mm	Negative No action†	Negative Give BCG†
2	5–14 mm	Positive No action‡	Positive Investigate?‡
3/4	15 mm plus	Strongly positive Investigate	Strongly positive Investigate

* Source: JCVI, 1996.
† Unless contact of case (repeat test in 6 weeks).
‡ Will vary with age and reason for test.

Non-pulmonary TB is more common in children, ethnic minorities and those with impaired immunity. The most commonly affected sites are lymph nodes, pleura, genito-urinary system and bones and joints. Constitutional or local systems may be reported. Diagnosis may be supported by tuberculin test and biopsy results: Over 90% of non-AIDS cases are tuberculin test positive (Table 3.79.2). New blood tests, such as ELISPOT or QuantiFERON may offer some advantages over tuberculin testing in vaccinated populations or in areas with high exposure to environmental mycobacteria, but their exact role is yet to be clarified.

Laboratory confirmation

Rapid presumptive diagnosis of infectious cases can be achieved by microscopy of sputum (preferably early morning) samples: *M. tuberculosis, M. bovis* and *M. africanum* all stain poorly with Gram stain, but staining with Ziehl–Neelson (ZN) stain reveals acid-fast (and alcohol-fast) bacilli (AFB). Many laboratories now use an auramine stain, which is more sensitive than ZN. As a general rule, sufficient bacilli in the sputum to be detectable by standard methods equates to sufficient to be infectious and three consecutive negative sputum smears is usually assumed to represent non-infectiousness. Although this test is usually sufficient to begin treatment and contact tracing, follow-up culture (preferably liquid culture) is essential as AFBs may occasionally be other species of Mycobacteria (see Box 3.79.1), culture also increases the sensitivity of diagnosis for cases of lower infectivity and allows antibiotic sensitivities to be checked.

In 2002, 7.7% of isolates of *M. tuberculosis* in the UK were resistant to at least one

---

Box 3.79.1 Mycobacteria other than tuberculosis (MOTT)

• Also known as atypical, environmental, anonymous, non-tuberculous, tuberculoid or opportunistic.
• Includes *M. avium, M. intracellulare* and *M. scrofulaceum* (collectively known as *M. avium* complex). Also includes *M. kansasii, M. malmoense, M. marinum, M. xenopi, M. fortuitum, M. chelonae, M. absessus, M. haemophilium, M. marinarum, M. paratuberculose, M. simiae,* and *M. ulcerans.*
• Common environmental contaminants. Occasionally found in water supplies, swimming pools or milk. Some cause nosocomial infections. Person-to-person spread rare.
• Rarely causes disease in immunocompetent individuals. *M. avium* complex and some others may cause disseminated disease in those with AIDS.

first-line drug and 1.1% were multidrug resistant ('MDR'). Culture and sensitivity testing has routinely taken around 6–12 weeks, but rapid culturing at reference laboratories may reduce this to 30 days. New molecular techniques may reduce this wait to 3–4 days when results are urgent. Genotyping is useful in identifying and investigating clusters of cases and should ideally be introduced into routine surveillance and control.

Transmission

Almost all TB in Europe is contracted by inhalation of *M. tuberculosis* bacilli in droplet nuclei. These nuclei derive from humans with pulmonary or laryngeal TB predominantly by coughing, although sneezing, singing and prolonged talking may contribute. Such nuclei may remain suspended in air for long periods. The risk of transmission depends upon the amount of bacilli in the sputum, the nature of the cough, the closeness and duration of the interaction and the susceptibility of the contact (Box 3.79.2). Without treatment, an average case of pulmonary TB would infect 10–15 people per year.

Bovine TB may be contracted by ingestion of raw milk from infected cows and occasionally via the air-borne route. Although *M. bovis* has increased in cattle in the UK and some other European countries in recent years, most human cases probably represent reactivation of infection acquired before routine treatment of milk supplies and testing of cattle.

Direct transmission, either through cuts in the skin or traumatic inoculation (e.g. prosector's wart) is now rare. Droplet aerosols may be generated in healthcare settings from surgical dressing of skin lesions, autopsy, bronchoscopy and intubation.

Acquisition

The incubation period, as defined by reaction to a tuberculin test, is usually 3–8 weeks (occasionally up to 12 weeks). The latent period may be many decades.

The infectious period is for as long as there are viable organisms in the sputum: cases are usually considered infectious if organisms demonstrable on sputum smear. Appropriate chemotherapy renders most patients non-infectious in 2 weeks.

Acquisition of an infective dose usually requires prolonged exposure and/or multiple aerosol inoculae, although some strains appear to be more infectious.

Immunity usually occurs after primary infection and involves several responses, including delayed-type hypersensitivity, the basis of the tuberculin test. Conditions such as AIDS, which affect cellular immunity, increase the risk of disease. Other risks are given in Box 3.79.2.

Prevention

Control of TB in developed countries has a number of components:
• Limitation of infectiousness by targeted case finding and early treatment.
• Limitation of antimicrobial resistance by multidrug therapy (e.g. British Thoracic Society guidelines) and measures to maximise compliance, such as directly observed therapy (DOTS) and patient-centred case-management, particularly in socially marginalised groups and those already identified as having drug-resistant infection. TB outcome surveillance is important to assess the effectiveness of control services.
• Identification and treatment of further cases by contact tracing in response to notifications of TB (see Chapter 4.9). Up to 10% of clinical cases in the UK are found by this method. In addition, potentially latently infected individuals can be offered chemoprophylaxis and non-immune contacts offered BCG immunisation.
• BCG vaccine was found to have an efficacy against TB of about 75%, lasting at least 15 years in British schoolchildren. It should offer similar protection against drug-resistant strains. Vaccination is recommended in the UK (provided the individual has no BCG scar, is tuberculin test negative and has no other contraindications) for:

Box 3.79.2 How to assess the likelihood of transmission of TB

1 How infectous is the source case?
- Sputum smear positive: infectious to any close contact.
- Smear negative, culture positive: possibly infectious to highly susceptible contacts.
- Sputum negative, bronchial washing positive: possibly infectious to highly susceptible contacts.
- Three consecutive sputum negatives: not infectious.
- Two weeks *appropriate* treatment: not infectious.
- Non-pulmonary/laryngeal disease: not infectious.
- Children, even if smear positive, are less infectious than adults.

2 How great is the exposure?
- Exposure to coughing is the most important risk, but sneezing, singing and long (more than 5 minutes) conversation can result in exposure to many infectious droplets.
- Prolonged or multiple indoor exposure usually needed to infect most contacts.
- Aerosols may persist after case leaves room.
- Dishes, laundry, etc., not infectious.
- Estimates of risk from specific exposures to infectious case in one review (although there may be reporting bias inflating some of these figures):
  Household: 1 in 3
  Dormitory: 1 in 5
  Bar or social club: up to 1 in 10
  Nursing home: 1 in 20
  School or workplace: 1 in 50 to 1 in 3
  Casual social contact: 1 in 100,000
  Background rate: 1 in 100,000

3 How susceptible is the contact to infection and disease?
- Susceptibility by age
  Neonates: Very high
  Age under 3 years: High
- BCG reduces risk by 50–80% in developed countries.
- Immunosuppressed at very high risk: includes AIDS, lymphoma, leukaemia, cancer chemotherapy and oral corticosteroids (equivalent to 15 mg prednisolone per day)
- Severe malnutrition leads to increased risk. Post-gastrectomy or jejunal-ileal bypass patients at risk if underweight.
- Silicosis or drug abuse increased risk.
- Diabetics and those with chronic renal failure have increased risk of reactivation of latent disease.

(i) schoolchildren between the ages of 10 and 14 years (may be discontinued).

(ii) higher risk occupations, e.g. those working in healthcare premises, prisons or certain hostels.

(iii) immigrants, students and refugees from high prevalence countries.

(iv) children born in the UK to ethnic minorities with links to high prevalence countries (e.g. Indian subcontinent or Africa, but not the West Indies) within a few days of birth.

(v) children born to families with a history of TB.

(vi) travellers to higher prevalence countries planning to stay over 1 month.

(vii) contacts of cases of active pulmonary disease.

- BCG is not recommended in many European countries.
- Screening of immigrants and refugees from high prevalence countries for active disease, latent infection and lack of immunity maybe offered as part of a total health package in their new district of residence, although the value of this has been questioned. Such individuals can be identified from a combination of Port Health forms, GP registers, school registers, refugee hostels and community groups.
- Infection control and occupational health services in hospitals to reduce exposure of patients to infected healthcare workers or potentially infectious patients, with particular care in units dealing with immunocompromised patients and units likely to admit patients with TB.
- Those contacts with evidence of infection (tuberculin test) but not disease can be protected by isoniazid prophylaxis to prevent later disease. Prophylaxis is also recommended for young children who are contacts of an infectious case of TB, even if tuberculin negative.

Surveillance

- All forms of clinical TB are notifiable in almost every European country, including the UK.
- The two main sources of surveillance data are notifications of clinical cases from clinicians (such as respiratory physicians) and positive reports from microbiology laboratories. Other potential sources are pathologists (histology and autopsy), surgeons and pharmacists. Reliance on only one source will lead to incomplete ascertainment.
- District TB registers are useful and may include data on
  (i) age, sex, ethnicity, country of birth, place of residence.
  (ii) type of disease, sputum status, antibiotic sensitivities.
  (iii) treatment outcome.

- Enhanced surveillance of TB was introduced into the UK in 1999. District co-ordinators collect a standardised dataset on all new cases, which is forwarded to regional and national databases.
- The 'EuroTB' programme collects data on TB from national centres throughout Europe. However, reporting systems differ substantially between contributing countries, making comparisons difficult.

Response to a case

- All TB cases should be notified to local public health departments.
- Investigate whether infectious by three early morning sputum samples for microscopy and culture.
- Ensure isolate tested for drug resistance.
- Early treatment with standard multidrug therapy. Consider appropriate measures to maximise compliance.
- Most cases can be treated at home: there is no need to segregate cases from other household members, unless they are neonates or immunocompromised.
- Those treated in hospital who are smear positive (or pulmonary or laryngeal disease with results pending) should be segregated in a single room, preferably with measures to reduce airflow to other patient areas. Particular care is needed in units containing immunocompromised patients or if the case is suspected to have drug-resistant TB.
- Adults with smear-negative disease, non-pulmonary disease or those who have been on appropriate treatment for 2 weeks do not require isolation. Persons visiting children with TB in hospital (one of whom may be the source case) should be segregated from other hospital patients until they have been screened.
- Screen household contacts of cases of pulmonary disease. Contacts of non-pulmonary cases need only be screened if the case is thought to have been recently infected (e.g. a young child).

• Casual contacts need only be screened if the case is smear positive and either

    (i) the contact is unusually susceptible to TB (e.g. young child or immunocompromised adult) or

    (ii) the case appears to be highly infectious (e.g. more than 10% of contacts infected).

• The recommendations of the British Thoracic Society for investigation and management of contacts are shown in Figure 3.79.1.

• Check that the index case and any secondary cases are not healthcare workers, teachers or others who work with susceptible people (see 3.79.3).

Investigation of a cluster

• Aim is to discover whether there is an unrecognised infectious source.

• Check diagnosis of cases. Are they confirmed microbiologically? Beware the occasional 'pseudo-outbreak' (e.g. if all cases confirmed by same laboratory).

• Liaise with reference laboratory for genotyping of all isolates to look for potentially linked cases.

• Any clinical or epidemiological clues as to whether cases have recent or old infection?

    (i) Age and previous residence abroad.

    (ii) Clinical and radiological signs.

    (iii) Risk factors for new infection (e.g. contact with case or travel to high prevalence country)?

    (iv) Risk factors for reactivation (e.g. diabetes, renal failure)?

• Obtain microbiological samples on all non-confirmed cases.

• Undertake hypothesis-generating study. Include family links, social networks, leisure and hobbies, links to institutions, especially those containing highly susceptible individuals and/or overcrowding (hospitals, nursing homes, schools, jail, homeless hostels) and for travel to (or visitor from) a high prevalence country.

• Check drug sensitivities and compliance with treatment for known respiratory cases associated with cluster.

Control of an outbreak

• Undertake contact tracing for known cases to identify and treat undiscovered infectious cases (and others with infection or disease who would benefit from treatment).

• In outbreaks linked to hospitals

    1 look for an unsuspected infectious source, e.g.

        patient with MDR TB remaining infectious despite prolonged therapy (check sensitivity results).

        smear negative cases infecting highly susceptible contacts (check culture results).

        delayed diagnosis in AIDS cases (do not rely on classic clinical picture).

        healthcare worker, patient or visitor with undiagnosed TB (chronic cough unresponsive to antibiotics?).

    2 consider breakdown in infection control procedures, e.g.

        procedures such as bronchoscopy, sputum induction and pentamidine inhalation may generate aerosols.

        inadequate isolation of sputum positive patients.

        inadequate decontamination of multiuse equipment.

Suggested case definition for use in an outbreak

Confirmed: clinically compatible illness with demonstration of infection with outbreak genotype.

Probable: culture or PCR positive or demonstration of acid-fast bacilli with clinically compatible illness and epidemiological link, but no genotype available.

Clinical: clinical diagnosis leading to initiation of antituberculous therapy in individual with epidemiological link to outbreak.

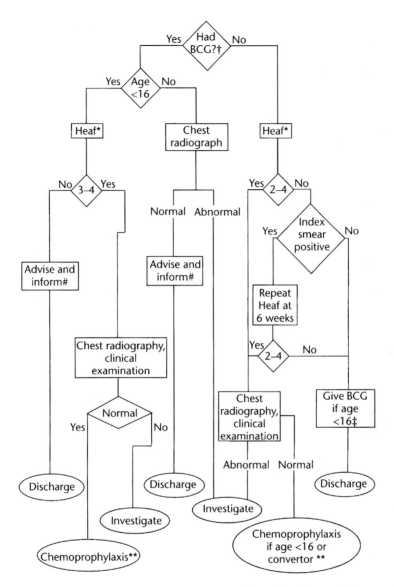

Fig. 3.79.1 Control and prevention of tuberculosis in the United Kingdom. Contact tracing: examination of close contacts of patients with pulmonary tuberculosis. Contacts of patients with non-pulmonary tuberculosis need not usually be examined. Note: children under 2 years who have not had a BCG vaccination and who are close contacts of a smear positive index patient should receive chemoprophylaxis irrespective of tuberculin status. †Previous BCG vaccination cannot be accepted as evidence of immunity in HIV-infected subjects. *A negative test in immunocompromised subjects does not exclude tuberculous infection. #Advise patient of tuberculosis symptoms and inform GP of contact. **Persons eligible for, but not given, chemoprophylaxis should have follow-up chest radiographs at 3 and 12 months. ‡See BTS guidelines. From the Joint Tuberculosis Committee of the British Thoracic Society, *Thorax*, 2000; **55**: 887–901, with permission.

Box 3.79.3 How to manage specific TB scenarios

1 If the case is a healthcare worker with patient contact (or a patient found to have TB after admission onto an open ward):
- Decide how infectious the case is:
  respiratory or laryngeal TB?
  cough or cavities on chest X-ray?
  sputum smear and/or culture positive?
  results of screening of close contacts?
- Decide how long case has been infectious, in particular duration of cough.
- If case thought to be infectious, convene Incident Management Team including:
  hospital control of infection staff,
  senior hospital manager,
  local public health officer (CCDC),
  physician with expertise in TB,
  contact tracing services (TB Health Visitor),
  medical records manager,
  manager of affected ward/unit,
  occupational health and
  press officer
- Draw up list of contacts. Consider:
  inpatients, outpatients, referrals from other consultants; other members of staff.
  classifying contacts by level of exposure (e.g. patients for which case was 'named nurse' could be classified higher exposure and other patients on ward as lower exposure).
- Decide whether any of these contacts are particularly susceptible to TB (see Box 3.79.2):
  ask medical and nursing staff who treat them;
  review case notes.
- Organise screening of highly susceptible contacts (remember incubation period of up to 2 months since last contact with case).
- Write to GPs of other contacts so that exposure is noted.
- Consider need for helpline and press release for worried patients.
- Reconsider actions when results of screening and culture results are known.

2 If case is a teacher or pupil at a school:
- Consider teacher potentially infectious even if only sputum culture positive (smear negative). Screen all children in relevant teaching groups (including games) and close staff contacts.
- Although children are rarely infectious, if child case is sputum smear positive, screen other children in same year.
- If more than one child infected, screen staff. Also consider potential staff source if no further cases found in screening household of child.

3 If the case has recently travelled on an aircraft:
- Check if patient sputum smear and culture positive.
- Was flight within last 3 months and over 8 hours in duration?
- Did the passenger have a cough at time of flight?
- If criteria above are satisfied, ask airline to identify passengers in the same compartment of the aircraft and contact them by letter.
- Letter to recommend passengers contact their own doctor and give a central telephone number for advice.
- Inform public health authorities for areas with affected passengers.

3.80 Tularaemia

Tularaemia (rabbit fever, deer-fly fever, Ohara disease, Francis disease) is a zoonotic disease caused by an infection with the bacteria *Francisella tularensis* normally transmitted to humans from animal hosts. It is also a potential bioterrorism agent.

Suggested on-call action
None usually required.

Epidemiology

Tularaemia is endemic in many parts of the world, including Eastern Europe, Scandinavia, North America, China and Japan. Large outbreaks in Europe were recently reported from Northern Europe (Finland in 2000 and Sweden in 2003) and the Balkans (e.g. Kosovo in 2000 and 2002).

Clinical features

A variety of clinical manifestations may occur (ulceroglandular, oropharyngeal, oculoglandular, pneumonic, septicaemic and typhoidal). They depend on the portal of entry into the human body. Symptoms include high fever, body aches, swollen lymph glands and difficulty in swallowing. Fatal outcomes are rare in Europe. Fatalities occur mainly from typhoidal or pulmonary disease. With appropriate antibiotic treatment, the case-fatality rate is negligible.

Laboratory confirmation

Diagnosis is mostly made clinically and confirmed by a rise in specific serum antibodies. Those are usually detectable after 2 weeks of the illness. Cross reactions with *Brucella* species occur. Two biovars can cause human disease. Type A are more virulent than type B (case-fatality rate 5–15% versus <1%). Type B strains occur across northern Europe and Russia, the more severe type A is generally restricted to North America.

Transmission

Tularaemia is a zoonosis; reservoirs include wild rabbits, hares and muskrats as well as some domestic animals and ticks. The most prevalent modes of transmission includes arthropod bites, drinking water or food contaminated by rodents, handling of under-cooked infected meat or inhalation of dust from contaminated hay. In Sweden and Finland, it is believed that tularaemia is transmitted to humans and animals via mosquitoes.

Acquisition

The incubation period varies depending on virulence of infecting strain and size of inoculum. It is usually 3–5 days, but may be as long as 2 weeks. The infectious dose is low and depends upon the portal of entry and the type of *F. tularensis*: approximately 10–50 type A organisms may cause infection by the inhalational route. Person-to-person transmission has not been reported.

Prevention

Health education to
• avoid tick bites;
• avoid untreated potentially contaminated water;
• ensure meat from rodents is cooked thoroughly.

Surveillance

• Tularaemia is notifiable in many countries (not UK).

• Cases should be reported to the Public Health Authorities so that assessments of risk can be made.
• Severe unexplained cases of sepsis or respiratory disease in otherwise healthy individuals should be reported to local public health authorities.

Response to a case

No public health action usually necessary.

Investigation of a cluster

• Search for a common source of infection related to arthropods, animal hosts, water or food.
• Consider deliberate release if two or more suspected cases linked in time and place or single confirmed case if either not explained by occupational risk or travel to endemic area.

Control of an outbreak

• Investigate and control identified source.
• Emphasise prevention.

Response to a deliberate release

• Report to local and national public health authorities.
• Define exposed zone and identify individuals exposed within it (some may have left scene).
• Cordon off exposed zone.
• Decontaminate those exposed: remove clothing and possessions, then shower with soap and water.
• Chemoprophylaxis (currently ciprofloxacin) as soon as possible for those exposed.
• Record contact details for all those exposed.
• Some health and emergency workers may also need prophylaxis.
• Police may take environmental samples.
• More general information in Chapter 4.14 and specific advice on HPA website.

Suggested case definition
Compatible clinical illness with laboratory confirmation of tularaemia.

3.81 Typhoid fever

Typhoid fever is a severe systemic infection caused by *Salmonella typhi*. A clinically similar, though usually less severe, illness may be caused by *S. paratyphi* (see Chapter 3.55). The collective name for these conditions is enteric fever.

Suggested on-call action
• Exclude cases and contacts who are food handlers or in other risk groups (see below).

Epidemiology

Infection occurs worldwide and is associated with poor sanitation. In underdeveloped countries the incidence of infection is around 50/100,000 per year and is more common in summer. This compares with around 200 cases a year in England and Wales most of which are imported, often from the Indian subcontinent.

Clinical features

The illness begins with fever; rigors may occur. Patients complain of headache, cough, malaise, myalgia and may be constipated. Later in the course diarrhoea, abdominal tenderness, vomiting, delirium and confusion may occur. A few inconspicuous pale red spots (rose spots), scattered over the trunk, are seen in less than 20% of cases and are undetectable in pigmented skin. The spleen may be enlarged and abdominal tenderness is common but not severe.

Complications typically arise in the third week. In the abdomen, ulceration of Peyer's patches may result in haemorrhage (1.7%) or intestinal perforation (1–4%). DIC and renal failure occur in severe cases. Osteomyelitis may develop, especially in those predisposed by sickle cell disease. Other rare complications include cholecystitis, meningitis and typhoid pneumonia. Relapses occur in 5–10% of cases, and may be more common following antibiotic treatment.

Laboratory confirmation

Definitive diagnosis of typhoid is by culture of the organism from a normally sterile site (e.g. blood). Blood, urine and faeces should be cultured; faeces are usually positive after the first week of illness and results should be available in 72 hours. Culture of a bone marrow aspirate may be positive when there is no growth from other sites. The Widal agglutination test detects antibody to the somatic 'O', flagellar 'H' and Vi antigens of typhoid bacilli. Acute and convalescent sera may provide a retrospective diagnosis when a fourfold rise in titre occurs. Interpretation of a single high positive (for rapid diagnosis) is difficult. Phage typing may be available for unexplained clusters.

Transmission

Infection results from the ingestion of water or food contaminated by faeces from a human case or occasionally, an asymptomatic carrier; this includes fruit or vegetables washed in water contaminated by sewage, and shellfish. Water-borne outbreaks may occur. Direct person-to-person spread is possible in poor hygienic conditions and, rarely, between homosexual men. Urinary carriers are rare in developed countries. *S. typhi* is extremely infectious; infection may occur with ingestion of fewer than 100,000 organisms. Achlorhydria and disturbance of bowel flora (e.g. by antibiotics) decrease the minimum infective dose.

Splenectomy (e.g. in sickle cell disease, or immune defects) makes it more difficult to eradicate *S. typhi*.

Acquisition

The incubation period ranges from 1 to 3 weeks. The infectious period lasts as long as bacilli are present in the stool. This usually begins in the first week of illness; approximately 10% of patients will be excreting bacilli 3 months after the onset. Approximately 3% of persons infected with *S. typhi* become chronic carriers; this carrier state may last many years and is more common in females and those with gallbladder disease.

Prevention

- Sanitation, clean water and personal hygiene.
- Vaccination has had a limited effect as a control measure, although it provides useful protection in individuals. Vaccination is recommended for travellers to endemic countries, including those visiting their country of origin.

Surveillance

- Typhoid is notifiable in most countries, including the UK.
- Report on clinical suspicion to local public health authorities.

Response to a case

- Check antibiotic resistance of isolate.
- Enteric precautions and hygiene advice for cases; isolation if hospitalised.
- Obtain food and travel history for the 3 weeks prior to onset of illness.
- Cases who have not visited an endemic country in the 3 weeks before onset should be investigated to determine the source of infection.

- Investigate household and other close contacts with a faecal specimen for culture. If positive, treat as case.
- Do not treat contacts in groups at risk for further transmission (Box 2.2.1) as negative until three consecutive negatives taken at weekly intervals commencing 3 weeks after last exposure to case. Exclude contacts who are food handlers until these results are known. Exclude others until formed stools for 48 hours and hygiene advice given.
- Quinolones may reduce the period of carriage in those for whom exclusion is producing social difficulties.
- Exclude cases who are
  food handlers (Box 2.2.1: risk group 1) until six consecutive negative stool specimens taken at one week intervals and commencing 3 weeks after completion of antibiotic therapy.
  Health/social care workers, children aged under 5 years and cases with poor personal hygiene (risk groups 2, 3 and 4) until three consecutive negative faecal samples taken at weekly intervals, commencing 3 weeks after completion of treatment.
- Exclude all other cases until clinically well for 48 hours with formed stools and hygiene advice given.
- Exclude contacts in risk groups 1–4 until two negative faecal specimens taken 48 hours apart and hygiene advice given.

Investigation of a cluster

- Investigate to ensure that secondary transmission has not occurred.
- Most clusters in developed countries will result from exposure to a common source abroad, or transmission within close family groups.
- Chains of transmission can be investigated through phage typing.

Control of an outbreak

- Outbreaks should be investigated as a matter of urgency.

- All cases and contacts should be investigated to identify the source of the outbreak.
- This could be due to contact with a chronic carrier, with faecal material, or with contaminated food, milk, water or shellfish.
- Contacts should be observed and investigated if they develop symptoms suggestive of typhoid after appropriate specimens are taken.

Suggested case definition

Probable: a clinically compatible case epidemiologically linked to a confirmed case in an outbreak.

3.82 Typhus, other rickettsial infections and ehrlichiosis

Rickettsia are small bacteria that replicate only intracellularly. Transmission is by means of an arthropod vector. The natural host is typically a rodent. Only epidemic typhus is primarily a disease of man. Ehrlichiosis is a recently recognised pathogen (in the USA) that causes an illness similar to the spotted rickettsioses. Transmission is probably tick-borne. There is no person-to-person spread.

Diagnosis

Following an infected arthropod bite, replication of the organism at the site may give rise to a characteristic skin lesion, a small painless ulcer with a black centre, called an eschar. The infection then becomes generalised and there is a fever; which in more severe infections is high and unremitting. If there is a rash, it appears around the fourth or fifth day of illness and may have either a dusky macular appearance or be petechial. In the most serious infections, multiple organ damage may develop, usually towards the end of the second week.

Table 3.82.1 Main diseases cause by Rickettsiae and Ehrlichiae

Disease and organism	Incubation period	Mode of transmission and epidemiology	Clinical
Epidemic typhus (louse-borne typhus) R. prowazeki	1–2 weeks	Natural reservoir: rodents. The illness reaches humans via infected dogs and their ticks. Transmitted directly between humans by the human body louse, which feeds on the body but lays its eggs in clothing. Now principally a disease of tropical highlands such as Ethiopia and the Andes. Infestation tends to occur where poverty and a cold climate coincide.	The illness is relatively mild in children; mortality increases with age; untreated, about 50% of 50-year-olds will die. There is no eschar, but there is usually a rash, often petechial. The high fever may be associated with severe headache, vomiting and epistaxis. Complications include diminished consciousness, pneumonia and renal failure.
Trench fever R. quintana	1–2 weeks	Louse borne.	Resembles epidemic typhus, but milder. The rash may be macular or maculopapular.
Murine typhus R typhi	1–2 weeks	Transmitted from rats to man by fleas. It occurs worldwide, but particularly in tropical Asia.	Resembles epidemic typhus, but milder.
Rocky mountain spotted fever R. rickettsii	3–14 days	Various reservoir hosts are described; rodents most significant. The principal vector is the dog tick, bringing the risk of infection close to humans. North American disease, occurs widely in the eastern US as well as in the Rocky Mountains.	It is a severe illness. The rash is typically petechial and complications, including pneumonia and myocarditis, are common. Untreated, the mortality is around 20%.
Boutonneuse fever R. conorii	5–8 days	Similar tick typhus syndromes, caused by R. conorii or its close relatives, occur in the Mediterranean, Asia, Australia and Brazil.	An eschar is usual, sometimes with regional lymphadenopathy, and a macular rash may occur. Fatality is rare.
Rickettsialpox R. akari	1–2 weeks	Transmitted naturally between rodents by mites. Man is usually infected in recently cleared ground where the mites abound in South and East Asia and in parts of Queensland, Australia. Also reported from Russia, eastern US and South Africa.	Disseminated vesicular rash that may be confused with chickenpox. Fatality is low.
Scrub typhus R. tsutsugamushi	6–21 days	Mite scrub typhus occurs over a vast area, including Japan, China, the Philippines, New Guinea, Indonesia, other islands of the southwest Pacific Ocean, southeastern Asia, northern Australia, India, Sri Lanka, Pakistan, Russia and Korea.	Only fever, headache and swollen lymph nodes and in some cases myalgia, gastrointestinal complaints or cough. Mortality about 5% untreated.
Ehrlichiosis (1) E chaffeensis	3–4 weeks	Transmission follows when the deer ticks bite human skin and inoculate organisms. Found in the US.	Illness similar to rocky mountain spotted fever.
Ehrlichiosis (2) E sennetsu	14 days	Found in US, Japan and Malaysia.	Illness similar to rocky mountain spotted fever.

Rickettsial infection should be considered if there is fever with either the typical rash or an eschar and an appropriate travel history. Diagnosis is usually clinical. To confirm serologically use assays that detect antibodies to rickettsial antigens (where available) such as the indirect fluorescence antibody test or latex agglutination rather than the non-specific, insensitive Weil–Felix test. PCR may be available.

Prevention and control

Tick-borne disease can be prevented by reducing the incidence of tick bite through wearing long trousers, tucking trouser legs into socks and using repellents (those containing permethrin can be sprayed on boots and clothing; those containing DEET (*N,N*-diethyl-*m*-toluamide) can be applied to the skin); conducting a body check and removing any ticks found. To remove attached ticks use fine-tipped tweezers or fingers shielded with a tissue, paper towel or rubber gloves. Grasp the tick as close to the skin as possible and pull upward with steady, even pressure, twisting may cause the mouthparts to break off and remain in the skin (If this happens, remove with tweezers). The tick (saliva, hemolymph, gut) may contain infectious organisms therefore do not squeeze or handle the tick with bare hands. After removing the tick disinfect the bite site and wash hands with soap and water.

For a louse-borne disease epidemic delousing measures with changing of clothes and impregnation with insecticide may be necessary.

Typhus is formally notifiable in many countries, including the UK.

3.83 *Vibrio parahaemolyticus*

Vibrio parahaemolyticus causes a gastrointestinal infection that is particularly associated with consumption of contaminated seafood.

> **Suggested on-call action**
>
> If you or reporting clinician/microbiologist know of other cases then consult Local Outbreak Plan.

Epidemiology

V. parahaemolyticus food poisoning is rare in north and west Europe, e.g. 20–25 cases per annum are reported in England and Wales. It is, however, responsible for over half of foodborne disease in Japan in summer months and is also relatively common during the summer in coastal areas of the US, the Caribbean, Bangladesh and Southeast Asia. Most cases in the UK are in travellers returning from warmer countries. All ages are affected.

Clinical features

Characterised by explosive watery diarrhoea, usually accompanied by abdominal cramps. Nausea, vomiting and headache are common. Fever and chills occur in a minority of cases as may bloody diarrhoea. The illness usually lasts 1–7 days (median of 3 days). Death is rare but may occur in very young children or elderly people with underlying disease.

Laboratory confirmation

Diagnosis is dependent upon isolation of the organism from culture of stool specimen or rectal swabs on selective media (i.e., warn the laboratory if organism suspected). Almost all pathogenic *V. parahaemolyticus* are 'Kanagawa-positive' (complete lysis of human erythrocytes) but most environmental isolates (and *V. cholerae*) are 'Kanagawa-negative'.

The organism may also be cultured from food: at least 10^3 organisms per gram would be expected. There are numerous serotypes but isolates from both food and faeces often contain a mixture of types.

Transmission

V. parahaemolyticus is ubiquitous in coastal waters of temperate and tropical countries (demonstrated in both the UK and the Netherlands). During the warm season (water >10°C), the organism is found in water, fish and shellfish.

Transmission to humans is food-borne via consumption of raw or undercooked seafood (particularly in Japan), or food contaminated after cooking, e.g. by washing with seawater. The organism multiplies rapidly at room temperature: most outbreaks appear to involve food being held for several hours without refrigeration, allowing formation of an infective dose. Fresh shellfish imported into Europe from Asia has been contaminated in the past.

The organism is killed by temperatures of 80°C for 15 minutes and refrigeration is effective at controlling multiplication.

Acquisition

The incubation period is dependent upon the ingested dose: extremes of 4–96 hours have been reported, with the median for most outbreaks being 13–23 hours. The organism is non-communicable between humans. The minimum infectious dose is 10^6 organisms; despite this, there is usually a high attack rate in common source outbreaks. Immunity does not appear to develop in response to infection.

Prevention

• Cook seafood so that all parts reach 80°C for 15 minutes, or irradiate before eating raw.
• Avoid cross-contamination from raw seafood in kitchen. Do not use raw seawater to wash food.

Surveillance

Report to local public health departments (notify as 'suspected food poisoning' in UK) and to national surveillance systems.

Response to a case

• Obtain details from case on foods consumed in 48 hours before onset, (especially seafood) and any history of travel.
• Although person-to-person transmission unusual, UK guidelines suggest cases in risk groups 1–4 (Table 2.2.1) excluded from work/school for 48 hours after first normal stool.

Investigation of a cluster

• Plot epidemic curve: if all cases within 48 hours then single exposure likely. If not, assume continuing source as secondary spread unlikely.
• Obtain food (especially seafood) and travel/recreation history for 48 hours before onset of each case.
• Organise laboratory testing of suspect foods.

Control of an outbreak

• Identify and rectify any of the following faults:
  (i) processes risking undercooking of seafood;
  (ii) processes risking cross-contamination from seafood;
  (iii) consumption of raw seafood without adequate temperature control;
  (iv) use of raw seawater.
• Reinforce food hygiene and handwashing.
• Report any suspected commercially produced food to relevant authority, e.g. Food Standards Agency in UK.

Suggested case definition
Confirmed: diarrhoea or abdominal cramps with *V. parahaemolyticus* identified in stool sample.
Clinical: watery diarrhoea and abdominal pain with onset 4–48 hours after exposure to suspect meal.

3.84 Viral haemorrhagic fevers

Viral haemorrhagic fevers (VHF) are severe, life-threatening viral infections of high mortality that commonly present with haemorrhagic manifestations. They are endemic in a number of parts of the world: Africa, South America and some parts of Asia, the Middle East and Eastern Europe. About 35 cases of VHF have been reported in England and Wales over the past 10 years. The environmental conditions in the UK and Western Europe do not support the natural reservoirs or vectors of these diseases. The risk of epidemic spread in the general population is negligible.

There is a risk of secondary infection from four types of VHF (Lassa, Ebola, Marburg and Crimean/Congo haemorrhagic fevers), particularly among those who might be exposed to body fluids, particularly from needlestick injury or by contamination of broken skin or mucous membranes. High rates of secondary disease in those caring for cases in developing countries have been reported.

Suggested on-call action

- Undertake risk assessment.
- Contact Infectious Disease Unit and discuss with consultant.
- Ensure malaria excluded.
- Ensure clinical case is isolated, if appropriate arrange transfer to high security unit with special expertise.
- Ensure precautions in place for body fluids.
- Identify contacts and place under observation.
- Arrange press contact details.

Epidemiology

Each of the viruses grouped together here have a different epidemiology (Table 3.84.1). They are found in rural areas.

Other haemorrhagic fevers caused by viruses that may be imported from the tropics and present with haemorrhagic manifestations; these include Rift Valley fever (central, east and southern Africa, spread by mosquitoes), Omsk (Siberia), Kyasanur (Southwest India, spread by ticks). Korean, Hantaan (Asia, Europe, Scandinavia, Kenya), Argentinian (rural areas), Bolivian (rural north east), Venezuelan, Brazilian (Amazonian region) are transmitted through excreta from rodents.

Surveillance

- VHFs are notifiable in most countries, including the UK.
- Local and national public health authorities should be informed of cases immediately on clinical suspicion.

Response to a case

- Many countries have specific guidelines for responding to a case or suspect case (in England and Wales the Guidelines of the Advisory Committee on Dangerous Pathogens; see Appendix 2).
- Strict infection control precautions are required to protect those who may be exposed.
- In England and Wales the Control of Substances Hazardous to Health (COSHH) Regulations 1994 require employers to assess risks to employees and others in the workplace including, when appropriate, an assessment of the risk of VHF infection occurring at work.

Patient assessment and risk categorisation

VHF should be considered in any patient presenting with a pyrexia of unknown origin (PUO) shortly after having returned from abroad, in most cases this can be dismissed on epidemiological grounds, most patients suspected of VHF will be suffering from malaria. Laboratory tests to exclude or confirm malaria should be undertaken as soon as possible for minimum and moderate risk patients. A checklist of enquiries to help

Table 3.84.1 Transmissible VHFs

Virus	Lassa fever virus	Ebola	Marburg	Crimean-Congo haemorrhagic fever [CCHF]
Family	Arenaviridae	Filoviridae	Filoviridae	Nairovirus
Epidemiology	Rural areas of west Africa	Rural areas of W and Central Africa	Exposure of laboratory workers to body fluids of tissues from African Green monkeys from Uganda.	Africa, Asia, former USSR and SE Europe.
Reservoir/transmission	Multi-mammate rat	Not known: Monkey? Primate?	Monkey?	Tick borne.
Clinical diagnosis	Gradual onset, malaise, fever, sore throat. Pharyngeal exudates common. Hypotension and shock. Albuminuria	Sudden onset, malaise, fever, myalgia, diarrhoea. Hypotension and shock.	Sudden onset, malaise, fever, myalgia, diarrhoea. Hypotension and shock.	Sudden onset, malaise, fever, headache, anorexia. Petechial rash, purpura.
Case-fatality rate	15–20% case fatality rate for hospitalised cases	50–90% case fatality rate for hospitalised cases.	50–90% case fatality rate for hospitalised cases.	2–50% case fatality rate for hospitalised cases.
Laboratory diagnosis	Virus can be isolated from blood, urine, and throat washings. IgM may be detectable by ELISA or IFA Specimens must be handled in a Category 4 laboratory	IgG detection by IFA, ELISA, Western blot viral nucleic acid detection in skin snip Specimens must be handled in a Category 4 laboratory	IgG detection by IFA, ELISA, Western blot Viral nucleic acid detection in skin snip Specimens must be handled in a Category 4 laboratory	Virus can be isolated from blood, urine, and throat washings. IgM may be detectable by ELISA or IFA Specimens must be handled in a Category 4 laboratory
Transmission	Person-to-person transmission via contact with bodily secretions (including sexual contact).	Person-to-person transmission via contact with bodily secretions (including sexual contact).	Person-to-person transmission via contact with bodily secretions (including sexual contact).	Person-to-person transmission via contact with bodily secretions (including sexual contact). Butchering infected animals
Incubation period:	6–21 days	2–21 days	3–9 days	3–12 days.
Infectious period:	Virus is present in body secretions, including the pharynx during the acute illness, and may be excreted in the urine for 2–3 months	Virus is present in body secretions, including the pharynx during the acute illness, may be excreted in semen for 2–3 months	Virus is present in body secretions during the acute illness.	Virus is present in body secretions during the acute illness.
Prevention	Avoid contact with rat excreta Strict isolation of clinical case Strict handling of body fluids	Strict isolation of clinical case Strict handling of body fluids	Strict isolation of clinical case Strict handling of body fluids	Avoid tick bites and contact with rat excreta. Strict isolation of clinical case Strict handling of body fluids

identify patients at risk is available in the guidelines. A risk assessment where patients are assigned to one of three risk groups, minimum, moderate or high, should be undertaken to ensure appropriate management for the patient and protection for the laboratory and clinical staff. Clinicians should seek the help and advice of a specialist in infectious diseases or tropical medicine.

Minimum risk

This category includes febrile patients who have
• not been in known endemic areas before the onset of illness;
or
• been in endemic areas, (or in contact with a known or suspected source of a VHF), but in whom the onset of illness was definitely more than 21 days after their last contact with any potential source of infection.

Moderate risk

This category includes febrile patients who have
• been in an endemic area during the 21 days before the onset of illness, but who have none of the additional risk factors that would place him or her in the high-risk category;
or
• not been in a known endemic area, but who may have been in adjacent areas or countries during the 21 days before the onset of illness and who have evidence of severe illness with organ failure and/or haemorrhage, which could be due to a VHF and for which no alternative diagnosis is currently evident.

High risk

This category includes febrile patients who
1 have been in an endemic area during the 3 weeks before illness and
• have lived in a house or stayed in a house for more than 4 hours where there were ill, feverish persons known or strongly suspected to have a VHF;
or
• took part in nursing or caring for ill, feverish patients known or strongly suspected to

have a VHF, or had contact with the body fluids, tissue or the dead body of such a patient;
or
• are a laboratory, health or other worker who has, or has been likely to have come into contact with the body fluids, tissues or the body of a human or animal known or strongly suspected to have a VHF;
or
• were previously categorised as 'moderate' risk, but who have developed organ failure and/or haemorrhage.
2 have not been in an endemic area, but during the 3 weeks before illness they
• cared for a patient or animal known or strongly suspected to have a VHF or came into contact with the body fluids, tissues or dead body of such a patient or animal;
or
• handled clinical specimens, tissues or laboratory cultures known or strongly suspected to contain the agent of a VHF.

Initial management

Decisions on the management of a suspected case should be taken with an Infectious Disease Specialist. An incident/outbreak control group should be convened to ensure that formal guidance is implemented correctly.

Minimum risk patients may be admitted (if requiring hospitalisation) under standard isolation and infection control procedures. Moderate risk patients should be admitted to a high security infectious disease unit or intermediate isolation facilities and, apart from the malaria test, specimens should only be sent to a high security laboratory. High-risk patients must be admitted to a High Security Infectious Disease Unit, samples should only be sent to a High Security laboratory and close contacts should be identified. Special precautions (ambulance category III) are required to transport moderate and high-risk patients.

The CCDC (local public health officer) will wish to ensure that
• the patient is in the category of accommodation appropriate to risk.

• any ambulance staff have been appropriately advised (liaise with Ambulance Control Unit).
• hospital staff have been appropriately advised (liaise with Infection Control Doctor).
• cases or contacts in other districts are followed up (liaise with other CsCDC).
• any specimens or contaminated material from before diagnosis suspected are dealt with appropriately.
• contacts are identified and followed up appropriately.
• any necessary disinfection of domestic and primary care premises is carried out.
• the body of any deceased case is appropriately dealt with.
• appropriate agencies (DH and CDSC in England) are informed.
• arrangements are made for dealing with the media.

Laboratory confirmation

Obtaining and handling laboratory specimens (blood, urine, etc.) is the most common cause of cases of VHF in healthcare settings. Blood and body fluids from high-risk VHF patients are likely to contain high concentrations of virus; therefore, most laboratory tests are discouraged in the initial assessment. Good laboratory practice guidelines must be in place and specimens must be taken and examined by experienced staff in appropriate facilities.

UK guidance is that specimens for virological investigations from moderate or high-risk cases must be sent to a viral diagnostic laboratory equipped to handle Hazard Group 4 biological agents. In the UK, appropriate high security laboratories are the HPA Laboratories at Colindale and Porton Down. The appropriate specimen and investigation should be discussed first. Virus can be detected in body fluids. Newer techniques involve the detection of viral nucleic acid.

Post-mortem examination is a potential risk: if further tests necessary to confirm the diagnosis, specialist advice should be sought.

Management of contacts

Close contacts of a high risk or confirmed case should be kept under daily surveillance for a period of 21 days from the last possible date of exposure to infection. Close contacts are those who after the onset of the patient's illness:
• had direct contact with the patient's blood, urine or secretions, or with clothing, bedding or other fomites soiled by the patient's blood, urine or secretions (not including saliva);
• cared for the patient or handled specimens from the patient, e.g., household members, nurses, laboratory staff, ambulance crew, doctors or other staff;
• had direct contact with the body of a person who had died of VHF, either proven or in high or moderate risk categories, before the coffin was sealed;
• had direct contact with an animal infected with VHF, its blood, body fluids, or corpse.

There need be no restriction on work or movement within the UK, but the contact's temperature should be recorded daily and enquiry made about the presence of any suspicious symptoms. Those suffering any rise of temperature above 38°C should be kept under observation at home and, if fever persists for more than 24 hours, advice should be sought from a consultant in infectious or tropical diseases regarding the need for admission to an isolation unit.

When contact with a VHF patient has not been close, the risk of infection is minimal. Therefore, there is no need to trace and/or follow-up contacts that are not in the categories listed above.

3.85 Warts and verrucae

Warts are caused by infection of the epidermis with human papillomavirus (HPV). Various HPV genotypes affect different sites influenced by environmental and host factors.

Suggested public health on-call action
Usually none required.

Table 3.85.1 Wart morphologies

Clinical type	Appearance	HPV type
Common warts (verrucae vulgaris)	Flesh coloured or brown, keratotic papules	1,2,4,57
Plane or flat warts (verrucae planae)	Smaller, flat topped, non-scaling, papules, cluster on hands, neck or face	3,10
Plantar warts (verrucae plantaris)	Grow inwards and are painful, common in adolescents and children	1,2,4,57
Condylomata acuminata (genital warts)	Occur in the genital tract, transmitted sexually (see Chapter 3.25)	6,11

Epidemiology

Most people will have warts at some time in their life. The prevalence increases during childhood, peaks in adolescence and declines thereafter. The prevalence in children and adolescents in the UK is 4–5%. Warts are more common in white ethnic groups. Warts clear spontaneously over time.

Clinical features

Various wart morphologies are recognised (see Table 3.85.1).

Laboratory confirmation

The diagnosis can be confirmed histologically.

Transmission

Warts spread by direct contact or indirectly via contact with fomites or contaminated floors and surfaces. The attack rate is thought to be low. Autoinoculation occurs as a result of scratching and shaving.

Acquisition

The incubation period rages from 1 month to 2 years. A person with warts is infectious for as long as the warts persist. Warts are more common in immunocompromised people.

Control

• Health education, environmental hygiene in swimming pools and other communal areas and avoiding direct contact with warts where practicable may reduce spread.
• Case reporting is not necessary.
• No single treatment is completely effective. Spontaneous regression is common and warts may be left untreated unless painful or unsightly.
• Children with warts do not have to stay away from school. Affected children can go swimming. Plantar warts should be covered if practicable in swimming pools, gymnasia and changing rooms.

3.86 West Nile virus

Introduction

A potentially serious encephalitis caused by the West Nile virus (WNV).

Suggested on-call action
None unless outbreak unrecognised in which case inform Public Health Authorities.

Epidemiology

Acquired from a mosquito bite. Most infections are mild febrile illnesses, and about 1 in 150 infections is severe. Recognised in Africa, the Middle East, south and east Europe (including Portugal and France), and recently (1999) seen in the US. Outbreaks reported in Romania, Russia and Israel.

WNV, or other arboviral diseases, should be considered in adults >50 years with encephalitis or meningitis and have visited endemic areas.

Clinical features

Usually asymptomatic or mild. Typically aseptic meningitis or acute encephalitis associated with fever (characteristic if with acute flaccid paralysis). Symptomatic and severe illness is more common in elderly. Symptoms and signs include fever, rash, pharyngitis, conjunctivitis, gastrointestinal symptoms, weakness, change in mental status, ataxia and extra pyramidal signs, optic neuritis, cranial nerve abnormalities, polyradiculitis, myelitis and seizures; myocarditis, pancreatitis, and fulminant hepatitis have been described. Case-fatality rates of 10–15%.

Laboratory confirmation

Virus-specific IgM can be detected in most CSF and serum specimens at the time of clinical presentation using IgM antibody capture enzyme-linked immunosorbent assay (MAC-ELISA). Paired serum samples should be tested. False positive results may be seen in those recently vaccinated against (or recently infected with) related flaviviruses (e.g. yellow fever, Japanese encephalitis, dengue).

Transmission

WNV is spread by the bite of a mosquito, infected when by feeding on an infected bird. Transmission through blood transfusion, transplant, breastmilk and transplacentally has been described.

Incubation period

The incubation period is thought to range from 3 to 14 days.

Prevention

Avoidance of mosquito bites (see Chapter 3.46), especially for the elderly during periods of transmission.

Surveillance

Surveillance of virus in bird flocks and mosquitoes can inform risk.

Response to a case

• Inform local and national public health authorities.
• If the first case clinicians should be alerted to the presence of circulating WNV.

Response to a cluster/control of an outbreak

• Ensure public health advice about avoiding mosquito bites.
• Mosquito control.

3.87 Whooping cough

Whooping cough (pertussis) is an acute bacterial respiratory infection caused by *Bordetella pertussis* (a related organism, *Bordetella parapertussis*, also causes a pertussis-like illness). Its public health importance lies in the severity of the disease, particularly in young infants, and its preventability by vaccination.

Epidemiology

Pertussis is well controlled in countries with good immunisation coverage. Where coverage is low, the disease has a cyclical pattern, with epidemics occurring at 3–4 yearly intervals. These epidemics affect young children; infants under 6 months are particularly at risk.

The incidence of pertussis varies widely across Europe and has changed over time in many countries. There were large epidemics in the UK during the 1970s and 1980s when vaccine coverage fell due to (unfounded) concerns about vaccine safety. Vaccine coverage has since risen to over 90%, and in 2003 only 409 cases were notified in England and Wales. Epidemics of pertussis also occurred in Sweden, where pertussis vaccine was discontinued altogether for some years. Germany, the Netherlands and France have also experienced resurgences of pertussis in recent years. The WHO target is to reduce pertussis incidence to less than 1 per 100,000 in Europe by 2010.

The reported case-fatality rate is 1 per 1000 overall, although it is higher than this in young infants, in whom pertussis is often not recognised. Enhanced surveillance using new laboratory methods such as PCR diagnosis can significantly improve detection rates.

Clinical features

The initial illness starts with cough, cold and a fever. Over the next week, the cough gradually becomes paroxysmal; there are bouts of coughing, which are terminated by the typical whoop or by vomiting. The cough often lasts for 2–3 months. Young infants do not usually whoop, and coughing spasms may be followed by periods of apnoea. Adults and vaccinated children have a milder illness that lasts 2–3 weeks. Pertussis is being increasingly recognised as a cause of chronic cough in adults.

Laboratory confirmation

The classical method is culture from a pernasal swab, although the organism is difficult to grow, so sensitivity is low (although specificity is high). The sensitivity has been greatly improved by the advent of PCR diagnosis. Serology (EIA) is also available.

Transmission

Man is the only reservoir. Transmission is by droplet spread from an infectious case, often an older sibling or parent. Carriers do not exist. Mild or subclinical cases among vaccinated individuals are also a source of infection.

Acquisition

The incubation period is 7–10 days, but may occasionally be up to 3 weeks. A case is highly infectious during the early stage of the illness, before the typical cough; infectiousness then decreases and the case is normally not infectious 3 weeks after the onset of paroxysmal cough, although in a proportion of cases (up to 20%) infectivity may persist for up to 6 weeks. The period of communicability may be shortened by erythromycin treatment. An attack of pertussis usually confers immunity, although second cases do sometimes occur.

Prevention

• Immunisation is highly effective at preventing illness, although its role in limiting transmission is less clear. Pertussis vaccine has also been shown to reduce the incidence of sudden infant death syndrome.

- There are two types of pertussis vaccine: killed whole-cell preparations and subunit acellular vaccines. Most countries in Europe, including the UK now use acellular vaccines because of the lower incidence of side-effects. The vaccines are given in combination with diphtheria, tetanus, polio and Hib antigens, and sometimes also hepatitis B. Booster doses are recommended at various ages, usually in the second year of life (although not in the UK where the booster is scheduled at 3–5 years).
- It is important that pertussis vaccine is not delayed in infants, and that older siblings and parents are fully vaccinated. The only true contraindication is a severe reaction to a previous dose.

Surveillance

- Pertussis is notifiable in most European countries, including the UK.
- Laboratories should also report all clinically significant infections to the local and national surveillance centres.
- Serotyping should be performed in the national reference unit; surveillance of serotypes is important to monitor vaccine efficacy.

Response to a case

- Isolate, with respiratory precautions, in hospital.
- Start antibiotic treatment (erythromycin) and exclude from nursery or school for 5 days after treatment has started (course to continue for 14 days).
- Arrange for laboratory confirmation.
- Check vaccination status of case and household contacts, and arrange for vaccination if any are unvaccinated; report vaccines failures to the national surveillance unit.
- Erythromycin prophylaxis may be of value for unvaccinated household contacts of suspected or confirmed pertussis, particularly infants under 6 months of age, if given within

21 days of onset of the first case. The dose is 125 mg, 6 hourly for children up to 2 years of age; 250 mg, 6 hourly for children 2–8 years of age; and 250–500 mg, 6 hourly for children over 8 years of age and adults. Treatment should be continued for 7 days.
- Casual contacts, including school contacts, would not normally be offered prophylaxis.

Investigation of a cluster

- Obtain laboratory confirmation, including serotyping.
- Check vaccination status of cases.
- Look for links to populations with low vaccine coverage (e.g. religious communities in the Netherlands).
- Consider potential sources of infection, e.g. unvaccinated adults.

Control of an outbreak

- Look for unvaccinated individuals and consider community-wide vaccination, if coverage is low (N.B.: Three doses of vaccine are required for protection, so vaccination is a long-term outbreak control measure).
- Treatment of cases and erythromycin prophylaxis for unvaccinated contacts as above.
- Look for undiagnosed cases.
- Outbreaks in institutions can be controlled by a combination of case finding, antibiotic treatment and case exclusion.

Suggested case definitions for an outbreak

Clinical: 14 days or more of cough plus one of
- epidemiological link to a confirmed case, *or* one of
- paroxysms, whoop, or post coughing vomiting.

Confirmed: compatible symptoms with *B. pertussis* infection confirmed by culture, PCR, or serology.

3.88 Yellow fever

An imported, acute flavivirus infection, which may be severe.

Epidemiology

Yellow fever is endemic in Central Africa and areas of South and Central America. The mosquito vector does not occur in Europe, but the disease is a potential risk to travellers to endemic areas.

Clinical features

Cases are classified as inapparent, mild, moderately severe, and malignant. Onset is sudden, with fever of 39–40°C. The pulse, rapid initially becomes slow for the fever. In mild cases, the illness ends after 1–3 days. In moderately severe and malignant cases, the fever falls suddenly 2–5 days after onset, and a remission of several hours or days ensues. The fever then recurs, and albuminuria and epigastric tenderness with haematemesis appear. Oliguria or anuria may occur and petechiae and mucosal haemorrhages are common. In malignant cases, delirium, convulsions and coma occur terminally.

Up to 10% of clinically diagnosed cases die, but overall mortality is actually lower, since many infections are undiagnosed.

Laboratory confirmation

Diagnosis is confirmed by virus isolation from blood, by a rising antibody titre (in absence of recent immunisation and after exclusion of cross reactions to other flaviviruses) or at autopsy. Antigen or genome detection tests may be available.

Transmission

In sylvatic yellow fever, the virus is acquired from wild primates and transmitted by forest canopy mosquitoes. In urban yellow fever, the virus is acquired from a viraemic patient within the previous 2 weeks and transmitted by the *Aedes aegypti* mosquito.

Acquisition

Incubation lasts 3–6 days.

Prevention

• Active immunisation with the live, attenuated vaccine effectively prevents cases.
• Vaccination requirements vary by country; information and addresses of vaccination centres can be obtained from public health authorities.
• Eradication of urban yellow fever requires widespread mosquito control and mass immunisation.

Surveillance

Yellow fever is a notifiable disease and should be reported to local public health authorities and to WHO.

Response to a case

• The case should be reported urgently to WHO (via national centre) and the country of origin.
• The case should be transferred to suitable isolation facilities and strict procedures such as those laid down by the Advisory Committee on Dangerous Pathogens (UK) be followed.
• In an area where there is potential for further mosquito transmission, patients should be isolated in a screened room sprayed with residual insecticide.
• Hospital and laboratory personnel should be aware of the risk of transmission from inoculation.

Investigation of a cluster and control of an outbreak

Not usually relevant to Europe, but check that cases have been to infected area in week before onset.

Control of an outbreak is through mass immunisation and vector control.

Suggested case definition
Clinically compatible illness with fourfold rise in antibody titres or demonstration of virus, antigen or genome.

3.89 Yersiniosis

Non-plague yersiniosis has emerged in recent years as an important cause of intestinal infection in many countries. *Yersinia enterocolitica* causes predominantly enterocolitis, whereas *Yersinia pseudotuberculosis* mainly causes an appendicitis-like illness.

Suggested on-call action
• Exclude symptomatic cases in high-risk groups. • If you or reporting microbiologist/ clinician know of other cases, consult outbreak control plan.

Epidemiology

Although documented in temperate regions in all continents, *Y. enterocolitica* is more common in northern Europe (particularly Scandinavia) and Canada, where it appears to be responsible for 2–4% of cases of diarrhoea. All ages are susceptible, but most cases occur in those under 10 years. Peak incidence in Europe is in autumn and winter. Infection may be more common in rural areas and amongst those exposed to pigs or their carcasses. Reported cases have fallen over the last decade in England and Wales (from over 500 in 1990 to under 40 since 2000), but this trend is not true for all European countries.

Y. pseudotuberculosis has a worldwide distribution but is more commonly reported from Europe. Most cases are aged 5–20 years and males are more commonly affected. Peak incidence is in winter.

Clinical features

Y. enterocolitica enteritis presents with diarrhoea accompanied by fever and abdominal pain in two-thirds of cases, and vomiting in one-third. The duration of illness is usually 2–3 weeks, slightly longer than for most enteric pathogens. Bloody diarrhoea occurs in approximately 20–25% of affected children. Sequelae include reactive arthritis and erythema nodosum. Other presentations include pharyngitis, appendicitis-like syndrome in older children and septicaemia in the infirm.

Y. pseudotuberculosis usually presents as mesenteric adenitis causing fever and right lower abdominal pain. Many cases result in appendicectomy. Erythema nodosum may occur, but enteritis and septicaemia are uncommon.

Carriage of *Yersinia* species in studies of asymptomatic individuals ranges from 0 to 2.9%.

Laboratory confirmation

Serological diagnosis is available for both species. *Y. enterocolitica* can be diagnosed by stool culture but grows slowly on routine culture media and may not be routinely ascertained by many laboratories. If yersiniosis is suspected on epidemiological grounds then enrichment and highly selective media can be used, but this takes several days. Small numbers of organisms may continue to be excreted for 4 weeks.

Y. enterocolitica are divided into 6 biotypes, of which types 2, 3 and 4 are the most common, and over 50 serotypes, of which O3 and O9 are the most common in Europe. A phage typing scheme also exists.

Y. pseudotuberculosis may be confirmed by isolation from an excised mesenteric lymph node. All strains are biochemically homogenous and, although there are 6 serotypes, most human cases are serotype 1. Genotyping may be available in some countries.

Transmission

The most important reservoir of *Y. enterocolitica* in Europe is asymptomatic carriage in pigs. Other hosts are rodents, rabbits, sheep, goats, cattle, horses, dogs and cats. *Y. pseudotuberculosis* is found in a number of mammals and birds, particularly rodents and poultry. Humans usually acquire the infection orally via following:
1 Food, especially pork or pork products. Pork is easily contaminated in the abattoir and if eaten raw or undercooked may cause illness. Refrigeration offers little protection as the organism can multiply at 4°C. Milk has also been implicated in *Y. enterocolitica* outbreaks, probably due to contamination after pasteurisation, although pasteurisation failure is possible. Vegetables such as tofu or bean sprouts become contaminated from growing in contaminated water. Outbreaks of *Y. pseudotuberculosis* in Finland have been linked to carrots and lettuce. The optimum temperature for growth is 22–29°C.
2 Person to person: evidence for transmission to household contacts is conflicting, but outbreaks have occurred in nurseries, schools and hospitals in which person-to-person spread is likely to have played a part. Respiratory transmission from cases with pharyngitis appears unlikely.
3 Direct contact with animals: human cases have been reported after contact with sick puppies and kittens.
4 Blood-borne: contaminated blood in blood banks has led to severe disease and several deaths in recipients. Not all donors were

unwell. The ability of the organism to replicate in refrigerators is likely to be relevant.

Acquisition

The incubation period is usually 4–7 days with a range of 2–11 days. The infectious dose is likely to be high, perhaps 10^9 organisms. Secondary infection appears to be rare, but it may be best to assume that the infectious period extends until 48 hours after the first normal stool. Natural infection confers immunity, although the extent and duration is unclear. Maternal antibodies protect the newborn.

Prevention

• Avoidance of consumption of raw meats, particularly pork products.
• Reduction of contamination of raw pork by improved slaughtering methods, improved husbandry or irradiation of meat.
• Avoidance of long-term refrigeration of meat (maximum 4 days). Growth should not occur at freezer temperatures under −2°C.
• Pasteurisation of dairy products and subsequent separation from unpasteurised milk-handling processes.
• Chlorination of drinking water.
• Washing of salad items to be eaten raw.
• Exclusion of blood donors with recent history of diarrhoea or fever.
• General measures to protect against gastrointestinal infection, including handwashing, safe disposal of human and animal/pet faeces, food hygiene and exclusion of cases with high risk of onward transmission.

Surveillance

• Cases of yersiniosis should be reported to local public health departments (notify as suspected food poisoning in UK) and to national surveillance systems.
• Clinicians should inform the local public health department of any increase in cases of mesenteric adenitis or appendicectomy, especially in autumn and winter.

Response to a case

• Give hygiene advice to case (enteric precautions).
• Exclude case and symptomatic contacts if in risk group (Box 2.2.1) until 48 hours after first normal stool. No microbiological clearance necessary.
• Obtain history of consumption of pork or pork products, raw or undercooked meat, milk, salad or water. Ask about sick pets, blood transfusions and exposure to animals/carcasses.

Investigations of a cluster

• Discuss case finding with local laboratory: need to change testing policy for routine specimens?
• Discuss further microbiological investigations of existing cases to discover if all one serotype or phage type.
• Conduct hypothesis-generating study. Questionnaire should include consumption of pork and pork products; consumption of raw or undercooked meats; salad items; source of milk; source of water; all other food consumed in last 11 days; contact with other cases; blood or blood product transfusions; hospital treatment; occupation; contact with animals (wild, agricultural or pet).

Control of an outbreak

• Exclude symptomatic cases in high-risk groups and ensure enteric precautions followed.
• Reinforce food hygiene and handwashing.
• Look for ways in which food could have become contaminated (especially cross contamination from raw pork), undercooked or stored too long in a refrigerator. Check that pasteurised milk could not become contaminated in dairy.
• Prevent use of unpasteurised milk. Prevent use of raw vegetables grown in untreated water, unless subsequently cleaned adequately.

> **Suggested case definition for outbreak**
>
> *Clinical*: diarrhoea or combination of fever and right lower abdominal pain with onset 4–7 days after exposure.
> *Confirmed*: isolate of outbreak strain or serological positive with one of diarrhoea, fever, abdominal pain or vomiting beginning 1–11 days after exposure.

3.90 Other hazards

3.90.1 Helminths

Intestinal roundworms
(see Table 3.90.1a)

Most intestinal nematodes are not passed directly from person to person, and so spread is rare in developed countries. Control is based on enteric precautions and early treatment of cases. The main exception is threadworm infection (see Chapter 3.74).

Tapeworms (cestodes)
(see Table 3.90.1b)

Humans are the only definitive host for the tapeworms *Taenia saginata* and *Taenia solium* and may also be accidental intermediate hosts for *T. solium*, giving rise to cysticercosis, and for *Echinococcus granulosus*, giving rise to hydatid disease.

Eggs, or whole detached segments (proglottids), are evacuated in the faeces of the definitive host and disseminate in the environment. Following ingestion by a suitable intermediate host they develop into invasive larvae in the gut, migrate through the tissues and settle as cysts at sites determined by the tropism of the parasite. When the intermediate host is eaten by a definitive host, allowing the cysts to develop into adults, the life cycle is completed.

Table 3.90.1a Nematodes: intestinal roundworms

Disease and organism	Mode of transmission	Epidemiology	Clinical	Investigation	Public health action
Ascariasis *Ascaris lumbricoides*	Humans are reservoir but transmission is indirect. Non-infective eggs excreted in faeces become infectious after 2–3 weeks in soil and may survive many months. Infective eggs ingested from soil or foods contaminated by soil. Eggs hatch in duodenum. Larvae migrate in blood and lymphatics to lung and oropharynx where swallowed to develop into adult worms in small intestine. Adults live 6–12 months.	Worldwide but concentrated in tropical and subtropical areas with poor sanitation. Estimated that more than 1 billion persons are infected, making ascariasis the world's most prevalent intestinal helminth infection.	Migrating larvae may produce an eosinophilic pneumonia Asymptomatic patient may pass an adult worm by vomiting or per rectum. Heavy infection may produce abdominal cramps and may cause intestinal obstruction. Even moderate infections can lead to malnutrition in children.	Diagnosis is made by detection of the eggs in stools. Occasionally, adult worms are passed in the stool or vomit.	Uncooked and unwashed vegetables should be avoided in areas where human faeces (night soil) is used as fertilizer. There is no risk of transmission from a case in Europe if basic hygienic precautions are taken.
Whipworm infection	Humans are the only reservoir, but transmission is indirect. Non-infective develop in soil over 10–14 days. Ingested from soil or via contaminated food or water. No migration to other tissues. Adult worms may live 7–0 years.	The parasite is found principally in the tropics and subtropics.	Infection is often asymptomatic. Heavy infections cause abdominal pain, anorexia and diarrhoea and may retard growth. Rarely weight loss, anaemia and rectal prolapse may occur.	Identification of the eggs in faeces. Eggs are excreted in faeces too.	Prevention rests upon adequate sanitation and good personal hygiene.

Hookworm infection *Ancylostoma duodenale* or *Necator americanus*	Eggs passed in human stool hatch in 1–2 days and release larvae, which mature over 5–8 days and may then penetrate human skin (often on feet), migrate to the lungs via blood vessels, ascend to epiglottis, and are swallowed. Adult worms may live 2–10 years. Occasionally cat and dog hookworms may infect humans.	*A. duodenale* is widely distributed in the Mediterranean, India, China, Japan and South America. *N. americanus* is the predominant hookworm of Central and South Africa, southern Asia, Melanesia, the Caribbean and Polynesia. About 25% of the world's population are infected with hookworms.	Most cases are asymptomatic. Migration of larvae may cause an eosinophilic pneumonia. Adult worms in the intestine may cause colicky pain and non-specific symptoms. Chronic infection may lead to iron-deficiency anaemia and hypoproteinaemia.	Depends upon recognition of the eggs in fresh stool.	Preventing defecation where others may come into contact with the stool. Avoiding direct skin contact with the soil. Wearing shoes. Periodic mass deworming may be effective in high-risk populations.
Strongyloidiasis *Strongyloides stercoralis*	Adult worms live in the duodenum and jejunum. Released eggs hatch immediately and release larvae that are passed in faeces. After a few days the larvae mature and can penetrate the skin of humans, migrate through the lungs and reach the intestine, where they mature in about 2 weeks. Filariform larvae can bypass the soil phase and directly penetrate the colon or the skin.	Endemic throughout the tropics and subtropics.	Most cases are asymptomatic. There may be non-specific abdominal symptoms. An enteritis, protein-losing enteropathy, urticaria and pulmonary symptoms are seen less frequently. Larva currens, a serpiginous, migratory, urticarial lesion, is pathognomonic.	Larvae can be identified in stool 25% of the time. Repeat examination of concentrated stool is necessary.	Prevention of primary infections is as for hookworms. To prevent the serious hyperinfection syndrome, patients with possible exposure to *Strongyloides* (even in the distant past) should undergo several stool examinations and, if necessary, a string test or duodenal aspiration before receiving immunosuppressive therapy, including steroids.

Continued p. 246

Table 3.90.1.a *Continued*

Disease and organism	Mode of transmission	Epidemiology	Clinical	Investigation	Public health action
	Transmission is often due to exposure of bare skin to larvae in contaminated soil in unsanitary conditions. Faecal–oral transmission may occur in institutions for mentally handicapped and day-care centres. Self-reinfection may occur and can result in extremely high worm burdens (hyperinfection syndrome).	Hyperinfection produces serious gastrointestinal symptoms including haemorrhage, pulmonary infiltration and hepatitis and may involve the CNS. Even with treatment the mortality is over 50%. The hyperinfection syndrome and disseminated stronglyoidiasis are seen in persons with impaired immunity. Immunosuppression may lead to overwhelming hyperinfection in persons with previously asymptomatic infection.			

Trichinosis *Trichinella* spp., especially *T. spiralis*	From eating undercooked meat from infected carnivores. Larvae develop in the small intestine, penetrate the mucosa and become adults in 6–8 days. Mature females release living larvae for 4–6 weeks, before dying or being expelled. Newborn larvae travel to striated muscle cells, where they encyst over 1–3 months. The cycle continues when encysted larvae are ingested by another carnivore.	Trichinosis occurs worldwide. The life cycle is maintained by animals that feed on (e.g., pigs) or that hunt (e.g., bears, boars) other animals whose striated muscles contain encysted infective larvae (e.g., rodents). There have been outbreaks in Europe associated with imported horsemeat.	Gastrointestinal symptoms are absent or mild; nausea, abdominal cramps and diarrhoea may occur during the first week. The characteristic syndrome of periorbital oedema, myalgia, fever and subconjunctival haemorrhages and petechiae appears in weeks 2–3.	There are no specific tests for the intestinal stage of trichinosis. Eosinophilia usually begins when newborn larvae invade tissues, peaks 2–4 weeks after infection and gradually declines. Muscle enzymes are elevated in 50% of patients. A muscle biopsy may disclose larvae, inflammation and cysts.	Trichinosis is prevented by cooking meat thoroughly (55°C [140°F] throughout). Larvae can also be killed by freezing at −15°C (5°F) for 3 weeks or −18°C (0°F) for 1 day. Meat should be inspected before being sold. There is no person-to-person spread. Investigate clusters for a common contaminated food source.

Continued p. 248

Table 3.90.1.a *Continued*

Disease and organism	Mode of transmission	Epidemiology	Clinical	Investigation	Public health action
			Soreness may affect the muscles of respiration, speech, mastication and swallowing. Heavy infection may cause severe dyspnoea, multisystem disease or fatal myocarditis. Most symptoms and signs resolve by the third month.	Serologic tests can give false-negative results, especially if testing is done early. Serologic tests are of most value if they are initially negative and then turn positive.	
Capillariasis Three of the *Capillaria* produce disease in man	*Capillaria phillipensis* Reservoir thought to be fish.	Endemic in Phillipines and Thailand.	Protein loosing enteropathy. May be fatal.	Identify parasite in fresh stool.	No person-to-person spread.
	Capillaria hepatica Reservoir rats and rodents.	North and South America, Africa, Eastern Europe, Southeast Asia, India. Larva Migrans Russia, North Africa.	Hepatitis, Eosinophilia.	Liver biopsy.	No person-to-person spread.
	Capillaria Aerophila Ingestion of contaminated soil.		Rare, fever, cough, wheeze	Eggs seen in sputum.	No person-to-person spread.

Table 3.90.1.b Tapeworms (cestodes)

Disease and organism	Mode of transmission	Epidemiology	Clinical	Investigation	Public health action
Taeniasis *T. saginata* *T. solium*	Infection is acquired by eating undercooked infected pork or beef.	Occurs in most countries where beef or pork is eaten undercooked. Rare in northwest Europe.	Adult *T. saginata* (beef tapeworm) may grow to 10 m and *T. solium* (pork tapeworm) to 4 m, but infection is usually asymptomatic. Abdominal pains are sometimes reported. Detached motile segments (proglottids) of *T. saginata* may be noticed as they emerge from the anus.	Infections are usually diagnosed because of eggs or proglottids in the faeces.	Basic hygienic precautions. Exclusion of cases of pork tapeworm in risk groups 1–4 (see Box 2.2.1) until 2 negative stools at 1 and 2 weeks post-treatment. Regular deworming of pets.
Dwarf tapeworm *Hymenolepsis nana*	Eggs excreted in human faeces are infectious. May spread faeco–orally or via contaminated food. May be autoinfection.	Imported from Asia, southeast Europe, Africa or Latin America. Occasionally found in institutions or immunocompromised.	Asymptomatic or mild abdominal discomfort. May be anorexia, dizziness, diarrhoea.	Identification of characteristic eggs in stool.	Basic hygiene precautions. Exclusion of risk groups 1–4 until treated. Consider screening household.
Fish tapeworm *Diphyllobothrium Latum*	Acquired by eating undercooked fish.	Worldwide, rare in northwest Europe.	Causes B12 deficiency.	Identification of eggs in the faeces.	Avoiding raw, smoked or undercooked fish.

Continued p. 250

Table 3.90.1.b *Continued*

Disease and organism	Mode of transmission	Epidemiology	Clinical	Investigation	Public health action
Cysticercosis: Disease due to the pork tapeworm (*T. solium*)	If eggs excreted by a human carrier of the pork tapeworm are ingested the cysticerci preferentially settle in skeletal muscle and CNS, where they act as space occupying lesions.	Occurs in most countries where beef or pork is eaten undercooked and person-to-person transmission occurs. Rare in northwest Europe.	Clinical features may include epilepsy, raised intracranial pressure and chronic basal meningitis.	Diagnosis has been much advanced by modern brain imaging techniques, which may be supported by serology or by evidence of cysticerci in other tissues. Definitive identification of parasite segments and eggs, and serology is available from reference laboratory.	
Hydatid disease: Disease due to the dog tapeworm *Echinococcus granulosus* or *E. multilocularis*	Humans acquire hydatid cysts, the metacestodes of *Echinococcus* spp. by ingesting eggs excreted in the faeces of an infected dog.	Found in most sheep- and cattle-raising parts of the word.	The commonest sites for hydatid cysts are liver, lung and bone. The cysts expand slowly over several years. Occasionally leaks occur, which may cause hypersensitivity phenomena such as generalised urticaria and can seed further cysts at distant sites. Symptoms are most often due to the mass effect of the lesion.	An appropriate imaging technique, such as ultrasound of the abdomen, will reveal the diagnosis, and may be supported by serology.	Treatment of hydatid disease and cysticercosis should be undertaken by specialists. Most cases will be acquired. Poor hygiene and close contact with infected animals and ingestion of undercooked infected meat are all risk factors.
Sparganosis *Spirometra*	Infection by larvae of *Spirometra* tapeworm.	Human infection results from use of flesh of an infected frog as poultice (Southeast Asia), or exposure to contaminated water.	Larvae develop into cysts in subcutaneous tissue.		Avoid frog poultices.

Filariae (see Table 3.90.1c)

Filariae produce larvae called microfilariae directly without an egg stage, and have a life cycle involving an arthropod intermediate host, usually a biting insect that acts as a vector for the dissemination of the disease. At least 10 species infect man. The incubation period is prolonged and may be more than a year. There is no person-to-person spread; individuals remain infectious for the insect vector if microfilariae are present. The insect vectors are not present outside the endemic range of the diseases.

3.90.2 Protozoa

(see Table 3.90.2)

Leishmaniasis oriental sore

Leishmania are flagellate protozoan parasites. The major species are *L. donovani*, the causative agent of kala-azar, *L. tropica* and *L. major*: causing Old World cutaneous leishmaniasis and *L. brazilienzis*, the agent of New world cutaneous (American) leishmaniasis.

Trypanosomiasis

There are three trypanosomes that are pathogenic to man. *T. brucei* gambiense and *T. brucei* rhodesiense are transmitted to man through the bite of a blood-sucking fly of the *Glossina* genus (tsetse fly). *T. cruzi* infects man by inoculation of faeces from its blood-sucking insect vector, the triatomid bug.

Babesiosis

Infection with bovine or rodent *Babesia* spp., which causes a malaria-like illness.

3.90.3 Fungi (see Table 3.90.3)

In addition to the common superficial fungal infections, a number of fungal species are implicated in deep-seated disease processes. These include ubiquitous organisms, such as *Candida* and *Aspergillus*, which are only invasive in an immunocompromised host, specifically in neutropenia or T-cell defects. Others occur as specific infectious entities in apparently otherwise healthy individuals, often within a confined geographical range; these primary deep pathogens are usually acquired by the respiratory route. Almost all fungal pathogens can cause opportunist infections. None of these agents spread person to person.

3.90.4 Rare viruses

(see Table 3.90.4)

Person-to-person spread is rare with these viruses. However it may occur in some of them (Monkeypox). Public health action comprises identifying the mode of transmission and reducing exposure. Expert advice should be sought.

3.90.5 Bites, stings and venoms

Epidemiology

Although western Europe has few indigenous venomous species, the pet trade has increased the likelihood of exposure to exotic animals, which may bite or sting.

Table 3.90.1c Nematodes: Filariae

Disease and organism	Mode of transmission	Epidemiology	Clinical	Investigation	Public health action
Lymphatic filariasis (elephantiasis) *Wuchereria bancrofti* *Brugia malayi*	Adult worms inhabit the lymphatics, and the microfilariae, which have a strong diurnal periodicity, appear briefly in the peripheral blood around midnight when they can be ingested by mosquitos, which are the vectors.	*Wuchereria bancrofti* has a widespread distribution in South Asia, the Pacific islands, tropical Africa and some parts of South America. Two species of *Brugia*, restricted to Southeast Asia, give rise to a similar syndrome.	Cause of elephantiasis. Fever and lymphangitis may occur early in the disease. The most serious consequences are the chronic sequelae of lymphatic damage caused by dying worms. Gross lymphoedema, most often of the legs or genitals, and chyluria are typical features.	Definitive diagnosis is by recognition of the microfilariae in a midnight sample of blood. Serology provides supportive evidence but there may be cross-reactions with other nematode infections.	Eliminating vector-breeding sites.
Onchocerciasis (river blindness) *Onchocerca volvulus*	Microfilariae in the skin are ingested by a black fly of the genus *Simulium*. These are the insect vectors.	Primarily an African disease although there are some foci in Central America.	The adult *Onchocerca* lives in the subcutaneous tissues. Clinical consequences are caused by the inflammation resulting from death of the microfilariae. In the skin this causes a chronic dermatitis Most significant is damage to the eye. The inflammatory process may involve all the structures between the cornea and the optic nerve. Blindness occurs after 20 years or more of heavy infection.	Diagnosis depends on detecting microfilariae in superficial snips of skin.	Eliminating vector-breeding sites.

Loiasis *Loa loa*, (African eye worm)	Adult *Loa loa* are migratory and roam widely in the subcutaneous tissues and may become visible on passing under the conjunctiva of the eye. The microfilariae appear with a diurnal periodicity in the blood around midday.	Rain forests of West and Central Africa.	Many cases asymptomatic, symptoms include 'Calabar swellings', diffuse areas of subcutaneous oedema, usually distally on the limbs, which last a few days.	Diagnosis is by recognising the microfilariae in midday blood.	Eliminating vector-breeding sites.
Dracontiasis *Dracunculus medinensis* (Guinea worm)	The disease is acquired by drinking water containing *Cyclops*, which harbour larvae. These invade, develop into adults and mate. The gravid female, about 60-cm long, then makes her way to the lower extremities where she penetrates to the surface, giving rise to an irritating ulcer. Contact with water causes her to release larvae through this defect where they may be able to infect new *Cyclops*.	Indian subcontinent, Africa.	The chronic ulceration, and associated secondary infection, may be a severe problem in conditions of poor hygiene. Death of the worm causes intense inflammation.	Recognition of larvae or adult worm.	Provision of clean drinking water.

Table 3.90.2 Protozoa

Disease and organism	Incubation period	Infectious period	Mode of transmission	Epidemiology	Clinical	Investigation	Public health action
Visceral leishmaniasis	Usually 2–4 months 10 days to 1 year.	As long as there are parasites present, this may be many years. Person-to-person spread is reported.	Transmitted to man by the bite of a sandfly. Infective blood meals may come from another man or an animal reservoir host. This may be a dog or rodent, depending on the species of *Leishmania*.	Tropical and subtropical areas. Mediterranean, Middle East, Indian sub-continent.	A primary lesion resembling cutaneous leishmaniasis may occur. The onset is usually insidious. Patients present with anorexia malaise and weight loss, and may complain of abdominal discomfort due to splenic enlargement. Anaemia and cachexia are present and the liver and spleen are enlarged. Fever is intermittent and undulant with often two spikes in 1 day. Untreated patients undergo a slow decline and die usually from secondary infections after about 2 years.	Amastigotes of *Leishmaniasis donovani* may be found by direct microscopy of bone marrow or splenic aspirate. Occasionally amastigotes may be demonstrated in the buffy coat cells. The leishmanin reaction is usually negative due to failure of cell-mediated immunity.	Measures to break transmission cycle. Cover the cutaneous lesion. No isolation required. Rare direct person-to-person spread.

Cutaneous leishmaniasis	A few days to more than 6 months.	Direct person-to-person spread.	The lesions begin as a small itching papule with increasing infiltration of the dermis. The lesion becomes crusted, which, when scratched, produces a shallow discharging ulcer. A variety of different clinical courses follow.	Laboratory diagnosis is made by split skin smear, with culture on Schneider's insect medium. Antibody titres using indirect fluorescent antibody test may also be helpful. Culture in special medium should also be performed.

Table 3.90.3 Fungi

Disease, organism, epidemiology, investigation and public health relevence	Clinical
Aspergillosis *Aspergillus fumigatus, A. flavus.* Also rarer Aspergiilli. Occurrence: Worldwide, including Europe. Incubation period: Days to weeks. Transmission: Inhalation of organism found in damp hay, decaying vegetation, soil, household dust, building materials, ornamental plants, items of food and water. Investigation: Serum precipitins, microscopy of sputum. Culture confirmation. Public health relevence: Clusters may occur where the immunocompromised are gathered together. Environmental investigation should be carried out to determine the source. Nosocomial infection may be associated with dust exposure during building renovation. Occasional outbreaks of cutaneous infection traced to contaminated biomedical devices.	Chronic pulmonary disease. Invasive disease in the immunocompromised, which most frequently involves the lungs and sinuses. This fungus may disseminate and involve the brain, kidneys, liver, heart, and bones. Neutropenia due to cytotoxic chemotherapy and systemic corticosteroids are predisposing factors for invasive aspergillosis. Also causes allergic sinusitis and allergic bronchopulmonary disease. If severe granulocytopenia persists, mortality rate can be very high (up to 100% in patients with cerebral abscesses). Patient outcome depends on resolution of granulocytopenia and early institution of effective antifungal drug therapy.
Blastomycosis *Blastomyces dermatitidis* Incubation: Weeks to many months. Occurrence: Central and southeast USA, Central and South Africa, India, Near and Middle East. Transmission: Inhalation, exposures to wooded sites and moist soil enriched with decomposing organic debris (farmers, forestry workers, hunters and campers at risk). Investigation: Microscopy, culture. Public health relevence: Identify likely exposure–often not determined.	Picture similar to TB. Symptomatic infection (50% of cases) usually presents as a flu-like illness with fever, chills, productive cough, myalgia, arthralgia and pleuritic chest pain. Some patients fail to recover and develop chronic pulmonary infection or widespread disseminated infection (affecting the skin, bones and genitourinary tract). Occasionally affects the meninges. Mortality rate is about 5%.
Candidiasis *Candida albicans* is the most common cause of candidiasis. Occurrence: Worldwide. Transmission: Endogenous organisms. Investigation: Microscopy and culture. Public health relevence: None unless contaminated devices considered.	Candidiasis may be classified as superficial or deep. Deep: The alimentary tract and intravascular catheters are the main routes of entry for visceral candidiasis. The main predisposing factors are prolonged courses of broad-spectrum antibiotics, vascular catheters, cytotoxic chemotherapy and corticosteroids. Superficial: Candidiasis of the mouth and throat, also known as 'thrush' or oropharyngeal candidiasis – Vulvovaginal candidiasis (VVC); women with VVC usually experience genital itching or burning, with or without a 'cottage cheese-like' vaginal discharge. Males may have an itchy rash on the penis. Pregnancy diabetes mellitus. Use of broad-spectrum antibiotics. Use of corticosteroid medications and immunosupression are risk factors.

Table 3.90.3 *Continued*

Disease, organism, epidemiology, investigation and public health relevence	Clinical
Chromoblastomycosis *Chromomycosis* Public health relevence: None.	A chronic localised infection of the skin and subcutaneous tissue following the implantation of the etiologic agent. The mycosis usually remains localised with keloid formation. Many different fungi may cause this disease.
Coccidioidomycosis *Coccidioides immitis.* Incubation: Weeks to years. Occurrence: North and South America arid and desert areas. Transmission: Inhalation of organism after disturbance of contaminated soil, occupational exposure in farmers, etc. Investigation: Microscopy, culture. Public health relevence: Antidust measures in endemic areas. Risk groups: Persons in areas with endemic disease who are exposed to dust (construction or agricultural workers and archaeologists). High-risk groups are African Americans and Asians, pregnant women during the third trimester and immunocompromised persons.	Symptomatic infection usually presents as flu-like illness. Some patients develop chronic pulmonary infection or widespread disseminated infection (affecting meninges, soft tissues, joints and bone). Severe pulmonary disease may develop in HIV-infected persons. Meningitis may lead to permanent damage. Mortality high in HIV-infected persons with diffuse lung disease.
Cryptococcosis *Cryptococcus neoformans.* Occurrence: Worldwide. Transmission: Inhalation of air-borne yeast cells, isolated from the soil, usually in association with bird droppings. Less common C. *neoformans var. gattii* isolated from eucalyptus trees in tropical and sub-tropical regions. Investigation: Direct microscopy with India ink staining; antigen detection is more sensitive. Public health relevence: None.	Principally a disease of the immunosuppressed and occurs most commonly in AIDS. Initial pulmonary infection is often asymptomatic. Most patients present with disseminated infection, especially meningoencephalitis. Resembles tuberculous meningitis with subacute onset and similar CSF findings. Meningitis may lead to permanent neurologic damage. Mortality rate is about 12%.
Histoplasmosis *Histoplasma capsulatum* Incubation: Weeks to years. Transmission: Found in soil and in bird and bat droppings. Infection is acquired by the inhalation of spores; bat caves are sometimes identified as the source. Occurrence: North and South America (Ohio and Mississippi river valleys) Africa, India and Southeast Asia. Investigation: Culture. Public health relevence: Identify likely exposure – often not determined.	Symptomatic infection usually presents as a flu-like illness with fever, cough, headaches and myalgias. Illness may resemble acute pneumonia, chronic, apical, chest infection mimicking tuberculosis or (in the immunocompromised) a fulminant disseminated infection. Asymptomatic infection is very common in endemic areas. Resolution may leave multiple miliary calcifications on the chest X-ray. Some patients develop chronic pulmonary infection or widespread disseminated infection.

Continued p. 258

Table 3.90.3 *Continued*

Disease, organism, epidemiology, investigation and public health relevence	Clinical
Mycetoma, Madura foot **Actinomycosis** *Madurella mycetoma* Actinomycetes are a group of bacteria that were formerly classified with fungi because they can be cultured on fungal media and they form long branching chains. Species of *Actinomyces* are amongst the causes of mycetoma (see below). Investigation: Microscopy, culture, biopsy. Public health relevence: None.	Localised chronic granulomatous infections with multiple discharging sinuses and slowly progressive destruction of underlying structures including bone occur in many tropical countries and are known collectively as mycetomas. They may be caused by true fungi such as *Madurella mycetoma* or by actinomycetes such as *Streptomyces somaliensis* or *Nocardia brasiliensis*. Organisms are inoculated through the skin, typically by thorns. After some delay, a painless swelling appears, which subsequently breaks down and discharges pus. A network of sinuses and chronic inflammatory tissue extends over a period of months, destroying surrounding structures. Bacterial secondary infection commonly exacerbates the problem. The commonest site for mycetoma is the foot. *Actinomyces israelii* typically causes multiple abscesses around the mouth, in the chest or at the terminal ileum. Drug treatment will differ markedly according to the organism so that accurate microbiological diagnosis is essential.
Mycotic keratitis Public health relevence: Investigate for contaminated contact cleaning fluid and iatrogenic transmission.	Corneal infection caused by fungi or yeast. The risk factors include trauma, contact lens usage, chronic ocular surface diseases, surgery and corneal anesthetic abuse. Fungal keratitis is a serious condition that requires prolonged treatment and close follow-up.
Nocardiosis *Nocardia asteroid* Public health relevence: None.	Causes severe systemic opportunistic infections and occasionally chronic chest infections in the immunocompetent.
Opportunistic mycoses Public health relevence: None.	Fungal infection is associated with immunosupression. Immunosupression may be due to underlying disease, malignancy, diabetes mellitus or HIV, or pharmacological. Fungi account for about 10% of all nosocomial infections in the US. The most common reported were *Candida* spp. (85.6%), followed by *Aspergillus* spp. (1.3%). *C. albicans* accounted for 76% of all *Candida* spp. infections. Other fungal pathogens (e.g., Malassezia, Trichosporon, Fusarium and Acremonium) represented 11% of the nosocomial fungal pathogens. Patients are being treated for an increasing variety of conditions with immunosuppressive agents. In these patients the diagnosis of fungal infection is frequently made post-mortem. Fungal infection should be considered in all immunosuppressed patients with an unexplained fever. Diagnostic tests for fungi are improving; mycological advice should be sought early so that appropriate specimens are sent. *Candida* septicaemia in a transplant recipient or periorbital mucormycosis in a diabetic require prompt treatment if the patient is to survive.

Table 3.90.3 *Continued*

Disease, organism, epidemiology, investigation and public health relevence	Clinical
Pityriasis versicolor. *Malassezia furfur* Investigation: View scrapings under Wood's lamp. Public health relevence: Avoid sharing of towels, etc.	*M. furfur* colonises oily areas of the skin, especially the scalp, back and chest causing characteristic discoloured or depigmented lesions of the skin. Young people around puberty are most commonly affected.
South American blastomycosis *Paracoccidioides brasiliensis* Occurrence: South America. Investigation: Microscopy, culture. Public health relevence: None.	Usually involves the skin, mouth, throat and lymph nodes, occasionally the lungs, liver or spleen. Lymph nodes become swollen and may drain pus; nodes most commonly infected are in the neck and axillae.
Sporotrichosis *Sporothrix schenckii.* Occurrence: Found in sphagnum moss, in hay, in other plant materials and in the soil. It enters the skin through small cuts or punctures from thorns, barbs, pine needles or wires. Incubation: 1–12 weeks. Investigation: Microscopy of swab, biopsy. Public health relevence: Outbreaks have occurred among nursery workers handling sphagnum moss, rose gardeners, children playing on baled hay and greenhouse workers. Wearing gloves and long sleeves when handling materials that may cause minor skin breaks. Avoid skin contact with sphagnum moss.	An infection of the skin; those persons handling thorny plants, sphagnum moss or hay are at increased risk. Usually starts with a small painless, red, pink or purple nodule resembling an insect bite, which appears on the limb where the fungus first entered through a break on the skin. This is followed by additional nodules that ulcerate and are slow to heal. Cases of joint, lung and CNS infection have occurred but are rare. Usually they occur in the immunocompromised.
Zygomycosis/Mucormycosis *Rhizopus, Rhizomucor, Absidia, Mucor* Transmission: Inhalation of spores. Investigation: Microscopy, biopsy. Public health relevence: None.	Invasive sinopulmonary infections such as the rhinocerebral syndrome, which occurs in diabetics with ketoacidosis present with pain, fever, orbital cellulites and proptosis. The palate, the facial bones and nasal septum may be destroyed. Mucormycosis (phycomycosis) is infection caused by a fungus of the group Mucorales. The other common site of infection is the lung. Rarely, the skin and digestive system are involved.

Table 3.90.4 Rare potentially imported viral infections

Viral species	Infection	Clinical	Incubation period	Vector/transmission	Geographical spread
Arenaviridae	Junin, Machupo, Sabia virus	Fever, prostration and haemorrhagic features	7–16 days	Wild rodents	South America
Bunyaviridae	Lymphocytic chroriomeningitis	Meningoencephalitis	8–13 days	Common house mouse, hamster, cell lines	US, South America, Europe
	Bunyamwera virus	Fever, headache, non-specific	3–12 days	Mosquito	All continents except Australia and Antarctica
	Oropouche	Fever, headache, non-specific	3–12 days	Midge	Central and South America
	Phleboviruses: Sandfly fever	Fever, headache, non-specific	3–12 days	*Phlebotomus* flies and mosquitoes	Africa and some parts of Asia and Mediterranean
	Rift Valley fever	Fever, haemorrhagic features	3–12 days	Handling animal tissues	Central Asia, Africa
	California encephalitis LaCrosse virus	Meningoencephalitis	5–15 days	Mosquito	Mid-west US
Flaviviridae	Powassan encephalitis (POW)	Fever, encephalitis	7–14 days	Tick borne (*Ixodes*)	US, Canada, Russia
	Russian spring–summer encephalitis	Fever, encephalitis	7–14 days	Tick borne (*Ixodes*)	Russia
	Louping Ill	Fever, encephalitis	7–14 days	Tick borne (*Ixodes*)	UK
	St. Louis encephalitis	Encephalitis, hepatitis	5–15 days	Mosquito	Americas
	Omsk haemorrhagic fever	Fever, diarrhoea, vomiting, haemorrhage	3–8 days	Tick bite	Far East
	Kyasanur Forest disease	Fever, diarrhoea, vomiting, haemorrhage	3–8 days	Tick bite	Far East
	West Nile fever	Fever, meningism	3–12 days	Mosquito	USA , East , Europe, East Mediterranean

Family	Virus	Symptoms	Incubation	Host/Vector	Distribution
Paramyxoviridae	Hendra virus Nipah virus	High fever, myalgia, respiratory disease, encephalitis	4–18 days	Horses Pigs ?Fruitbats	Australia, Malaysia
Poxviridae	Monkeypox	Fever, rash	?	? Monkeys and squirrels	Central Africa
Togaviridae	Eastern equine Encephalitis Western equine Encephalitis	Fever, encephalitis	5–15 days	Mosquito	US and Canada
	Venezuelan equine Encephalitis	Fever, chills, encephalitis	2–6 days	Mosquito	South and Central Americas
	Barmah Forest Ross River Chickungunya Sindbis	Fever, arthritis, rash	3–11 days	Mosquito Mosquito Mosquito Mosquito	Australia Australia, South Pacific Africa Southeast Asia Widespread not America

Bites

Human, dog and cat

These bites frequently become infected. The bite should be cleaned and dead tissue removed. Infecting organisms are usually derived from the oral flora; these may include streptococci, *Pasteurella* and anaerobes. Antibiotics covering the likely organisms should be given if there is evidence of infection.

Venomous snakes

There are few venomous snakes in Europe; however, bites may arise from imported snakes. Venomous snake bites are medical emergencies; a poisons centre should be contacted. The symptoms and signs depend upon the species and size of snake, the volume of venom injected, the location of the bite (central bites tend to be more severe than peripheral), the age, size and health of the victim.

The victim should avoid exertion and be urgently moved to the nearest medical facility. Rings, watches and constrictive clothing should be removed and the injured part immobilised in a functional position just below heart level. Tourniquets, incision and suction are contraindicated.

Attempts should be made to identify the snake so that the appropriate antivenom can be provided.

Spiders

Venomous spiders may be introduced as novelty pets. In the event of a bite every attempt should be made to identify the spider and a poisons centre should be contacted.

Other arthropods

There are a large number of other biting arthropods, mosquitoes, fleas, lice, bedbugs, sandflies, horseflies; none of these are venomous. The lesions produced vary from small papules to large ulcers, dermatitis may also occur, bites can be complicated by sensitivity reactions or infection; in hypersensitive persons, they can be fatal.

Ticks

Ticks may transmit infection such as Lyme disease or relapsing fever. Ascending flaccid paralysis may occur when toxin-secreting ticks remain attached for several days. Symptoms and signs include anorexia, lethargy, weakness, incoordination and ascending flaccid paralysis. Tick paralysis may be confused with Guillain–Barré syndrome, botulism, myasthenia gravis or spinal cord tumour. Bulbar or respiratory paralysis may develop.

Tick paralysis is rapidly reversible on removal of the tick (or ticks) and may require only symptomatic treatment.

Mites

Mite bites are common. Chiggers are mite larvae that feed in the skin, causing a pruritic dermatitis. There may be sensitisation.

Centipedes and millipedes

Some centipedes can inflict a painful bite, with some localised swelling and erythema. Lymphangitis and lymphadenitis are common. Millipedes may secrete a toxin that can cause local skin irritation and, in severe cases, marked erythema, vesiculation and necrosis. Some species can spray a secretion that causes conjunctival reactions.

Stings

Bees, wasps

The average person can tolerate approximately 20 stings/kg body weight. One sting can cause a fatal anaphylactic reaction in a hypersensitive person.

Stings may remain in the skin and should be removed. An ice cube will reduce pain. Persons known to be hypersensitive should carry epinephrine with them.

Scorpions

Stings from pet scorpions should be treated as potentially dangerous as the species may be difficult to determine. The victim should be observed. Information on antivenoms should be obtained from a poisons centre.

3.90.6 Chemical food-borne illness

Scombrotoxin fish poisoning

Caused by excess histamine, leading to diarrhoea, flushing, headache and sweating, sometimes accompanied by nausea, abdominal pain, burning in the mouth, tingling and palpitations. Onset is 10 minutes to 2 hours after consumption and symptoms usually resolve over 12 hours. Antihistamines may reduce severity. Excess histamine typically results from inadequate refrigeration of tuna, mackerel and other fish. Histamine level of fish can be tested.

Paralytic shellfish poisoning

Caused by saxitoxins produced by certain algae. Causes neurological symptoms: dizziness, tingling, drowsiness and muscular paralysis. Severe cases may suffer respiratory failure and death. May occasionally be gastrointestinal symptoms. Onset is 30 minutes to 2 hours after consumption. Usually because of the consumption of filter-feeding bivalve shellfish or crustacea (e.g. mussels, clams, oysters, scallops and crabs) that have consumed the algae, sometimes after 'red tides'. Saxitoxins can be measured in shellfish by specialist laboratory.

Diarrhetic shellfish poisoning

Caused by okadaic acid and other toxins in algae. Causes diarrhoea, nausea, vomiting and abdominal pain, with onset 30 minutes to 12 hours after consumption. Illness lasts 3–4 days. Usually associated with eating shellfish, often after 'red tides'. Toxin may be detected in shellfish.

Phytohaemagglutinin poisoning

Because of inadequate preparation of pulses such as red kidney beans, butter beans and lentils. Causes nausea and vomiting, followed by abdominal pain and diarrhoea, with onset 30 minutes to 12 hours after consumption.

Mushroom poisoning

Because of cyclopeptides and amatoxins consumed in *Amanita phalloides* (death cap), *Amanita verna*, *Amanita virosa* and some *Galerina* and *Lepiota* species. Causes colic, nausea, vomiting and diarrhoea, which after apparent recovery may be followed by liver or kidney failure with appreciable mortality. The advice of a regional poisons centre is vital for both investigation and treatment.

Others

• Gastrointestinal illness due to heavy metal poisoning (e.g. from food containers).
• Intoxication (alcohol-like) due to mushrooms.
• Gastrointestinal, liver and renal illness due to aflatoxins (e.g. fungal contamination of cereals).
• Neurological illness due to pesticides.
• Ciguatera fish poisoning (Americas, Australia, Pacific).
• Amnesiac shellfish poisoning (North America).
• Puffer fish poisoning (Japan).

Section 4
Services and organisations

4.1 Administrative arrangements for communicable disease control

Communicable disease control in England depends on joint working between many different agencies and individuals (Table 4.1.1). The arrangements in individual European countries are described in Section 5.

Health protection and the Health Protection Agency

Health protection describes the subset of public health activities aimed at protecting individuals, groups and populations from infectious diseases and environmental hazards such as chemical contamination and radiation. Historically, in the UK, the National Health Service (NHS) was the main provider of health protection services such as immunisation programmes, hospital infection control teams and in particular consultants in communicable disease control (CCDC). Since 1988 CCDCs have been appointed by each health authority to provide local leadership for the control of communicable disease and the health effects of environmental hazards. In April 2002 following the changes to NHS organisation described in *Shifting the Balance of Power,* health authority responsibilities for health protection passed to Primary Care Trusts.

The Health Protection Agency for England was established on 1 April 2003 following the publication of a Government's strategy document *Getting Ahead of the Curve.* The HPA, which has national, regional and local tiers, combines CCDCs and their staff with a number of specialist organisations (Table 4.1.1). The role of the HPA is to provide support and leadership to the NHS and other agencies to protect people from infectious diseases, poisons and chemical and radiological hazards. The HPA advises government on health protection policies and programmes, it provides authoritative information and advice to professionals and the public and it responds to emerging threats to public health and health protection emergencies, including outbreaks and deliberate release incidents. The HPA also has a role in health emergency planning.

Health Protection Units

The local tier of the HPA in England comprises 39 Health Protection Units (HPUs), each covering a population of about one million people. Each unit is staffed by CCDCs (now sometimes called consultants in health protection), health protection nurses and other support staff. The HPU works directly with PCTs, hospital trusts and local authorities on surveillance, investigation and management of incidents and outbreaks and the delivery of national action plans.

The NHS, Department of Health and Strategic Health Authorities

The UK National Health Service (NHS) was set up 56 years ago and is now the largest organisation in Europe. The overall aim of the Government's Department of Health (DH) is to improve the health and well-being of the population by supporting activity to protect, promote and improve health and securing the provision of high quality health and social-care services. There are 28 Strategic Health Authorities (SHAs), which are responsible for planning services, achieving national priorities and monitoring the performance of local services.

Primary Care Trusts

There are 302 Primary Care Trusts (PCT) in England, covering populations ranging in size from 60,000 to over 300,000. PCTs are local health organisations that are responsible for health services and improving health in their areas. PCTs carry out most of the functions that

Table 4.1.1 The organisations that formed the HPA

Organisation	Function
Public Health Laboratory Service (PHLS)	A network of about 50 public health laboratories, the Central Public Health Laboratory (CPHL) and the Communicable Disease Surveillance Centre (CDSC). The management of most of the laboratories has now reverted to the hospitals where they are located leaving nine regional HPA laboratories, which undertake public health and reference microbiology. The CPHL is the main British reference centre for microbiology, offering specialised tests, identification of unusual organisms and epidemiological typing. CDSC is the national surveillance centre.
The Centre for Microbiology and Research (CAMR)	Research on microbiological hazards associated with health care, work on the development and manufacture of diagnostic, prophylactic and therapeutic products.
The National Focus for Chemical Incidents (NFCI)	Support and advice to local NHS bodies and Government health departments on the management of major chemical incidents. Surveillance of environmental hazards.
The Regional Service Provider Units (RSPUs)	Expertise and support to health authorities on the management of chemical incidents and integrated pollution prevention and control (IPPC).
The National Poisons Information Service	Information and advice to healthcare professionals in the NHS on the diagnosis, treatment and management of patients who have been poisoned.
Health Emergency Planning Advisers (HEPA)	Guidance on all aspects of emergency planning, including hazard identification, risk assessment, preparation of plans, training, exercising of plans and performance monitoring
The National Radiological Protection Board (will join with HPA in April 2005)	Advice on all aspects of radiation hazards.

were previously the responsibility of health authorities including assessing health needs and ensuring that a full range of services is provided (Table 4.1.2). PCTs are also responsible for health protection and health emergency planning but receive assistance from the HPA to do this. PCTs are responsible for the delivery of immunisation services, HIV prevention services and infection control services in their community facilities. Some PCTs provide genitourinary medicine (GUM) services and tuberculosis services, while in other areas they commission these services from acute trusts.

Local government authorities

Local government in England and Wales is based on elected councils, which are accountable to the residents that they serve.

There are 39 county councils whose functions include police, fire, education, social services, waste disposal, civil defence, highways, consumer protection and planning, and there are around 400 district councils whose functions include environmental health, housing, planning, refuse collection, cemeteries and crematoria, markets and fairs, licensing activities and leisure and recreation. Some district councils, particularly those covering the large cities also carry out county council functions (unitary authorities). Councils consist of elected members or councillors and exercise their powers through committees, subcommittees or delegation to salaried officers. Officers acting on behalf of a council must ensure that the powers and responsibilities they exercise have been lawfully delegated to them by the elected members. Often legislation requires that the council exercises its power through a specific

Table 4.1.2 Local Health Services

Primary care services	General practitioners (GP), dentists, opticians and pharmacists. GPs care for patients with infection including diagnosis and treatment. They notify cases of infection to the local authority proper officer (usually the CCDC). They advise on hygiene, other infection control measures and travel health and deliver immunisation programmes.
Community health services, including community-based healthcare workers, clinics and community hospitals and nursing homes	Community nurses and other community-based healthcare workers usually work as members of a primary healthcare team, they manage infection problems and require access to infection control advice. Community trusts vary but they should have an infection control doctor (ICD) now called Director of Infection Prevention and Control and one or more community infection control nurses (CICN).
NHS walk-in centres	Prompt access to health advice and treatment.
NHS Direct	24-hour phone line, staffed by nurses, healthcare advice to the general public.
Care Trusts	NHS and local authorities work together to provide health and social-care services.
Mental Health Trusts	Specialist mental health services, in-patient and out-patient.
Acute (hospital) Trusts	NHS hospitals are run as non-profit making trusts. Hospitals are required to have satisfactory infection control arrangements.
Foundation Trusts	A new type of NHS hospital run by local managers, staff and members of the public; it has greater financial and operational freedom.
Ambulance Trusts	Emergency access to healthcare.

Table 4.1.3 Other agencies with a role in infectious disease control

The Department for the Environment, Food and Rural Affairs (DEFRA)	Promotes sustainable development and a better environment, protect public health in relation to food-borne disease and zoonoses.
The Drinking Water Inspectorate (DWI)	Safety of public water supplies, performance of water companies.
State Veterinary Service (SVS)	Control of animal health.
Environment Agency (EA)	Assessing, monitoring and reporting on waste disposal and human health and environment.
Health and Safety Executive (HSE)	Improve health and safety at work; reduce risks to workers and the public from work activities; control and investigation of Legionnaires' disease; enforcement of Control of Substances Hazardous to Health Regulations; infectious disease risks in the workplace.
The Food Standards Agency (FSA)	Protect the public from risks connected to the consumption of food; protect the interests of consumers; provide government response to outbreaks of food-borne disease; operate food hazard warning system; policies for microbial hazards associated with food; target to reduce food-borne disease by 20% by April 2006.
Occupational Health Services	Advise managers and employees about the effect of work on health and of health on work; minimise infectious hazards at work including advising on immunisation.

Table 4.1.4 Agencies, individuals and organisations involved in health protection

Health Protection Agency	Consultant for Communicable Disease Control
	Health Protection Nurse
	Regional HPA laboratory
	Centre for Infection (CDSC/CPHL)
	Centre for Radiation, Chemical and Environmental Hazards
	Centre for Emergency Preparedness and Response
Primary Care Trust	Director of Public Health
	Director for Infection Prevention and Control
	Community Infection Control Nurse
	Health visitors, district nurses, school health nurses
Hospitals	Director for Infection Prevention and Control
	Infection Control Doctor
	Medical microbiologist
	Infection Control Nurse
	Infectious disease specialist
	TB specialist, TB nurse advisers
	GUM specialist, GUM health adviser
Local authority departments (environmental, the health, education, social services)	Environmental Health Officers
	Trading Standards Officers
	Proper officer (usually CCDC)
	Teachers, social workers, home carers
	Residential home managers, safety managers
Primary care	General practitioners, practice nurses and other practice staff, community pharmacists, general dental practitioners
Private nursing homes, residential homes	Managers, nursing staff, carers
Occupational health departments	Occupational health doctors and nurses
Day nurseries	Managers, nursery nurses
General public	Citizens, consumers, newspapers, radio, TV
Food Standards Agency	See Table 4.1.2
The Department for the Environment Food and Rural Affairs	State Veterinary Service
	Drinking Water Inspectorate
Water companies	Quality managers
Environment agency	See Table 4.1.2
Health and Safety Executive	See Table 4.1.2

Table 4.1.5 Responsibilities of local health protection teams

Core activities	Non-core activities
Setting up and maintaining surveillance systems	District Immunisation Co-ordinator
Analysing trends in infectious disease incidence	District HIV Prevention Co-ordinator
Response to individual cases of infection	Tuberculosis contact tracing
Investigation and control of outbreaks	Port health
Proper officer for public health legislation	Emergency planning
Liaison with others involved in control of infectious disease	
Advice to local authorities, primary care staff and public	
Infection control advice and support to nursing and residential homes and schools	
Investigation of environmental hazards	
Chemical incident planning and management	
Advice on commissioning services to prevent, control and treat infection	
Prevention and health promotion programmes	
Teaching and training	
Continuing education, audit and research	

officer, usually referred to as the proper officer. For some public health legislation the proper officer would be the CCDC.

Environmental health departments and environmental health officers

The responsibilities of environmental health departments include food safety, air quality, noise, waste, health and safety, water quality, port health controls at air and sea ports, refuse collection and pest control. Environmental health officers (EHOs) investigate outbreaks of food- and water-borne infections, advise on and enforce food safety legislation, inspect food premises and investigate complaints and provide food hygiene training. EHOs liaise with a wide range of other professionals including the CCDC, general practitioners, teachers, microbiologists and veterinarians.

4.2 Surveillance of communicable disease

The effective management of infectious disease depends on good surveillance, which has been defined as the continuing scrutiny of all aspects of the occurrence and spread of a disease through the systematic collection, collation and analysis of data and the prompt dissemination of the resulting information to those who need to know so that action can result.

The purpose of surveillance

• Surveillance allows individual cases of infection to be identified so that action can be taken to prevent spread.
• Surveillance measures the incidence of infectious disease. Changes in incidence may signal an outbreak, which may need further

investigation and the introduction of special control measures.
• Surveillance tracks changes in the occurrence and risk factors of infectious disease and can indicate if sections of the population are at increased risk of infection as a result of environmental or behavioural factors. This allows specific interventions to be targeted at those groups.
• Surveillance allows existing control measures to be evaluated, and if new control measures are introduced, continuing surveillance will allow their effectiveness to be measured. A fall in the incidence of an infection may allow existing control measures to be relaxed.
• Surveillance allows the emergence of new infections of public health importance to be detected. It allows the epidemiology of these infections to be described and will produce hypotheses about aetiology and risk factors.

The principles of surveillance

A good surveillance system consists of the following key steps.
• There should be a case definition, which includes clinical and/or microbiological criteria.
• Cases of infection are identified from a variety of sources including reports from clinicians and laboratories. The case or an informant, who may be a relative, friend or medical or nursing attendant, is contacted by telephone, visit or letter, depending on the degree of urgency. A data set is collected for each case. The data that are collected depend on the nature of the infection. For all infections, the following minimum data set is usually collected: name, date of birth, sex, address, ethnic group, place of work, occupation, name of GP, recent travel, immunisation history, date of illness and clinical description of illness. For food-borne infections, food histories and food preferences may be recorded. For infections that are spread from person to person, the names and addresses of contacts may be requested, and for infections with an environmental source such as Legionnaires' disease, places visited and routes taken may be recorded. For some infections where intervention is required, additional data are

collected. For example, in the case of meningococcal infection the names of close household contacts may be recorded so that chemoprophylaxis and immunisation may be offered. For rare or novel infections, or where there is a need to find out more about the epidemiology, an enhanced data set may be collected or there may be a request for laboratory data to confirm the diagnosis. An example of this is the serological confirmation of clinical reports of measles, mumps and rubella using salivary antibody testing.

• Data are recorded on specially designed data collection forms and collated in a computerised database (e.g. CoSurv). Data may also be downloaded from databases used for patient management.

• One of the first uses of the data is to ensure that the cases satisfy the case definition. The database then allows analysis of the data and the production of summary statistics including frequency counts and rates, if suitable denominators are available. This permits the epidemiology of the infection to be described in terms of person, place and time and the detection of clusters of outbreaks. Local data can be shared and merged to produce data sets at national or even international level.

• Interpretation of the data and summary statistics leads to information on trends and risk factors, which are disseminated so that action can be taken. Dissemination can take place in a variety of ways. Increasingly data is available online but may also be found in local and national newsletters and journals (see Section 5 for country-specific details).

• Feedback to local data providers is important. It demonstrates the usefulness of the data and creates reliance on it. This in turn will lead to improvement in case ascertainment and data quality. Local data may be sent to GPs, hospital clinicians, microbiologists and EHOs.

• There should be continuing surveillance to evaluate the effect of interventions.

Sources of surveillance data

A number of data sources are available for the surveillance of infectious diseases. Many cases of infection are subclinical. These cases can only be detected by serological surveys. Clinical infection that does not lead to a medical consultation can be measured by population surveys. Cases that are seen by a doctor may be reported via a primary care reporting scheme or statutory notification system. Cases that are investigated by laboratory tests may be detected by a laboratory reporting system, and those that are admitted to hospital will be counted by a hospital information system. Finally the small proportion of infections that result in death will be detected by the death notification system. When designing a surveillance system, it is important to ensure that the most appropriate data source is utilised. For example it is not sensible to rely on laboratory reports for the surveillance of pertussis, which is only rarely diagnosed by the laboratory. In England and Wales the main routine data collecting systems are as follows.

Statutory notifications of infectious disease

The system for each European country is described in the relevant chapter of Section 5. The current list of notifiable infectious diseases in England and Wales is shown in Table 4.2.1. Any clinician suspecting these diagnoses is required to notify the proper officer of the local authority, who is usually the CCDC. The proper officer sends a weekly return to the Health Protection Agency (HPA) CDSC and the data are collated and published on their Website. Statutory notifications are an important way of monitoring trends in infectious disease, such as whooping cough, where the diagnosis is rarely confirmed by laboratory test.

Laboratory reporting system

HPA laboratories, NHS hospital laboratories and private laboratories should be able to offer a full diagnostic service for all common pathogenic microorganisms. If the laboratory is unable to carry out the work, then specimens are forwarded to a suitable reference laboratory. Medical microbiologists ensure that results of clinical significance are notified to

Table 4.2.1 Statutorily notifiable infectious diseases in England and Wales

Very rare infections	Rare infections	Common infections
Anthrax	Leptospirosis	Food poisoning
Leprosy	Yellow fever	Viral hepatitis
Typhus	Cholera	Whooping cough
Relapsing fever	Diphtheria	TB
Plague	Poliomyelitis	Malaria
Smallpox	Typhoid fever	Meningitis
Viral haemorrhagic	Paratyphoid fever	Meningococcal septicaemia
Fever	Rabies	Ophthalmia neonatorum
	Tetanus	Measles
	Encephalitis	Mumps
		Dysentery (amoebic and bacillary)
		Rubella
		Scarlet fever

the requesting clinician. Microorganisms of public health significance are also notified to the CCDC in accordance with previously agreed arrangements. This should be covered by a written policy. Typical arrangements for reporting to the CCDC are shown in Table 4.2.2. The method of reporting will vary depending on the urgency with which public health action is required. Increasingly, electronic reporting is in use but reporting by telephone, facsimile and letter are alternatives. In England reports are also sent to

Table 4.2.2 Reporting of infectious diseases to the CCDC in England

During working hours

Telephone CCDC as soon as possible for the following:

Typhoid fever	Paratyphoid fever	*Escherichia coli* O157
Meningococcal infection	All meningitis	Hib infection
Acute hepatitis B	Legionnaires' disease	Diphtheria

Also, less commonly:

Acute poliomyelitis	Anthrax	Botulism
Psittacosis	Cholera	Leprosy
Relapsing fever	Tetanus	Typhus
Viral haemorrhagic fever	Yellow fever	

CoSurv, telephone, fax or send notification form to CCDC or Environmental Services Department for the following:

Campylobacter	Shigellosis	Salmonellosis
Other food poisoning	Amoebic dysentery	Malaria
Mumps	Rubella	Measles
TB	Ophthalmia neonatorum	Pertussis
Viral hepatitis (other than 'B')	Cryptosporidium	

Out of hours and at weekends

Contact on-call Public Health staff member as soon as possible for the following infections:

Typhoid fever	Paratyphoid fever	Hib infection
Meningococcal infection	Toxin-producing diphtheria	

CDSC via the HPA Regional Surveillance Units (RSU). These data are collated and analysed and are published regularly in the Communicable Disease Report available weekly on the HPA Website. Although the data are usually of high quality, they are limited to infections for which there is a suitable laboratory test and infections that are easy to diagnose clinically tend to be poorly covered. Trends are difficult to interpret, since the data are sensitive to changes in testing or reporting by laboratories. In addition, because data are based on place of treatment rather than place of residence, denominators are not usually available and because negatives are not reported, neither the number of specimens tested nor the population at risk is known with certainty.

Reporting from primary care

In England the Royal College of General Practitioners (RCGP) Weekly Returns Service (WRS) is a network of 78 general practices that collect data on consultations and episodes of illness diagnosed in general practice. The data can be related to a defined population so that rates can be calculated for a selection of common diseases which are not notifiable, for which laboratory confirmation is not usually obtained and which do not usually result in admission to hospital. WRS is particularly useful in the surveillance of influenza and influenza-like illness. WRS data can be accessed via the HPA Website.

NHS Direct is a nurse-led telephone helpline with 22 call centres in England and Wales. Data on calls about selected symptoms are collated daily. Significant increases in symptoms that may be due to the deliberate release of a biological or chemical agent or more common infections are automatically detected and reported.

Hospital data

Data are available from hospital information systems on infectious diseases that result in admission to hospital. This is a useful source of data on more severe diseases likely to result in admission to hospital, although data are often

not sufficiently timely for some routine surveillance functions.

Sexually transmitted diseases

See Chapter 2.7 and Table 3.37.1.

Death certification and registration

Mortality data on communicable disease are of limited use since communicable diseases rarely cause death directly. Exceptions are deaths due to influenza, AIDS and TB. However, not all deaths due to infection are coded as such, and data may not be sufficiently timely for all surveillance functions.

International surveillance

International surveillance data can be found on the website of the WHO (http://www.who.int/en/). Surveillance is undertaken by individual European countries and summary data is available through Eurosurveillance, a multiformat journal (http://www.eurosurveillance.org). See also Table 5.1.1.

Enhanced surveillance

In England, CDSC has established enhanced surveillance systems for infections and hazards of particular public health importance. These systems may collect a more detailed data set from informants, they may combine epidemiological and microbiological data including typing or they may use multiple sources of data. Such systems have been established for meningococcal disease, TB, antimicrobial resistance, travel-associated legionella infection, zoonoses, influenza, infections in prisons, outbreaks of infectious intestinal disease and water-borne infections and water quality.

Other sources of data

The Medical Officers of Schools Association reports illness in children in approximately 55 boarding schools in England and Wales weekly to CDSC. This is useful in the surveillance of influenza.

The British Paediatric Surveillance Unit of the College of Paediatrics and Child Health co-ordinates surveillance of uncommon paediatric conditions. A reporting card is sent each month to consultant paediatricians in the UK. They indicate if they have seen a case that month and return the card. An investigator then contacts the paediatrician for further information. Conditions of infective origin that are under surveillance include congenital cytomegalovirus infection, congenital rubella, congenital toxoplasmosis, HIV/AIDS infection in childhood, complications of varicella, invasive fungal infection in low-birth-weight infants and neonatal herpes simplex virus infection. Similar schemes operate in other European countries.

Active surveillance of selected occupationally acquired infections is carried out by the Surveillance of Infectious Diseases at Work (SIDAW) Project at the Centre for Occupational Health at the University of Manchester (http://www.coeh.man.ac.uk/thor/sidaw.htm).

Other local reporting arrangements may include histopathology laboratories (for TB), haematology laboratories (for malaria), pharmacies, GUM clinics, chest clinics and drug teams. The CCDC should agree a local surveillance protocol, publicise case definitions and remind clinicians annually of their responsibility to report infections.

4.3 Managing infectious disease incidents and outbreaks

An infectious disease incident may be defined in one of the following ways:
• Two or more persons with the same disease or symptoms or the same organism isolated from a diagnostic sample, who are linked through common exposure, personal characteristics, time or location.
• A greater than expected rate of infection compared with the usual background rate for the particular place and time.

• A single case of a particular rare or serious disease such as diphtheria, rabies, viral haemorrhagic fever or polio.
• A suspected, anticipated or actual event involving exposure to an infectious agent (e.g. HIV infected healthcare worker, white powder incident, failure of decontamination procedures).
• Actual or potential microbial or chemical contamination of food or water.

The first two of these categories may also be described as an outbreak. The control of an outbreak of infectious disease depends on early detection followed by a rapid structured investigation to uncover the source of infection and the route of transmission. This is followed by the application of appropriate control measures to prevent further cases. Outbreaks of infectious disease are usually investigated and managed by an informal team comprising the local public health physician, a medical microbiologist from the local hospital or HPA laboratory and an EHO from the local authority. If the outbreak affects a large number of people, if it is a serious infection, if it affects a wide geographical area or if there is significant public or political interest, then consideration should be given to convening an outbreak control team to oversee the management of the episode. A written outbreak control plan detailing the steps that should be taken is an essential requirement. Incident management may be more effective if an incident control room is established. Potential areas for use as incident rooms within local authority or health premises should be identified in the outbreak control plan. In circumstances where there are likely to be significant numbers of enquiries from members of the public—for example during a look-back exercise following identification of a healthcare worker infected with hepatitis B—a dedicated telephone helpline may be established. Telephone helplines can deal with large numbers of people needing information, counselling or reassurance and they can be used for case finding. Setting up an incident room and telephone helpline are useful parts of an outbreak exercise or simulation (see Box 4.3.1).

In England CDSC co-ordinates a national surveillance scheme for general outbreaks of

Box 4.3.1 Setting up an incident room and telephone helpline

The incident room
- Dedicated use
- 24-hour access and security
- Large enough for the incident team, their equipment and files
- Sufficient telephone lines
- A dedicated fax machine
- Computer with access to the internet and e-mail
- Access to photocopying facilities
- Filing systems for storing all communications, minutes of meetings, notes of decisions, etc.

Helpline
- Decision taken by the outbreak control team
- Part of the local emergency plan
- A subgroup should take responsibility for planning and establishing the help lines
- The group should include a public health physician, a person with the authority to make financial decisions, a telecommunications expert and administrative support
- The purpose of the helpline must be clear
- List of staff needed to staff the line
- Needs of minority ethnic groups and the hearing impaired should be considered
- Early liaison with clinical specialists to ensure that staff are properly briefed
- Question and answer and frequently asked question sheets should be developed
- Mechanisms to deal with unexpected calls or complex queries
- Training to deal with obscene, silent or threatening calls
- Staff may have to deal with anxious and distressed callers and should be properly supported
- Facilities to call back may be required
- Briefing materials and procedures should be reviewed regularly to identify any inadequacies
- All calls should be logged
- A minimum data set would include date and time of call, sex, age and postcode of caller and the appropriateness of the call
- Further data collection would depend upon the nature of the helpline
- Headsets rather than handsets should be provided so that helpline workers can keep their hands free to make notes or use computer terminals
- Media can be used to publicise the helpline
- It can be difficult to estimate the number of telephone lines required; the limiting factor may be the number of people available to staff the lines. Most calls arrive in the first few days, so the maximum number of lines should be available at the start of an incident; excess lines can then be closed down
- Calls can first be screened by an experienced person who then allocates them appropriately-or calls can be taken by a first-line person, who passes on difficult calls
- Four-hour shifts are generally used, some may be able to do two shifts
- A supervisor is needed for each shift to deal with briefings and administration and cover staff breaks.
- The hours that the helpline is open will depend on circumstances
- It should include the evening so that those working in shifts or with children can call for example from 8 a.m. to 9 p.m.
- Hours may need to be adjusted to cope with anxieties raised by media coverage, e.g. keeping the helpline open until midnight if the issue is covered in the evening
- An answering machine message giving the opening hours should be available when closed
- After the incident the helpline should be reviewed; lessons learned can be recorded and a formal report prepared for the health authority

infectious intestinal disease. These are outbreaks affecting members of more than one private residence or residents of an institution. They are distinct from family outbreaks, which affect members of the same private residence only. When an outbreak is over, the CCDC or lead investigator is asked to complete a structured questionnaire. The output from this scheme is reported regularly on the HPA Website.

Detection

An outbreak will be recognised by case reports, complaints or as a result of routine surveillance.

An outbreak of haemorrhagic colitis due to consumption of cold turkey roll contaminated with E. coli O157 was discovered when several people who had attended the same christening party were admitted to the infectious disease ward at a local hospital.

An outbreak of gastroenteritis resulting from Salmonella panama infection due to the sale of contaminated cold meats from a market stall was detected when the local public health laboratory isolated this unusual organism from several faecal samples sent in by GPs from patients with diarrhoea.

An outbreak of food-borne viral gastroenteritis affecting people who had attended a wedding reception at a hotel came to light when affected guests complained to the local environmental health department.

An outbreak due to the common strain of Salmonella enteritidis PT4 was uncovered when environmental health officers questioned several people, initially reported as sporadic cases by clinicians and laboratories, with this infection in a Midlands town. They all reported buying and eating bakery products from a mobile shop. Further investigations revealed that custard mix used in the preparation of trifle had become contaminated with raw egg.

Systematic investigation

The reasons for investigating an outbreak are to identify and control source of infection and route of transmission to prevent further cases, to prevent similar outbreaks in the future, to describe new diseases and learn more about known diseases, to teach and learn epidemiology, to address public concern and to gather evidence for legal action.

A systematic approach to the investigation of an outbreak comprises eight stages.

1 Establishing that a problem exists: A report of an outbreak of infection may be mistaken. It may result from increased clinical or laboratory detection of cases, changes in reporting patterns, changes in the size of the at-risk population or false-positive laboratory tests.

Increases in the number of cases of tuberculosis in recent years following many years of decline may be due to increases in the size of certain population subgroups that are at increased risk of tuberculosis. These would include the elderly, the homeless and those that have migrated from areas of the world where the incidence of tuberculosis remains high.

An outbreak of cryptosporidiosis was due to false-positive laboratory tests. The microbiology technician mistook fat globules for oocysts of the protozoon Cryptosporidium parvum in faecal smears.

Other pseudo-outbreaks due to laboratory contamination were recognised because cases, despite having identical microbiological results, had no detectable epidemiological links, inconclusive clinical diagnoses and were only reported by one laboratory.

2 Confirming the diagnosis: Cases can be diagnosed either clinically or by laboratory investigations. At an early stage it is important to produce and adhere to a clear case definition. This is particularly important with previously unrecognised diseases in which proper definitions are needed before epidemiological studies can proceed.

In 1989, an investigation was started into an outbreak of atypical pneumonia affecting men of working age in the Birmingham area. Four weeks elapsed before the laboratory confirmed the diagnosis as Q fever and progress could be made with the epidemiological investigation. Cases of Q fever were defined as patients with onset of an acute febrile illness between 27 March and 3 July and a

fourfold rise in titre of complement fixing antibod-
ies to phase II antigen of C. burnetii, a sustained
phase II titre of ≥ 256, or the presence of specific
IgM on an indirect immunofluoresence test.

3 Immediate control measures: Control
measures involve either controlling the source
of infection, interrupting transmission or protecting those at risk.

4 Case finding: In an episode of infection,
the cases that are first noticed may only be a
small proportion of the total population affected and may not be representative of that
population. Efforts must be made to search
for additional cases. This allows the extent of
the incident to be quantified, it allows a more
accurate picture of the range of illness that
people have experienced, it allows individual
cases to be treated and control measures to be
taken, and it provides subjects for further descriptive and analytical epidemiology. There
are several ways of searching for additional
cases:

- Statutory notifications of infectious disease.
- Requests for laboratory tests and reports of
positive results.
- People attending their GPs, the local accident and emergency department, hospital
inpatients and outpatients.
- Reports from the occupational health departments of large local businesses.
- Reports from schools of absenteeism and
illness.
- Household enquiries.
- Appeals through TV, radio and local newspapers.
- Screening tests applied to communities
and population subgroups.

In a local outbreak of Salmonella panama in-
fection, a fax message was sent to all microbiolo-
gists in the region asking them to report isolates of
Salmonella panama to the investigating team.

In the 1989 outbreak of Q fever, local GPs were
telephoned and local occupational health depart-
ments were contacted to enquire about cases of
atypical pneumonia or unexplained respiratory
disease.

CCDCs and microbiologists can be alerted
by fax or e-mail. In the past they have been
asked to report cases of Legionnaires' disease

associated with a Midlands industrial site,
cases of meningitis associated with a university hall of residence and food-borne infection
associated with hotels and social gatherings.

5 Collection of data: A set of data is collected from each of the cases. This includes
name, age, sex, address, occupation, name of
GP, recent travel, immunisation history, date
of illness and clinical description of illness.
Data should also be collected about exposure
to possible sources of the infection. In the
case of a food-borne infection this would include a recent food history. In the case of infection spread by person-to-person contact,
the case would be questioned about contact
with other affected persons. In the case of
an infection spread by the air-borne route,
cases would be questioned about places they
had visited. It is preferable to collect these
data by administering a detailed semistructured questionnaire in a face-to-face interview.
This allows the interviewer to ask probing questions, which may sometimes uncover previously unsuspected associations between cases.
Telephone interviews or self-completion questionnaires are less helpful at this stage of an
investigation.

In an investigation of a possible national out-
break of Salmonella newport infection that was
thought to be food-borne, very detailed questioning
was undertaken about the food that had been con-
sumed in the 7 days prior to illness. This included
asking specifically what food items had been eaten
at each meal. In addition respondents were asked if
they had eaten particular food items and if so where
these had been purchased and the brand that had
been purchased.

In the investigation of an outbreak of Legion-
naires' disease thought to have an environmental
source, cases were asked to indicate on a map the
exact places they had visited in the 10 days prior to
illness. In addition they were asked specifically if
they had visited particular locations that had been
mentioned by other respondents.

It may be necessary to re-interview early
cases to ask about possible exposures that are
reported by later cases.

In the investigation of the Salmonella panama
outbreak, it was not until the seventh case was in-
terviewed that the market stall was mentioned for a

second time. The early cases were questioned again and all but one reported buying or receiving items that could be traced to this stall.

6 Descriptive epidemiology: Cases are described by the three epidemiological parameters of time, place and person. Describing cases by person includes clinical features, age, sex, occupation, social class, ethnic group, food history, travel and leisure activity. Describing cases by place includes home address and work address. Describing cases by time involves plotting the epidemic curve, a frequency distribution of date or time of onset. This may allow the incubation period to be estimated which, with the clinical features, may give some clues as to the causative organism (see Table 2.2.1). The incubation period should be related to events that may have occurred in the environment of the cases and which may indicate possible sources of infection.

In a national outbreak of Salmonella ealing infection, those affected were mainly infants. This suggested a connection with a widely distributed infant food. Dried baby milk was subsequently found to be the source of infection. A national outbreak of Salmonella napoli infection affecting mainly children was found to be due to contaminated chocolate bars.

Figure 4.3.1 is the epidemic curve that would occur in a milk-borne *Campylobacter* outbreak due to delivery and consumption of contaminated milk on one particular day (point source outbreak). Figure 4.3.2 is the epidemic curve in a similar outbreak in which contaminated milk was consumed at the school over several days (continuing source outbreak). Figure 4.3.3 is the epidemic curve in a community outbreak

of measles where the infection is spread from person to person (propagated outbreak). There is a smooth epidemic curve with distinct peaks at intervals of the incubation period.

7 Generating a hypothesis: A detailed epidemiological description of typical cases may well provide the investigators with a hypothesis regarding the source of infection or the route of transmission. A description of atypical cases may also be helpful.

8 Testing the hypothesis: Finding that consumption of a particular food, visiting a particular place or being involved in a certain activity is occurring frequently among cases is only a first step. These risk factors may also be common among those who have not been ill. To confirm an association between a risk factor and disease, further microbiological or environmental investigations may be required, or an analytical epidemiological study may be necessary. This can be either a cohort study or a case–control study.

- Case–control study: A case–control study compares exposures in people who are ill (the cases) with exposure in people who are not ill (the controls). These studies are most useful when the at-risk population cannot be accurately defined (e.g. when cases are laboratory reports of infection in the general population). Controls can be selected from a GP's practice list, from the PCT patient register, from the laboratory that reported the case, from people nominated by the case or from neighbours selected at random from nearby houses.

- Cohort study: The cohort study is a type of natural experiment in which a proportion

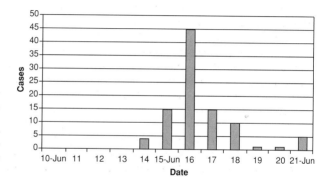

Fig. 4.3.1 Outbreak of *Campylobacter* gastroenteritis associated with consumption of unpasteurised milk (point source).

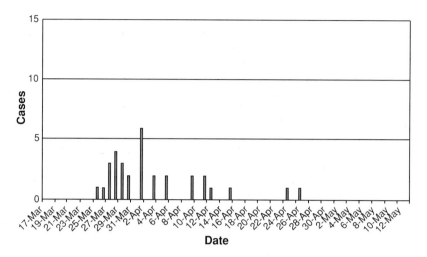

Fig. 4.3.2 Outbreak of *Campylobacter* gastroenteritis associated with consumption of unpasteurised milk (continuing source).

of a population is exposed to a factor, while the remainder is not. The incidence or attack rate of infection amongst exposed persons is compared with the rate amongst unexposed persons. For example, following a food poisoning outbreak at a social gathering, thought to be due to consumption of contaminated chocolate mousse, the cohort (all those who attended) is divided into those who ate the mousse (the exposed) and those who did not (the unexposed).

• Collecting the data: A set of data is collected from both cases and control or from the exposed and unexposed persons within the cohort. A case definition should be

agreed and sample size calculation should be performed to ensure that the study has adequate statistical power. To avoid any bias the data must be collected from each subject in exactly the same way. Usually this is done by questionnaire. Unlike the hypothesis-generating questionnaire, the questionnaire for an analytical study is often shorter, more structured and uses mostly closed questions. It may be administered at interview, by telephone or it may be a self-completion postal questionnaire. Questionnaires should be piloted before use. If several interviewers will be used they should be adequately briefed and provided with instructions to ensure the

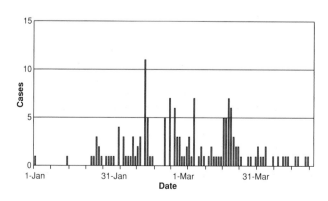

Fig. 4.3.3 Outbreak of measles in a community (propagated outbreak).

questionnaire is administered in a consistent way.

• Analysis: In both cohort and case–control studies initial analysis is by a 2 × 2 table. In cohort studies the ratio of incidence in exposed to incidence in unexposed is calculated. This is the relative risk. In case–control studies the odds of exposure in the cases is compared with the odds of exposure in the controls. This is the odds ratio, which usually approximates the relative risk. Confidence intervals for these estimates can be calculated and tests of statistical significance applied. Computer programmes (e.g. Epi-Info) are freely available, which will perform these calculations.

In an outbreak of cryptosporidiosis in Kent at the end of 1990, the hypothesis was that infection was associated with the consumption of cold drinking water supplied by the local water company. This was tested using a case–control study. Cases were defined as people living locally who had a diarrhoeal illness between 1 December 1990 and 31 January 1991, with oocysts present in a faecal sample. Cases were excluded if they had travelled abroad or if another household member had diarrhoea in the 4 weeks before the onset of their illness. The names and addresses of controls were obtained from the patient list held by the health authority. They were matched with the cases for sex, age group and GP or health centre. They were excluded if they had been abroad within 4 weeks of the onset of illness in their matched cases or if they themselves had diarrhoea since 1 December 1990. Five names and addresses of controls were obtained for each case. For each case and control a questionnaire was completed by a member of the investigating team during a telephone interview. The questionnaire asked about illness and consumption of various food items, including milk, salad, meat and cheese. Participants were also asked about the consumption of cold tap water both at home and outside the home, consumption of untreated, filtered or bottle water and exposure to recreational water. The results are given in Table 4.3.1. There was a dose–response relationship with the quantity of tap water consumed.

Table 4.3.1 Cryptosporidiosis in Kent, December 1990. Odds ratios for exposure to select factors

	Case		Control			
	Y	N	Y	N	Odds Ratio*	95% CI on odds ratio
Unpasteurised milk	0	29	0	80	N/A	N/A
Lettuce	16	11	51	29	0.83	0.31–2.22
Fresh raw vegetables	2	6	56	23	1.51	0.5–5.12
Unpasteurised cheese	0	29	10	69	0	0–1.15
Contact with farm animals	0	27	0	80	N/A	N/A

Tap water
    Y = >1 cup/day
    N = <1 cup/day
	19	7	33	47	3.87[†]	1.35–12.03[‡]

Water consumed outside the home	15	10	23	51	3.33	1.18–9.49
Water filtered	0	29	8	72	0	0–1.57
Bottled water	0	29	16	64	0	0–0.63[§]
Swimming pool	5	23	16	64	0.87	0.22–2.87
Rivers	2	26	1	79	6.08	0.3–363

* The odds ratio is the odds of exposure in the cases divided by the odds of exposure in the controls. An odds ratio of 1 indicates no association.

[†] Consumption of tap water is nearly four times as likely in cases as in controls.

[‡] The 95% confidence interval does not include 1, indicating that this is a significant association that is unlikely to be due to chance.

[§] Controls are significantly more likely than cases to have been exposed to bottled water, i.e. there is a protective effect.

Table 4.3.2 Salmonella infection in a south coast hotel, Christmas 1988. Relative risk of infection for consumption of selected foods (significant items only)

	Ill		Not ill			
Food	Ate	Did not eat	Ate	Did not eat	Relative risk*	95% CI on relative risk
Chocolate mousse	66	2	21	14	6.07[†]	1.65–2.31[‡]
Lemon mousse	60	4	25	12	2.82	1.2–6.67[§]
Crème caramel	55	9	24	13	1.7	1.01–2.57[§]

* The relative risk (RR) is the risk of illness in the exposed divided by the risk of illness in the unexposed. A RR of 1 indicates no difference and therefore no association between illness and exposure. The relative risk can only be calculated for cohort or cross-sectional studies.
[†] Illness is six times more likely in those who ate chocolate mousse.
[‡] The 95% confidence interval does not include 1, so the results are unlikely to have occurred by chance.
[§] There are weaker but none the less significant associations between illness and lemon mousse and crème caramel.

An outbreak of Salmonella enteritidis phage type 4 infection affected a party of 136 elderly people staying at a hotel on the south coast of England over Christmas and New Year 1988/89. The hypothesis was that illness was associated with consumption of contaminated food items served in the hotel restaurant. This was tested with a cohort study. The cohort was guests and staff at the hotel. Cases were defined as members of staff or guests who had gastrointestinal symptoms between 23 and 29 December. All members of the cohort were asked to complete a questionnaire during an interview with an EHO, which enquired about symptoms and food eaten in the hotel. Attack rates for those who did and didn't eat certain food items were compared and relative risks were calculated. Consumption of three food items (Table 4.3.2) were significantly associated with illness. All these items contained fresh egg, the presumed source of infection in this outbreak.

9 Further control measures and declaring the outbreak over: Once source and route of transmission are known further control measures may be required. Surveillance to detect new cases and continuing to plot the epidemic curve will allow the outbreak control team to set criteria for declaring the end of the outbreak. Generally for common source outbreaks the elapsed time since the latest case must be at least three times longer than the mean incubation period to declare the outbreak over at the 0.05 level of significance.

4.4 Community infection control

The community is defined as all environments that are outside hospital. This includes nursing and residential homes, hostels, day-care centres, schools, colleges and nurseries, factories, offices and other workplaces, leisure centres, hotels, restaurants, shops, cinemas, theatres and other places of entertainment, open spaces and communal areas, transport and finally people's own homes and gardens. These settings may bring together susceptible persons or provide opportunities for population mixing.

Control measures for community infection

To control infection, measures can be directed to the source of infection and the route of transmission or susceptible people can be offered protection with antibiotics or immunisation. The measures may involve the person or case, his or her contacts, the environment and the wider community. Ideally control measures should be evidence based or at least based on consensus and best practice.

Person

The case is contacted by visit, telephone or letter and details are recorded on a specific case report form. Diagnostic samples may be requested, e.g. faecal samples in the case of suspected gastrointestinal infections.

Control measures are based on an assessment of the risk that the case may spread infection. Guidelines are available to assist with this risk assessment. For example, with gastrointestinal infections the case may be assigned to one of four risk groups: food handler, health or social-care worker, child aged less than 5 years or older child or adult with low standards of personal hygiene (Box 2.2.1). Factors such as type of employment, availability of sanitary facilities and standards of personal hygiene should also be considered.

The case may be isolated until no longer infectious. The extent of this isolation will vary. Usually isolation at home will be sufficient. However, strict isolation for highly infectious or virulent infections that spread by both the air-borne route as well as direct contact may necessitate admission to an infectious diseases unit. It may be necessary to exclude infectious cases from school or work.

The case may be kept under surveillance, examined clinically or undergo laboratory investigations. He or she may be treated to reduce the communicable period or family and household contacts and medical and nursing attendants may be advised to adopt certain precautions to reduce the risk of transmission. Precautions that are advised to prevent transmission of blood-borne pathogens include not to share personal items, careful use and disposal of needles and other sharp instruments, careful disposal of clinical waste, safe sex and careful attention to blood spillages. Enteric precautions for gastrointestinal infections comprise use of gloves and gowns, sanitary disposal of faeces and babies' nappies, attention to personal hygiene including handwashing, regular cleaning and use of appropriate disinfectants. The case may be advised to restrict contact with young children and others who may be particularly susceptible to infection. He or she may be advised not to prepare food for other household members. Advice should be reinforced with written material such as leaflets, or a video may be available. Legal powers are available, but these are rarely used.

Public health law

The Public Health (Control of Disease) Act 1984 and the Public Health Infectious Diseases Regulations 1988 give UK local authorities powers to control communicable disease. These powers are exercised either directly or through the *proper officer* who, for CDC issues, is usually the CCDC. Some powers, such as those which deal with the notification of diseases, are purely administrative. However, there are other powers to control things, premises and people. This includes preventing the sale of infected articles, preventing infected people from using public transport, cleaning and disinfection of premises, excluding people from work and school, offering immunisation, compulsory examination, removal to hospital and detention in hospital and obtaining information from householders and schools in order to prevent the spread of disease.

There are four pieces of legislation concerned with diseases that can be transmitted sexually. The Venereal Disease Act 1917 makes treatment and advertising treatment for STDs other than by designated clinics an offence. The National Health Service (Venereal Diseases) Regulations 1974 and the National Health Service Trusts (Venereal Diseases) Directions 1991 give limited confidentiality to patients and the AIDS (Control) Act 1987 requires information about AIDS to be sent to the Secretary of State. There are public health regulations covering aircraft, ships and international trains that pass through the Channel Tunnel (see Chapter 4.15). These deal with infectious persons or infectious animals or material on board.

Contacts

Contacts of a case of infectious disease may be at risk of acquiring infection themselves, they may risk spreading infection to others, or they may be the source of infection. It is important to have a definition of a contact and conduct a risk assessment. For example, a contact of a case of gastrointestinal infection is someone who has been exposed to the excreta of a case. With typhoid this definition would be extended to those exposed to the same source as the case, such as those who were on the same visit abroad. A contact of a case of meningococcal infection is someone who has spent a night under the same roof as the case in the 7 days before onset, or has had mouth-kissing contact. Contacts may be subjected to clinical or laboratory examination. For example, in the case of diphtheria and typhoid, they may be offered advice, placed under surveillance, asked for laboratory specimens or offered prophylaxis with antibiotics or immunisation. In some circumstances contacts may be excluded from school or work (legal powers are available).

Environment

In some circumstances it may be appropriate to investigate the environment of a case of infection. This may involve inspection and laboratory investigation of home or work. Examples are food-borne infections, gastrointestinal infections and Legionnaires' disease. There are legal powers to control the environment, including powers to seize, destroy and prohibit the use of certain objects. This may be necessary in the event of infection caused by a contaminated foodstuff. It may be appropriate to advise on cleaning and disinfection.

Community

The occurrence of cases of infection will have an effect on the wider community. For example, a case of Legionnaires' disease or tuberculosis may generate considerable anxiety in the workforce. Meningitis and hepatitis B will have a similar effect in schools on staff, pupils and parents. Scabies in day-care centres and head lice in schools are other examples. It is helpful to keep all sections of the community informed about certain cases of infection. This can be done by letter or public meeting. In some cir-

cumstances it may be appropriate to set up a telephone advice line or Website. In addition it can be helpful to inform local newspapers, radio, television and politicians. All sections of the community have information needs with respect to the prevention and control of infectious disease. Advice is available from a range of health professionals. This can be reinforced by leaflets, videos and through the media. In community settings such as schools, nursing homes, residential homes and primary care it is helpful to make available written guidelines on infection control in the form of a manual or handbook. These materials can subsequently from the basis for training and audit in infection control.

Prevention of infectious disease

Activity to prevent infection can be directed at the host or the environment.

Host

Risk behaviour may be changed by health education campaigns. These may be national or local, and may be aimed at the general population or targeted at those who are particularly at risk. Infections that have been the subject of national health education campaigns include HIV infection, STIs, *Salmonella*, *Listeria* and VTEC infection. For example, the Chief Medical Officer has given the following food safety advice:

Avoid eating raw eggs or uncooked dishes made from eggs. Pregnant women, the elderly, the sick, babies and toddlers should only eat eggs that have been cooked until both the yolk and the white are solid. To avoid listeriosis, pregnant women and those people with decreased resistance to infection are advised to avoid eating soft ripe cheeses such as Brie, Camembert and blue vein varieties and to avoid eating paté. These groups are also advised to re-heat cook-chilled meals and ready-to-eat poultry until piping hot rather than eat them cold. Beef burgers should be cooked thoroughly throughout until the juices run clear and there are no pink bits inside.

Health services offer diagnosis, screening, treatment, prophylaxis and immunisation. Examples are routine and selective immunisation, services for tuberculosis screening, treatment for newly arrived immigrants and services for STI diagnosis and treatment.

Environment

Local authority environmental health departments have legal powers to control aspects of the environment that could be a source of infection, including supplies of food and water, disposal of sewage, waste management and pest control.

The Food Safety Act 1990 provides a framework for a range of regulations that govern the activity of food businesses, the composition and labelling of foods, chemical safety, food hygiene and the control of specific foodstuffs. The enforcement of food law is the responsibility of local authority environmental health officers (EHO). There are statutory codes of practice that provide guidance. EHOs have powers to inspect any aspect of the food chain including production, manufacturing, distribution and retail stages. They inspect food businesses at a frequency of once every 6 months to once every 5 years depending on risk, they take samples of food for testing and investigate food complaints from consumers. They have powers to take action against food premises that do not comply with food law. Enforcement action ranges from warnings, improvement or prohibition notices to prosecution.

The Food Standards Agency (FSA) was established by the Food Standards Act 1999. The FSA has powers to strengthen enforcement of food standards by managing the performance of enforcement authorities. *Food Alerts* are the FSA's way of letting local authorities and consumers know about problems associated with food and, in some cases, provide details of specific action to be taken. The Local Authorities Coordinators of Regulatory Services (LACORS) acts as a link between local food enforcement and central Government, giving advice and guidance to local authorities as well as advising the FSA on food enforcement issues.

The Food Safety (General Food Hygiene) Regulations 1995 place obligations on food businesses to ensure their activities are carried out in a hygienic way, including arrangements governing food handlers' fitness to work. Food-handling staff must report to management any infectious or potentially infectious conditions and immediately leave the workplace if they have such a condition. The conditions are diarrhoea and vomiting, gastrointestinal infections, enteric fever and infected lesions of skin, eyes, ears and mouth. Before returning to work following illness due to gastrointestinal infection there should be no vomiting for 48 hours, a normal bowel habit for 48 hours and good hygienic practices, particularly handwashing.

4.5 Healthcare-associated infection

Healthcare-associated infections (HCAI) are infections that occur in patients or healthcare workers as a result of healthcare interventions. Hospital-acquired infections are those acquired during a stay in hospital. Most HCAIs relate to hospitals, although in future as the dependency of patients who are cared for outside hospitals increases more HCAIs may be seen in community settings. HCAI include bacteraemias, urinary infections, chest infections, skin infections and surgical wound infections. The microorganisms that cause HCAI include MRSA, *Clostridium difficile*, gram-negative organisms such as *Acinetobacter, Enterobacter, Escherichia coli, Klebsiella, Proteus* and *Pseudomonas* and gram-positive organisms such as *Enterococcus, Staphylococci*, pyogenic streptococci and *S. pneumoniae*. Infections that are more typically community acquired such as TB, norovirus and influenza can also spread in healthcare settings and may present management challenges. Most cases of HCAI are sporadic but outbreaks and clusters can occur.

The impact of HCAI

The emergence of HCAI as a problem is explained by the classic balance between host, agent and environment. Patients are more susceptible because of age and underlying conditions, organisms may be resistant to antibiotics, treatment is more invasive and more intensive and hospitals are busier.

HCAI have an impact because they complicate other medical and surgical conditions, add to length of stay and treatment costs, cause anxiety and discomfort and may lead to disability and even death. Various estimates have been made of the cost of HCAI. In England it is estimated that there are 300,000 new episodes of HCAI each year giving a prevalence amongst hospital patients of 9%.

Risk factors for HCAI

Hospital patients with underlying disease, particularly the old and young and those with weakened immune systems are at greatest risk of HCAI. Invasive devices and procedures including surgery, pressure sores, intensive care, previous exposure to antimicrobial agents and previous hospital admission add to the risk.

Surveillance of HAI

Voluntary surveillance schemes have been in place in England for some years based on laboratory reporting of alert organisms. Recently mandatory schemes have been introduced for MRSA bacteraemia, *C difficile* diarrhoea, GRE bacteraemia, orthopaedic surgical site infection and serious untoward incidents. Most European countries have HCAI surveillance programmes. Although variations in protocols and hospital participation make direct comparisons unreliable, national HCAI prevalence rates are between 4 and 10% compared with 9% in the UK. In the UK there is a perception that HCAI is increasing, it has attracted public and media attention and has become a political priority. However, data suggest that in the past 3 years, levels of HCAI may be stabilising.

Control of HCAI

Control measures for HCAI comprise a range of activities that aim to prevent HCAI and limit the spread of community-acquired infection in healthcare settings. In a large US study, programmes of HCAI surveillance and control were associated with a 32% reduction in infection rates. In the UK there is agreement that a 10–15% reduction in HCAI is achievable. Such a reduction would result in the release of considerable resources that could be used for other aspects of patient care. Control of HCAI is an important part of risk management and clinical governance programme. HCAI is also an indicator of the quality of patient care and HCAI incidents may result in adverse publicity. Control of HCAI comprises surveillance and infection control practice (Table 4.5.1). Evidence-based guidelines have been published on handwashing, use of personal protective equipment, handling sharps, care of urinary catheters, enteral feeding and care of central venous catheters. Guidelines, recommendations and summaries of best practice from a wide range of authoritative sources are available on nearly all aspects of the control of HCAI.

Management arrangements for the control of HCAI

Overall responsibility rests with the chief executive and the trust board and the recently created post of Director of Infection Prevention and Control (DIPC). There should be an infection control team (ICT) comprising an ICD, one or more infection control nurses (ICN) and clerical support. There should also be a multidisciplinary infection control committee (ICC). In acute hospitals the ICD is usually a medical microbiologist. Roles and responsibilities for HCAI are summarised in Table 4.5.2.

Relationships between hospitals and community health services

HCAI may present after a patient has been discharged from hospital. Hospitals are

Table 4.5.1 Surveillance and control of HCAI

Surveillance
Laboratory-based surveillance of alert organisms detected in clinical specimens

Data should be collated using a computerised database to allow data retrieval and analysis. Weekly, monthly and annual totals and antibiotic resistance patterns should be reported. Infection rates may be calculated using appropriate denominators (admissions, discharges, occupied bed-days, days of device usage). Surveillance data should be widely circulated and discussed. An annual report should be compiled.	MRSA and other highly resistant *S. aureus* *S. pyogenes* Penicillin-resistant *S. pneumoniae* Beta-lactamase producing enterococci *Clostridium difficile* and/or detection of its toxins *Legionella* spp. (including serology results) *E. coli* O157 Salmonella or Shigella species Resistant gram-negative rods Other bacteria isolates with unusual antibiotic resistance (e.g. *Haemophilus influenzae* resistant to ampicillin and trimethoprim) *Pseudomonas aeruginosa* *Strenotrophomonas maltophilia* (*Xanthomonas maltophilia*) Viral isolates/positive antigen tests: Rotavirus, RSV, Varicella-zoster, Parvovirus B19 Fungi: In special units, Candida species, Aspergillus
Other laboratory-based surveillance	Blood cultures, CSF, vascular catheters, postoperative wound swabs, urine samples, etc
Surveillance by ward staff of alert conditions.	Diarrhoea and vomiting, food poisoning, pyrexia of unknown origin, soft tissue infections, childhood exanthemata, etc.
Targeted surveillance.	Liaison with special units and wards (intensive care, oncology, etc.) or particular subgroups of patients to enquire about infections, incidents and outbreaks.

Infection control measures

Developing and implementing policies	• hand washing • policies and procedures. • Personel Protective Equipment (PPE) • handling sharps
Written policies should be collated in an infection control manual. Policies should be audited, reviewed and updated regularly. Outbreak and incident control plans should be exercised if not in regular use.	• antibiotic usage • clinical procedures • disposal of waste • outbreaks and incidents • decontamination, sterilisation and disinfection • management of patients at risk of acquiring or transmitting infection • use of isolation facilities • management of specific communicable diseases • laundry • catering (including food hygiene) • domestic cleaning • mortuary procedures • engineering and building services (including Legionella infection) • equipment purchasing

---

Continued

Table 4.5.1 *Continued*

	• new building • staff immunisation (hepatitis B, influenza, BCG) • other aspects of occupational health (sharps injuries) • operating theatres • transfer and discharge of patients • pest control
Staff training and education	Induction Annual update
Carrying out audits	• hand hygiene • clinical practices (isolation, protective clothing, catheter care) • environmental cleaning and hygiene • ward kitchen areas • waste disposal • sharps management • care of linen • decontamination of equipment
Advice	• proposed building constructions • purchase of equipment and consumables • tenders for other services

responsible for passing relevant information to the GP and to community nursing staff. In turn they should provide feedback to the hospital, both to the ICT and the consultant who has treated the patient, both for surveillance purposes and to alert the ICT when a potentially infected patient is to be admitted to hospital. Collaboration between community staff, the ICT and the CCDC is encouraged by the appointment of a community ICN.

Outbreaks of infection in hospital

Infectious diseases can spread readily within hospitals, amongst staff and patients who may be more susceptible to infection as a result of illness or treatment. Despite high standards of infection control practice, outbreaks of infection or infectious disease incidents may occur.

Recognition of an outbreak

An outbreak is an incident in which two or more people who are thought to have a common exposure experience a similar illness or proven infection. Outbreaks in hospital are either detected by the laboratory or by nursing or medical staff. Cases of infection and outbreaks are reported to the infection control team (ICT).

Action

Hospitals should have written plans for responding to infectious disease incidents. These should cover the following:
• Recognition of an outbreak.
• Circumstances in which the ICD or CCDC would take the lead.
• Initial investigation by ICD and ICN, which determines whether or not an outbreak exists.
• If the outbreak is confined to hospital, whether it can be dealt with by the ICT or if an outbreak control group is needed. A major outbreak is one in which large numbers of people are affected, where the organism involved is particularly pathogenic or where there is potential for spread within the hospital and the community.

Table 4.5.2 Roles and responsibilities for HCAI

Department of Health	• Sets overall policy • Publishes guidance • Provides expertise • Provides public information
Strategic Heath Authorities	• Manage performance of NHS Trusts
Trust Chief Executive	• Ensures effective arrangements for HCAI • Core part of governance and patient safety • Promotes low levels of HCAI • Appoints DIPC
Director of Infection Prevention and Control	• Oversees policies and work of ICT • Reports directly to CE and board • Challenges poor practice • Assesses impact of policies • Produces annual report
Infection Control Committee	• Endorses policies • Advises and supports implementation • Oversees work of ICT • Agrees annual programme and monitors progress
Infection Control Team	• 24-hour advice on control of HCAI • Annual programme of activity • Surveillance of HCAI • Audit of compliance with policies • Education and training
Modern Matron	• Champion importance of HCAI • Promotes handwashing and hospital hygiene
Primary Care Trusts	• Same responsibilities as acute trusts • Advises on infection control in community premises • Appoint DIPC, community ICN, set up ICC • As commissioners of health services ensure that hospitals have arrangements for HCAI
Health Protection Agency	• Delivers national surveillance programmes • Monitors and assists in management of HCAI outbreaks
Consultants for Communicable Disease Control and team (employed by HPA)	• Surveillance, prevention and control of infection • Management of outbreaks • Advice to PCTs • Liaison with ICTs • Epidemiological advice
Healthcare Commission	• Reviews infection control arrangements in trusts
NHS Modernisation Agency	• Supports NHS to improve services and outcomes
Medicines and Healthcare related products Regulatory Agency	• Investigates adverse incidents including those associated with decontamination problems
National Institute of Clinical Excellence	• Guidance on current 'best practice'
NHS Estates	• Guidance on design and maintenance of buildings and equipment
NHS Purchasing and Supplies Agency	• Purchasing polices
National Patient Safety Agency	• Reporting system for adverse incidents affecting patients • Patient safety initiatives
NHS Litigation Authority	• Clinical Negligence Scheme for trusts • Framework for clinical risk management

- Outbreak to be reported to HPA and SHA.
- If the outbreak is not confined to hospital, the CCDC would be involved and the district outbreak plan would be implemented as appropriate
- Outbreaks of limited extent will be dealt with by the ICT along with the relevant clinicians and nurses.
- It would be usual for the CCDC to be informed, although he or she may already know of the outbreak through regular contact with the ICD.
- If the disease involved is statutorily notifiable, the medical staff responsible for the patient(s) must notify the CCDC as proper officer of the local authority.
- In any infectious disease incident where food or water is implicated, a local authority environmental health officer should be informed.

Initial investigation of a hospital outbreak

This should consist of the following:

1 Collect information on all cases occurring on all wards and units.
2 Establish a case definition; request laboratory tests.
3 Ensure provision of medical and nursing care for affected patients, including appropriate precautions to prevent secondary spread.
4 Consider antibiotic prophylaxis or immunisation, if appropriate (not usually applicable for gastrointestinal infections).
5 Consider catering arrangements, disinfection, handwashing, laundry, food samples, environmental samples and microbiological or serological screening of those at risk.
6 If a food-borne or water-borne infection is suspected, the EHO will conduct an environmental investigation, including inspection of kitchen, food handling and storage practices, review of illness amongst staff, requesting faecal samples from members of staff if necessary, review of menus, waste handling and pest control.

7 Implement control measures, e.g.
- patient isolation/cohort nursing;
- restriction of transfers and/or discharges;
- staff education in infection control procedures;
- clear instructions and information for ward staff, cleaners, etc.;
- information to patients' relatives and visitors.

8 Decide when the outbreak is over.
9 Communicate with SHA, HPA and media as appropriate.

Community outbreak affecting the hospital

Hospitals should have plans for responding to a major community outbreak affecting the hospital. Major outbreaks of infectious disease in the community may place heavy demands on hospital services. Acute outbreaks developing over a few hours are generally toxin mediated. Non-acute outbreaks, due, e.g. to influenza, develop over days or weeks. The ICT role would include advising on the collection of microbiological samples and advising on any control of infection measures. The hospital may activate its Major Incident Plan and convene an outbreak control group. The hospital response will involve clinical and managerial staff. Consideration should be given to: admissions policy; appropriate management of patients; opening up additional beds; consequences of staff illness; communications with media, community staff and general practitioners.

4.6 Risks to and from healthcare workers

Healthcare workers (HCWs) are at risk of acquiring infectious disease because of exposure during their work. They are also a potential source of infection for those whom they are caring for, particularly when working with those with impaired resistance to infection.

HCWs are an important sentinel group. Unexplained illness amongst HCWs may be an early sign of an unusual or novel outbreak, as occurred with SARS.

HCWs can be considered according to the level of probable exposure to infectious disease risks. Target groups for preventative interventions can then be identified following a risk assessment based upon the likelihood of transmission (See Tables 4.6.1 and 4.6.2.

Table 4.6.1

Category I	Clinical and other staff, including those in primary care, who have regular, clinical contact with patients.
Category II	Laboratory and mortuary staff who have direct contact with potentially infectious clinical specimens.
Category III	Non-clinical ancillary staff who have social contact with patients, but not usually of a prolonged or close nature.
Category IV	Maintenance staff, e.g. engineers, gardeners.

Table 4.6.2

Infection	Target group	Rationale	Comments
Diarrhoea	Category I	Personal and patient protection	Staff with diarrhoea should report to occupational health.
Diphtheria	Category I staff caring for patients with diphtheria Category II staff	Personal protection	National immunisation programme should ensure immunity. Category II staff should have immunity checked.
Hepatitis A	Category I staff working in institutions for patients with learning disabilities. Category II laboratory staff who may handle the virus. Category IV maintenance staff exposed to sewage	Personal protection	Immunisation may be offered following a risk assessment.
Hepatitis B	Category I & II staff with exposure to blood, blood stained body fluids and tissues	Personal and patient protection	Immunisation may be offered to other groups of staff following a risk assessment.
Hepatitis C	Category I & II staff with exposure to blood, blood-stained body fluids and tissues	Personal and patient protection	See section on lookback exercises.
HIV	Category I & II staff	Personal and patient protection	See section on lookback exercises. Risk assessment to be undertaken, particularly if exposure to TB.
Influenza	Category I staff	Personal and possibly patient protection	Annual immunisation should be offered by occupational health service.
Poliomyelitis	All HCWs	Personal protection	National immunisation programme should ensure immunity.

Continued

Continued

Infection	Target group*	Rationale	Comments
Rabies	Those directly caring for rabid patients	For their own protection	Immunisation
Rubella	Category I HCWs working in maternity departments	For patient protection	National immunisation programme should ensure immunity. HCWs in high-risk areas should have documented immunity.
SARS	Important for all Category I & II staff.	Personal and patient protection	Ensure surveillance of HCW in contact with SARS patients is in place.
TB	Important for all Category I & II staff	Personal and patient protection	Staff without a BCG scar or documented BCG immunisation should be tuberculin tested and offered BCG. Staff should report possible TB symptoms promptly.
Tetanus	Category IV staff at higher risk of tetanus-prone wounds, e.g. gardeners	Personal protection	National immunisation programme should ensure immunity.
Varicella	Category I, II, III HCWs with patient contact, especial attention to those working in high-risk clinical areas such as maternity and oncology	Patient protection; Varicella vaccine recommended for all nonimmune HCWs with patient contact (i.e. categories I, II, III)	Varicella-zoster vaccine now licensed in many European countries (including UK). Varicella-zoster antibodies to be checked. Nonimmune staff to be excluded from high-risk areas between days 7 and 21 following exposure.

* Categories of risk as used in UK.

Lookback studies

Purpose

The purpose of lookback studies is to
• determine those at risk of acquiring a communicable disease following an exposure, usually related to healthcare.
• inform exposed individuals about the risk to which they have been exposed.
• determine whom, amongst those exposed, have been infected.
• prevent further transmissions and/or clinical disease.
• provide appropriate interventions (treatment, counselling etc) for those exposed, both infected and uninfected.

• advance understanding about reducing and quantifying exposure risks.

Context

Lookback exercises are usually carried out following exposure, or suspected exposure to blood-borne viruses (hepatitis B, hepatitis C virus or HIV) within a healthcare setting. Similar exercises may be recommended for potential exposures to other infections, such TB and CJD. When lookback studies are being undertaken there may well be heightened media interest. Procedures for dealing with this should be established early. The importance of preserving the confidentiality of the HCW and contacts should be emphasised. There may well be concerned from the 'worried well' and mechanisms for providing reassurance may need to be established.

HIV (See Table 4.6.3)

Guidance on lookback exercises is given by the UK Expert Advisory Group on AIDS (EAGA) (see Appendix 2).

Table 4.6.3

When to carry out a look back:	EAGA recommends 'that all patients who have undergone an exposure prone procedure (EPP) where the infected health care worker was the sole or main operator should, as far as practicable be notified of this'.
What is an EPP?	A procedure in which there is a risk that injury to the HCW may result in exposure of the patient's open tissues to the blood of the HCW. This usually involves operations in which the HCWs fingers are not visible whilst exposed to sharp objects.

Risk of Exposure*	Definition	Examples
Higher	Major operations	Vaginal or abdominal hysterectomy, caesarean section, prolapse repair, salpingectomy
Low	Other procedures, suturing or sharp instruments	Laparoscopy, forceps delivery, episiotomy repair, incision of Bartholin's abscess
None	Procedures that do not involve suturing or sharp instruments	Manual removal of placenta, dilatation and curettage, cystoscopy, spontaneous vaginal delivery

Methods	Establish incident management team.
	Ensure overall co-ordination is clear.
	Establish helplines.
	Ensure GPs kept informed.
	Define EPP. It may be necessary to define high- and low-risk procedures in order to concentrate resources on those most at risk.
	Identify those exposed. This may involve extensive searches through hospital records, operating theatre registers, etc.
	Contact exposed patients. This may be personally by GPs or their staff or by letter. The method will need to be sensitive to the risk, and to the need of those contacted for support and counselling.
	It is important to ensure that helplines/counselling is in place, and that there are clear algorithms for the care of those identified.
	Ensure close liaison with press office throughout.
Transmission Risk	A number of lookback studies have been carried out following exposure to HIV infected HCWs. Studies of over 30,000 patients (about half of whom have undergone testing) have shown no evidence of transmission of HIV to patients. Two incidents, a Florida dentist who transmitted infection to 6 patients and a French orthopaedic surgeon who infected 1 patient, have been reported. The risk of transmission from an HIV-infected HCW to a patient following an EPP is likely to be low.
Sources of further advice	Expert Advisory Group on AIDS, CDSC, Department of Health Advisory Panel

* Source: *Commun Dis Public Health,* 1999, **2**: 127.

Hepatitis B (See Table 4.6.4)

HCWs who carry hepatitis B virus may infect patients who become exposed to their serum.

The UK Health Departments require all HCWs who undertake exposure-prone procedures to be vaccinated against Hepatitis B virus, and their subsequent immunity to be documented. Non-responders to vaccination should be investigated for evidence of chronic HBV infection.

HCWs who are hepatitis e antigen positive may not undertake EPPs because of the significant risk they pose to patients.

In spite of the recommendations for immunisation and restriction placed upon practice, a number of events have still occurred where patients have been exposed to an infected HCW, or to the risk of transmission in a health-care setting.

Hepatitis C (See Table 4.6.5)

HCWs who carry hepatitis C virus may infect patients who become exposed to their serum; however, the risk of transmission is much lower than the risk of transmission for Hepatitis B from an e antigen positive surgeon. HCWs are not restricted in carrying out exposure-prone procedures unless they have been shown to transmit hepatitis C. They should be advised on adherence to precautions for the control of blood-borne infection by the occupational health department.

Table 4.6.4

When to carry out a look back:	There is no formal guidance. However the recommendations given by EAGA for HIV lookback exercises are helpful.
	Notification exercises should not extend beyond 12 months unless high rates of transmission have been documented.
What is an EPP?	A procedure in which gloved hands may be in contact with sharp instruments, needle tips and sharp tissues (spicules of bone or teeth) inside a patients open body cavity, wound or confined anatomical space where the hands or fingertips may not be completely visible at all times.
Methods	As above
	The incubation period for hepatitis B virus (2–6 months) is such that exposed patients may be identified during the period before seroconversion.
	Serum should be taken from patients on identification and they should be retested 6 months after exposure to identify seroconversions.
	DNA sequencing of fragments of HBV DNA may be useful to establish transmission.
Interventions	Hepatitis B Immunoglobulin is effective up to 1 week after exposure and should be offered to individuals at risk.
	The value of Hepatitis B vaccination is unclear and there is probably little merit in using Hepatitis B vaccine more than 2 weeks after exposure.
	Systems will need to be put in place for ensuring that those who do not clear the virus are followed up and if appropriate offered treatment for chronic hepatitis B.
Transmission risk	Transmission rates identified in incidents involving surgical staff in the UK from 1975 to 1990 have ranged from 0.9 to 20% depending on the procedures and other factors.
Sources of further advice	Expert Advisory Group on Hepatitis
	HPA/CDSC
	Department of Health

Table 4.6.5

When to carry out a look back:	As for Hepatitis B
What is an EPP	As for Hepatitis B
Methods	Serum should be taken from those exposed on identification. Advice should be sought on the when repeat testing should be performed. It is recommended that serum is obtained from HCWs exposed to a known positive source at baseline, 6, 12 and 24 weeks and tested for HCV RNA at 6 and 12 weeks and anti-HCV at 12 and 24 weeks. Genotyping may be useful to establish transmission.
Interventions	Although there is some disagreement over the effectiveness of early treatment in preventing progression of disease most experts favour treatment of patients with acute hepatitis C.
Sources of further advice	Expert Advisory Group on Hepatitis HPA/CDSC Department of Health See Appendix 2 for guidance on the risks and management of occupational exposure to hepatitis C.

4.7 Co-ordination of immunisation services

The role of the immunisation co-ordinator

Effective immunisation services require the co-ordination of the inputs of many different professionals and agencies. Each local health authority, e.g. Primary Care Trusts (PCTs) in England, should delegate a particular person (or persons) to take on special responsibility for implementing improvements to immunisation programmes at local level. The main functions of the immunisation co-ordinator are as follows:

• To ensure that an appropriate strategy, with the aim of ensuring that every child (in the absence of genuine contraindications) receives immunisation, is devised and implemented.
• To ensure that appropriate resources are in place to support the strategy.
• To ensure that appropriate local policies and procedures, based on models of good practice, are in place to support the strategy.
• To act as a local source of advice and information on immunisation issues for both the public and professionals.

• To co-ordinate the role of all those involved with immunisation in primary care, child health services, hospitals, educational establishments, and elsewhere, and to gain their commitment to the strategy and its aim.
• To chair the District Immunisation Committee and ensure delivery of its' identified responsibilities (see below).
• To ensure that training and updating of all staff involved in immunisation is available.
• To ensure that up to date and reliable figures on immunisation uptake rates are available.
• To ensure that nonimmunised children are identified and followed up.
• To investigate the reasons for poor uptake figures and to promote appropriate methods to overcome identified problems.
• To ensure that appropriate audit is carried out on the availability effectiveness and efficiency of local immunisation services.

The separation of functions in the UK National Health Service from recent reorganisations means that some of those mentioned in the above list may be delegated to other individuals. In England, the functions may be split as follows:

• PCT – Assume overall responsibility for delivery of service and national targets, including provision of services, training, public information and collection of vaccine uptake data.

• Health Protection Agency (HPA) local team – Provide strategic leadership, co-ordination, expert advice and support to all PCTs in area in discharging their responsibilities.
• Paediatric and community health services – Provision of expert clinical advice, supporting clinical services for complex cases and, where appropriate, maintenance of the child health (immunisation) database.

The District Immunisation Committee (DIC)

The immunisation co-ordinator should be supported by a DIC. An appropriate membership might be as follows:
• HPA local immunisation lead/co-ordinator (Chair)
• PCT immunisation leads/co-ordinators
• Community paediatrician
• Information manager (child health/immunisation database)
• Community services manager

• Community services commissioner
• General practitioner
• Community nurses, including practice nurse
• Pharmacist
• Health promotion officer
   The terms of reference of the DIC could be as follows:
• To review and advise on immunisation policies within the district and to develop an integrated district wide strategy in order to achieve the maximum immunisation uptake within the district, in line with national guidelines.
• To implement and monitor the local immunisation programme.
• To ensure accurate information is maintained to support the immunisation programme and shared appropriately.
• To ensure the organisation of an efficient and effective recall system.
• To ensure an accurate record of all immunisations given to any child in the district is provided to any professional caring for that child and the parent/carer.

Box 4.7.1 UK immunisation schedule

Age	Vaccine
Neonates	BCG (high-risk groups only)
	Hepatitis B (high-risk groups only)
2, 3 + 4 months	3 dose primary course of:
	Diphtheria/tetanus/pertussis/polio/Hib (DTPa-IPV-Hib)
	Meningococcus C
12–15 months	1 dose primary course of:
	Measles/mumps/rubella (MMR1)
3–5 years	1 dose booster of:
	Diphtheria/tetanus/pertussis/polio (dTPa-IPV or DTPa-IPV)
	Measles/mumps/rubella (MMR2)
10–14 years	BCG
13–18 years	1 dose of booster of:
	Diphtheria (low dose)/tetanus/polio (Td/IPV)
Adult	Boosters for tetanus and polio if appropriate
	Vaccines for occupational or lifestyle risks
65 years plus	Influenza
	Pneumococcus
Any age	Influenza, pneumococcus (medical risk groups only)
	Travel vaccines

Box 4.7.2 How to rectify a poor vaccine uptake rate

First check how accurate the figures are. In our experience recorded figures can underestimate true uptake by as much as 3–4%.

• Check denominator against most up-to-date register of population. The immunisation database should be regularly updated from the GP register in the UK.

• Check the numerator by sending lists of apparently unvaccinated children to their GPs to verify. In the UK, the dates for calculating uptake rates for payment of family doctors do not exactly match those for calculating 'official' uptake figures. It may be useful to carry out this exercise every quarter.

• Is information being received on children who are immunised in neighbouring districts (e.g. resident of district A registered with GP in district B)?

Consider the following actions to increase the number vaccinated:

• Calculate uptake rates by each general practice. Low performers may benefit from assistance with organising routine clinics or opportunistic vaccination (e.g. prompts on medical notes or automatic electronic reminders) or input from a facilitator.

• Look for GPs with good uptake for most vaccines, but low uptake for pertussis or MMR. These practices may benefit from a visit by a community paediatrician (e.g. to educate on true contraindications) and access to an advice line or special clinic for children with 'problem histories'.

• Encourage other staff (e.g. hospital paediatricians, A & E staff, health visitors) to identify and refer non-vaccinated children.

• Consider domiciliary vaccination and opportunistic vaccination at routine health checks for non-attenders. This may also reduce inequalities in vaccine uptake.

• Organise CPD sessions for staff from targeted practices.

• Ensure nurses are trained to give immunisations without a doctor present.

• Organise public education on severity of illness and safety of vaccines via local media.

• Systems generally associated with good uptake involve a computerised system of routine appointments, personal letters from the patients' own doctor, target payments for GPs and arrangements for opportunistic or domiciliary immunisation. GP clinics tend to have higher uptake than Health Authority clinics.

Other points of interest:

• For children, a major predictor of low uptake of MMR and pre-school vaccinations is failure to attend for the primary immunisation course; a reminder card based on the health belief model led to a higher uptake in one Australian study; a collaborative immunisation programme has been shown to improve uptake in Ireland; and interventions need to concentrate on the most deprived in order to avoid widening inequalities.

• Particular problems may be identified with late immunisation of preterm infants and low uptake of BCG and hepatitis B in target groups. These problems are usually due to organisational failures. There also may be language difficulties for parents of some of the targeted groups. Ethnic-based targeting needs to address mixed race children.

• Accelerated schedules may help with difficult to reach groups (e.g. hepatitis B in intravenous drug users).

• Not all European countries monitor immunisation uptake rates in the elderly. Where measured they range from 25 to 81% of the elderly population. Many of the principles for improving childhood uptake also apply: predictive factors in UK include previous vaccination, recommendation by a health professional, belief that vaccine works and lack of concern of side-effects. Telephone appointing for elderly patients increases uptake. For 'at-risk' patients, computerised marking of patients, computerised selection and sending personal reminders all increased uptake in the Netherlands.

- To ensure appropriate training and updating is available on an ongoing basis for all staff involved in the immunisation programme.
- To ensure that advice is given on the appropriate systems for the storage of vaccines.
- To co-ordinate health promotion activities within the district on immunisation issues.
- To ensure organisation of an efficient patient recall system.
- To ensure that a source of clinical management advice concerning the immunisation programme is available within the district.
- To ensure that a rapid response is possible should a particular immunisation need arise.

Immunisation uptake rates

The theoretical aim of immunisation services is to achieve herd immunity against those diseases transmitted from person to person (e.g. measles) and to protect everyone against those with other sources (e.g. tetanus). Many countries have set general targets for immunisation uptake based on the WHO approach. In the UK, these are

- 95% uptake of all primary immunisations (including MMR) by the child's second birthday and
- 70% uptake of annual influenza immunisation in those over 65 years of age.

Many districts fail to achieve these targets. These districts are often those with the highest population density and therefore where a higher than average uptake is needed to achieve herd immunity. Many districts also vaccinate a significant proportion of their children much later than the target age: this further increases the pool of susceptibles allowing transmission to continue. A further consequence of late vaccination is the exposure of infants to pertussis and Hib at an age at which severity of disease is highest.

Contributing reasons for low or late immunisations may be

- reduced public confidence in certain vaccines after media scares, e.g. MMR and pertussis. Concern may be highest in higher social class parents.

- confusion amongst health professionals as to safety and true contraindications of vaccines, particularly pertussis.
- factors related to social deprivation, particularly high population mobility, lone parenthood, and large family size.
- factors relating to religion (particular problems in the Netherlands), lifestyle and ethnicity. Immigrant children are often not up to date with vaccination.
- problems with the way programmes are organised, delivered and remunerated.

4.8 Co-ordination of services for HIV infection in the UK

Prevention and control of HIV is complex both sociologically and organisationally and so co-ordination and leadership of all the various agencies that can play a part is essential.

In England, PCTs are responsible for ensuring that there is a full range of treatment, care and prevention services for HIV. PCTs may nominate an HIV co-ordinator to oversee this work. Services are delivered by a range of providers including specialist hospital based infectious disease services, GUM clinics (Chapter 2.9), GPs, community-based sexual health services, health promotion services, social services departments and voluntary organisations. PCTs should ensure that investment in HIV services is based on a sound understanding of the epidemiology of HIV at both local and national level. Accurate and timely HIV surveillance data is the key to this. HIV features in PCTs' Local Delivery Plans, which are local plans to improve health and modernise services. National and local targets to tackle priorities may be agreed.

The UK Department of Health published a National Strategy for Sexual Health and HIV in 2001 and followed this up with an action plan in 2002 (Table 4.8.1) much of which is

Table 4.8.1 UK Government priorities for HIV services

Surveillance	Maintain existing surveillance systems.
Delivery	PCTs identify a sexual health and HIV lead.
	Strategic Health Authority ensures PCTs are performance managed on commissioning arrangements.
	Sexual health and HIV Commissioning Toolkit published.
	Identify performance indicators (undiagnosed HIV, newly acquired HIV and gonorrhoea, uptake of hepatitis B vaccine).
	Monitor levels of investment following mainstreaming of the HIV budgets.
	Mechanism to enable service users to influence policy.
	Set up Independent Advisory Group on implementation of the sexual health and HIV strategy.
Prevention	National information campaign about risks of unprotected sex, targeting young adults.
	Review evidence base for local HIV and STI prevention.
	Review quality and accessibility of public information about sexual health and HIV (particularly gay men, African and other minority ethnic communities).
	Improve quality of telephone helplines and web-based resources.
	Improve education in schools about sex and relationships.
	Target groups at special risk through partnership (African communities, asylum seekers, gay men, people living with HIV, young injecting drug misusers, prisons and Young Offender Institutions, looked after children, people with learning disabilities).
Services	Publish set of recommended service standards for HIV treatment.
	Implement different levels of services (GPs, nurses, primary care teams, NHS walk-in centres, one stop shop, GUM clinics).
	HIV care services framework for African communities.
	Increase offer and uptake of HIV and STI testing.
	Improve GUM services.
Reduce the stigma associated with HIV and STIs	Tackle the stigma and discrimination that can be associated with HIV and STIs.
Improve social care for people living with HIV	Meet support needs of adults living with HIV and develop standards.
Workforce development	Develop national sexual health training strategy.

applicable to other similar areas of Europe. An Independent Advisory Group for Sexual Health and HIV monitors progress towards implementation of the plan.

Health service arrangements vary between countries in Europe. For example, in the Netherlands and Germany, municipal health services offer HIV testing and health education; treatment and care for HIV and AIDS is financed by health insurance; and treatment is provided by hospitals and individual physicians.

4.9 Services for tuberculosis control

Control of tuberculosis (TB) requires co-ordination and leadership of the various agencies and professions involved in the surveillance, prevention and control of TB. This requires a team approach with close working relationships between those involved in the care of patients with TB including the TB (thoracic medicine or infectious disease) physician, the microbiologist, the hospital infection control team, the TB nurse specialists, the CCDC and in some cases the HIV or GUM physician. In England, PCTs are responsible for ensuring that this occurs at local level.

Good TB programmes can reduce the transmission of tuberculosis and the incidence of drug-resistant disease. Failure to maintain such programmes contributed to loss of TB control in the late 1980s in some parts of the world. In England the Chief Medical Officer has recently published a TB Action Plan – *Stopping Tuberculosis in England*.

Key UK guidance documents for TB are listed in Appendix 2. There should be a written local policy for tuberculosis prevention and control (Table 4.9.1).

Table 4.9.1 Local policy for the prevention and control of tuberculosis

Policy area	Details
Aims and objectives	To reduce and eliminate TB by • reducing the risk of exposure and transmission, • providing quality treatment and care services and • preventing emergence of drug resistant TB.
Surveillance	A detailed data set should be collected on all cases of TB. A computerised register should be maintained. Regular reports should be made to national surveillance centres. A local TB annual report should be published.
Identification of cases	A high level of clinical suspicion for TB should be encouraged amongst health professionals, high-risk groups and those that work with them, teachers and members of the public. Surgeons, radiologists and microbiologists should discuss possible cases with the TB physician.
Diagnosis	All isolates must be sent to the regional TB reference laboratory. HIV testing should be offered where appropriate.
Notification	All cases of TB (including those associated with HIV infection) must be reported to local public health authorities.
Management of cases	Treatment of all cases must be supervised by a TB physician and a specialist TB nurse. Accurate prescribing is important. There should be early recognition and management of drug-resistant TB. Particular skills and tactics are needed with patients who are non-compliant or who have disorganised lifestyles. Directly observed treatment (DOT) should be used if necessary. Compulsory admission to hospital for treatment is not usually practicable.
Contact tracing	Contact tracing should be undertaken promptly to minimise the risk of continuing transmission. Contacts are managed according to national guidelines.
Control of infection	All hospitals that may admit patients with TB should have a tuberculosis control plan drawn up in conjunction with the infection control team covering assessment of risk of infection and transmission, including HIV-related and drug-resistant TB, isolation room requirements, measures for the protection of healthcare workers and other contacts, including use of masks and disinfection of equipment.

Table 4.9.1 *Continued*

	When patients in a hospital have been exposed to a healthcare worker or another patient with infectious tuberculosis, the infection control team, TB physician, occupational health department and the CCDC should work jointly to agree appropriate control measures.
Case finding	Case finding should be carried out by screening population groups at risk of infection and offering chemoprophylaxis and BCG where appropriate.
	High-risk groups include contacts of TB cases, new immigrants, refugees and asylum seekers, rough sleepers and hostel dwellers.
BCG immunisation	Local immunisation policies should follow national guidelines. In the UK, immunisation is recommended for school children aged between 10 and 14 years, high-risk neonates, contacts of cases with active pulmonary TB, new immigrants from high-prevalence countries, those at risk of occupational exposure and those planning to travel to and stay in a high-prevalence country for more than a month.
Occupational health	Employers are required to assess the risk of TB for their employees and select appropriate control measures. These may include pre-employment screening and use of BCG. Staff should be made aware of the symptoms of TB so that they can seek advice early if problems arise. This is particularly important for agencies that deal with vulnerable groups, e.g. health and education.
Prisons and other institutions where residents may be at higher risk of tuberculosis	The local health protection unit should liaise with medical staff at prisons and other relevant institutions where residents may be at higher risk of TB to agree appropriate policies for staff and prisoners.
Arrangements for outbreak, recognition and investigation	The identification of a single case of TB in a school or hospital or a cluster of cases of TB in a community setting requires a co-ordinated response, as with any other infectious disease incident or outbreak.
Education and training	There should be appropriately targeted educational material for the general public and healthcare staff and others at higher risk of tuberculosis.
Monitoring and audit	Performance targets should be set. There should be an audit of completeness of notification.
Resources	The local health protection unit requires resources for data collection and collation in order to undertake the core functions of surveillance, outbreak investigation and policy co-ordination.
	For control services, the British Thoracic Society suggests a minimum of one full-time equivalent health visitor or nurse plus appropriate clerical support for every 50 notifications. Some higher incidence districts and those with a large immigrant, refugee or homeless population may require more than this. Some elements of the TB control programme such as managing non-compliant patients, contact tracing and screening new arrivals are labour-intensive and require staff with appropriate training and expertise.

4.10 Travel health and illness in returning travellers

Over 600 million people spend a night in a foreign country each year. Fifty per cent of those travelling to the less-developed world for 1 month will have a health problem associated with the trip. These are mostly minor and fewer than 1% require hospitalisation. Individuals carry their epidemiological risk with them; hence cardiovascular disease is the most common causes of death in travellers from Europe. Injury and accidents (particularly motor vehicle), drowning, etc., are the next most common cause of serious morbidity and mortality. Infection contributes substantially to this morbidity in travellers, particularly diarrhoeal disease, but only about 1% of deaths.

Infectious disease complications of travel depend on the destination, and travel to ever more exotic locations has increased the contact between people and organisms that they would not routinely meet. Public health advice is relevant to the prevention of illness and the response to illness in travellers.

Prevention of ill health in travellers

Travel health clinics, which provide up-to-date advice on risk and risk reduction, can be effective in preventing ill health through simple precautions. The epidemiology of infection risks to the traveller changes rapidly and continuously, and thus those running travel clinics must have access to current information and recommendations. Giving appropriate advice to those with complex itineraries may be a difficult task. Opportunities should be taken to ensure that those who travel at short notice have their vaccination status reviewed regularly.

Advice should cover the following:
• Basic food, water and personal hygiene
• Avoiding insect vectors

• Safe sex and avoidance of potential blood-borne virus exposure
• Avoiding dog bites and other potential rabies exposures
• Malaria prophylaxis
• Vaccination against specific diseases as appropriate

Traveller's diarrhoea

Diarrhoea, usually short-lived and self-limiting is a major cause of illness in travellers; in 20% the person is confined to bed. The main risk factor is the destination; incidence rates vary from 8% per 2-week stay in industrialised countries to over 50% in parts of Africa, Central and South America, and Southeast Asia. Infants and young adults are at particularly high risk.

The likelihood of diarrhoea is related to dietary indiscretions; however, few travellers take sufficient care. The risk of traveller's diarrhoea and other faeco–orally transmitted diseases (e.g. hepatitis A and typhoid) in those who travel to developing countries can be reduced by the following precautions:
• Washing hands after toilet and before preparing or eating food.
• Using only sterilised or bottled water for drinking, cleaning teeth, making ice and washing food (e.g. salads).
• Avoiding uncooked food, (unless you can peel it or shell it yourself), untreated milk or milk products (e.g. ice cream), uncooked shellfish, food that may have been exposed to flies and any other potentially contaminated food.
• It is usually safe to eat freshly cooked food that is thoroughly cooked and still hot; also to have hot tea and coffee and commercially produced alcoholic and soft drinks.

Malaria (see Chapter 3.46)

It has been estimated that more than 30,000 American and European travellers develop malaria each year. The risk varies by season and place, it is highest in sub-Saharan Africa and Oceania (1:50 to 1:1000). An average of

7 deaths per year is reported in travellers from England and Wales.

Compliance with antimalarial chemoprophylaxis regimens and use of personal protection measures are key to the prevention of malaria. However, fewer than 50% of travellers at-risk adhere to basic recommendations for malaria prevention.

Measures to reduce the risk of mosquito bites:

• Sleep in screened rooms, use knockdown insecticide in evening and use an electrical pyrethroid vaporiser overnight.

• If the room cannot be made safe, use impregnated bednets.

• Wear long-sleeve shirts and long trousers in evening. Use insect repellent.

Advice on chemoprophylaxis has been made more difficult by the increase in chloroquine- and multidrug-resistant falciparum malaria, and primaquine- and chloroquine-resistant strains of *Plasmodium vivax*. The recommended regime will depend upon the proposed itinerary: most situations will be covered by the latest published guidance (see Appendix 2), with the HPA Malaria Reference Laboratory able to advise on specific problems (see Appendix 1).

Travellers to endemic countries should be aware of the symptoms of malaria and the need to seek urgent medical attention. Those who will be out of reach of medical services can be given stand-by therapy.

Immunisation and travel

Many countries and the WHO produce recommendations for vaccination of travellers (see Appendix 2) and these should be consulted.

Diphtheria, tetanus and polio

Foreign travel is an ideal opportunity to have these immunisations updated. Diphtheria is a problem worldwide, with large outbreaks recently in those states that were previously part of the Soviet Union. There are low levels of tetanus antitoxin and immunity to polio serogroups in many adults.

Hepatitis A

Hepatitis A is a common vaccine-preventable infection in travellers. It is endemic in many parts of the world, including southern Europe. The risk is especially high for those who leave the usual tourist routes. Immunisation is recommended for travellers to countries in Africa, Asia, Central and South America and the Caribbean, where hygiene and sanitation may be poor, and for some countries in Eastern Europe, although it may be less important for short stays in good accommodation.

Hepatitis B (HBV)

Immunisation against HBV should be given to all those who may come into contact with body fluids (e.g. those planning to work as healthcare workers). The incidence also appears raised in other long-stay overseas workers, perhaps as a result of medical and dental procedures received abroad or sexual transmission. Immunisation is not necessary for short-term business or tourist travellers, unless their sexual behaviour puts them at risk.

Typhoid

The risk of typhoid is especially high for those leaving the usual tourist routes, or visiting relatives or friends in developing countries. Typhoid vaccine is recommended for the same groups as hepatitis A vaccine. Vaccination against paratyphoid is not recommended.

Cholera

The risk of cholera is extremely low (approximately 1 case per 500,000 journeys to endemic areas). Cholera vaccine is not indicated for travellers. No country requires proof of cholera vaccination as a condition for entry.

Yellow fever

A yellow fever vaccination certificate is required for entry into most countries of sub-Saharan Africa and South America in which the infection exists. Many countries require a certificate from travellers arriving from, or who have been in transit through, infected areas. Some countries require a certificate from all entering travellers.

As the areas of yellow fever virus circulation exceed the officially reported zones, vaccination is strongly recommended for travel to all countries in the endemic zone (particularly if visiting rural areas), even if these countries have not officially reported the disease and do not require a vaccination certificate. The vaccination has almost total efficacy, while the case fatality rate for the disease is more than 60% in nonimmune adults. In recent years, fatal cases of yellow fever have occurred in unvaccinated tourists visiting rural areas within the yellow fever endemic zone.

Rabies

Rabies vaccination should be considered in all those who are likely to come into contact with animals where the disease is present (e.g. veterinarians) and those undertaking long journeys in remote areas.

Japanese B encephalitis

Immunisation should be considered in those staying for a month or greater in rural areas of endemic countries in Southeast Asia and the far East.

Meningococcal disease

Immunisation should be considered in those going to areas of the world where the incidence is high (e.g. the 'meningitis belt' of sub-Saharan Africa and areas in the north of the Indian subcontinent), or to events where there may be significant exposure, such as the Hajj in Saudi Arabia.

Tick-borne encephalitis

Vaccination is recommended for those who are to walk, camp or work in late spring and summer in warm, heavily forested parts of Central and Eastern Europe and Scandinavia. They should also cover arms, legs and ankles and use insect repellent.

Pregnancy, infection and travel

Dehydration resulting from diarrhoea can reduce placental blood flow; therefore, pregnant travellers must be careful about their food and drink intake. They should also be aware of infections such as toxoplasmosis and listeriosis, with potentially serious sequelae in pregnancy. Women should be encouraged to breastfeed if travelling with a neonate. A nursing mother with traveller's diarrhoea should not stop breastfeeding, but should increase her fluid intake.

The theoretical risks to the foetus from vaccination mean that in general women should avoid becoming pregnant within 3 months of receiving a live vaccine and avoid them during pregnancy. However, a risk/benefit approach will have to be taken if a pregnant woman who is not immune has to travel, and expert advice should be sought. Malaria during pregnancy carries a significant risk of morbidity and death. Pregnant women should be advised of this increased risk if intending travelling to endemic areas. If travel is essential, then chemoprophylaxis and avoidance of bites are essential, and expert advice should be sought.

The HIV-infected traveller

The HIV-infected traveller may be at risk of serious infection. Those with AIDS, CD4+ counts of <200/L and those who are symptomatic should seek specialist advice, particularly before going to the developing world. Those with a CD4+ cell count above 500 probably have a risk similar to a person without HIV infection.

Gastrointestinal illness: The HIV-infected traveller needs to be particularly careful about the foods and beverage consumed. Traveller's diarrhoea occurs more frequently, is more severe, protracted and more difficult to treat when in association with HIV infection. Infections are also more likely to be accompanied by bacteraemia. Organisms particularly associated with severe chronic diarrhoea in HIV-positive travellers include *Cryptosporidium* and *Isospora belli*.

Immunisation: All of the HIV-infected traveller's routine immunisations should be up to date. In general, live attenuated vaccines are contraindicated for persons with immune dysfunction. Live oral polio vaccine should not be given to HIV-infected patients or members of their households. Inactivated polio vaccine (IPV) should be used. Live yellow fever vaccine should not normally be given to HIV-infected travellers; however, if travel in an endemic area is absolutely necessary, vaccination may be considered after a risk assessment and consideration of the CD4 count. BCG should not be given because of disseminated infection in HIV-infected persons.

4.11 Non-infectious environmental hazards

Environmental health comprises aspects of human health and quality of life that are determined by physical, biological and social factors in the environment. Some physical and chemical factors in particular have the potential to adversely affect health and are described as environmental hazards (Table 4.11.1). However, there are other equally important environmental determinants of health, including regeneration, transport policy, sustainable development, energy policy, housing policy, social inclusion, planning policy, food policy and industrial accidents and occupational health and safety. Other determinants are natural disasters such as flooding, weather, climate change, war and famine. Environmental health practice is concerned with assessing, controlling and preventing environment factors that can adversely affect health now or in the future. Of relevance to the work of the local health protection team are surveillance of disease and environmental determinants of disease to identify unusual or novel patterns, the possibility of a disease cluster or a longer term

increase in the incidence of a disease in a particular area, possibly associated with a point source of pollution or contamination, and the response to an acute incident or other accident.

Investigating the health effects of environmental hazards

Communities living near potential sources of pollution such as industrial sites, contaminated land and other environmental hazards are often concerned about possible effects on health. They may link locally observed health effects with exposure at these sites. Clusters are defined as the aggregation of a number of similar illnesses in space and time and the perception that the number is excessive. Most types of health event may cluster, but cancer clusters receive the most attention. Greater significance is attached to a cluster when a site of industrial pollution is involved. The local health protection team may be asked to investigate possible clusters and other health problems associated with environmental hazards. A systematic approach should be adopted (Table 4.11.2). Dealing with the concerns of the public and media is fundamental to investigating clusters. Risk communication, risk perception and skills in handling enquiries from the public and the media are all important. From a public health perspective, addressing the community's perception of a cluster may be more important than epidemiological or statistical arguments.

Examples of environmental health investigations

Investigation of the possible effects of environmental hazards uses methodology similar to that used for CDC.

Case study one: opencast mining and poor health

In a large study to determine whether particulates from opencast coal mining had an effect on children's respiratory health, five communities close to opencast sites were compared with five control communities matched for

Table 4.11.1 Environmental hazards

Hazard	Notes
Factories and industrial processes	These may cause nuisance as a result of soiling of the environment, noise, odour or road traffic. Potential health effects may arise from chemical releases, fumes and particulates.
	The system of Integrated Pollution Prevention and Control (IPPC) established under a European Commission (EC) Directive regulates the environmental effects of industrial activities including emissions. There are two parallel systems: the 'Part A' regime of IPPC and the 'Part B' regime of Local Air Pollution Prevention and Control (LAPPC). The Environment Agency regulates Part A(1) installations, while Part A(2)and Part B installations are regulated by the local authority. As part of the regulation process, the regulating authorities consult with Statutory Consultees including PCTs in England. The Health Protection Agency supports PCTs in fulfilling their responsibilities. Operators are required to use Best Available Techniques (BAT) to avoid or reduce Emissions.
	The Control of Major Accident Hazard Regulations 1999 (COMAH) implement an EC Directive. COMAH is implemented jointly by the Health and Safety Executive (HSE) and the Environment Agency. Its aim is to prevent major accidents involving dangerous substances and limit the consequence to people and the environment. It applies to approximately 1200 establishments that have the potential to cause major accidents. COMAH site operators must prepare emergency plans.
Chemicals	There are 11 million known chemicals; 70,000 are in regular commercial use and 600 new chemicals enter the market place each month. Most chemicals have had little or no toxicological assessment. Large-scale industrial releases with serious effects are rare, but smaller scale events do occur including leaks and fires. Local environmental exposures due to drifting pesticide sprays can occur and some natural phenomena such as volcanic eruptions can present serious risks to health. It is helpful to identify local sites that may represent sources of major chemical hazard. This will allow action to be taken in the event of a release. The Control of Substances Hazardous to Health Regulations 1999 (COSHH) are made under the Health and Safety at Work, etc. Act 1974. They require employers to control exposure to hazardous substances to prevent ill health.
Outdoor air quality	Concentrations of outdoor air pollutants vary from region to region and from day to day. When concentrations are significantly raised, adverse effects on health occur. In the UK health-based air quality standards are available for a range of pollutants. These represent concentrations at which there should be little or no threat to human health at a population level. Air quality improvement targets have been published. There is an extensive network of air quality monitoring stations throughout the UK and real-time data from this can be found in the national archive of UK air quality data (http://www.airquality.co.uk/archive/index.php). Pollutants such as benzene and 1,3-butadiene are carcinogens. Other air pollutants may have chronic effects on health during infancy, and may have an effect on life expectancy as a result of long-term exposure throughout life. Particulate matter, ozone and sulphur dioxide may have acute effects on susceptible members of the population, leading to premature mortality and hospital admissions in those with pre-existing respiratory disease.

Table 4.11.1 *Continued*

Indoor air quality	Rates of respiratory disease and incidence of allergic responses such as asthma have increased in recent years, and there is concern that some of this increase may be linked to changes in the indoor environment, including allergens, tobacco smoke, oxides of nitrogen and formaldehyde.
Drinking water	Over 99% of the population in the UK receives mains water supplies; the quality of these supplies is very high and all are safe to drink. The basic unit of water supply is the water supply zone, which is designated by the water company, normally by reference to a source of water, and which covers a population of about 50,000 people. There are water quality standards, which include microbiological, chemical, physical and aesthetic parameters. Water in some water supply zones is temporarily permitted to exceed these statutory standards for certain chemicals such as lead, polycyclic aromatic hydrocarbons and pesticides. The most important source of lead in tap water in the UK is dissolution from household plumbing systems. Private water supplies are regulated by the local authority, but are subject to a much-reduced sampling regime. Whilst covering a much smaller proportion of the population than public water utilities in the same area, substantial numbers may receive water from private supplies.
Sewerage systems	The UK has the highest percentage connection rate to sewers of any country in the EU and it also has one of the highest levels of provision of sewage treatment.
Water resources management	Under the Water Resources Act 1991 in England and Wales, the Environment Agency regulates any discharges to water to improve the quality of bathing waters.
Solid waste	About 500 million tonnes of waste are produced each year in the UK. Waste is classified as controlled waste and non-controlled waste. The former, which may arise from household, commercial or industrial settings and which is further classified into hazardous and non-hazardous waste, is regulated and licensed by the by the Environment Agency according to the Environmental Protection Act 1990. Non-controlled waste includes waste arising from agriculture, mines and quarries.
Contaminated land	In the UK a long industrial history has resulted in a substantial legacy of land contamination. Since April 2000 there have been new arrangements for the identification and remediation of contaminated land. Contaminated land is defined as land which by virtue of contamination may cause harm or water pollution. The local authority is the main regulator of contaminated land. Liability for contaminated land is based on the *polluter pays* principle.
Ionising and non-ionising radiation	Activities involving the use of radioactive material result in radioactive waste that has to be regulated. Radioactivity also occurs naturally. Exposure to man-made radiation gives rise to greater public concern, although natural sources, such as radon, have greater health effects. The body that advises on standards of protection against ionising radiation is the International Commission on Radiological Protection (ICRP). Advice on radiological issues in the UK is the statutory responsibility of the National Radiological Protection Board (NRPB) now part of the Health Protection Agency. In the UK, workplace exposure is regulated by the Ionising Radiations Regulations 1985, made under the Health and Safety at Work, etc. Act 1974. Protection of the public and the environment from the storage, discharge or disposal of radioactive waste is covered in the UK by the Radioactive Substances Act 1993, which is policed by the Environment Agency.

Continued

Table 4.11.1 *Continued*

	A national survey of exposure to radon in homes has shown that while radon exposure in most homes is low, there are some in which it can pose a risk to health. Monitoring should identify homes above the radon action level so that appropriate remedial action can be taken.
Noise	Noise has an important effect on the quality of life. Prolonged exposure to very loud noise can cause permanent hearing damage, but the relationship between noise and aspects of mental health is complicated. Road traffic noise is the most widespread form of noise disturbance, but people object most to neighbour noise. Annoyance, anger, anxiety and resentment are the most frequently reported personal consequences of exposure to noise in the home.

Table 4.11.2 Investigation of clusters of disease

1. Initial enquiry	
Initial report	Use standard form to record details
Initial case definition	What is the disease/health event or symptoms?
Define the problem	Where is the affected area/population?
	Who are the index cases?
	When did the particular health event occur?
	What are the suspected exposures?
Follow up with the informant	The investigation may be resolved at this stage. The disease may be common, affected persons may only recently have moved to the area, there may not be a single plausible environmental factor, there may be no data on exposure and the increase in cases may be a chance occurrence.
Review	Further investigation may be indicated if there is an unusually high number of cases, a biologically plausible exposure(s) or community concern. As a minimum a report should be written and the results disseminated.
2. Confirm diagnosis and exposure	
Confirm diagnosis	Involve informant, clinicians and others. Examine records such as death
Specific case definition	certificates, e.g. birth certificates, hospital case notes, cancer and birth
Assess exposure	defect registries, occupational health records, GP records. Consent of the index case may be needed.
	Exposure via personal contact, food, water or drug consumption can be assessed by questionnaire. Exposure via water, air, soil or dust is more difficult to assess.
	Company records, aerial photographs, maps, records of water, soil and air quality monitoring, meteorological data and planning records about previous industrial sites and property uses may be used.
	The assistance of an environmental health specialist or an occupational hygienist may be needed, but measurement of exposure is usually not necessary at this point.
Review the literature	Review previously reported clusters of the disease, known associations with environmental exposure and any other epidemiological and toxicological information.

Table 4.11.2 *Continued*

Review	On review: • There may not be an excess number of cases, the apparent excess may be due to inward migration to an area or the cases may have different diagnoses. • The cluster may be explained because it involves a common disease or because of the characteristics of the local population • The nature of the disease and exposure, the size of the cluster and the plausibility of a disease/exposure relationship may require further investigation.
3. Intensive case finding	Identify further cases by examining the following data sources: hospital episode statistics, death certificates, cancer and birth defect registrations, occupational health records. Collect a minimum data set on each case: name, date of birth, ethnic group, sex, age at diagnosis, residence and length of residence at diagnosis, past residence, diagnosis, family history, exposures, confounding factors such as smoking, occupational history. Ethical approval may be required.
Analyse data	Use population data to calculate expected numbers of cases and compare with observed cases. Mapping the data may be helpful, a geographical information system (GIS) can be used. Plume dispersion modelling may be helpful. Allow for confounding factors such as smoking and socio-economic factors. Statistical significance may not be aetiologically important.
Review	If there is an excess of cases, further investigation may be needed if there is continuing concern, if the exposure is biologically plausible, if there has been a recent increase in cases or if the cases are concentrated around suspected environmental hazards or in particular occupational groups. As a minimum a report should be written and the results disseminated.
4. Surveillance or epidemiological study	A surveillance programme over several years will allow the epidemiology to be described. A registry or reporting system may have to be established. A case-control, cohort or cross-sectional study may be feasible.

socio-economic and other confounding variables. There were approximately 400 children aged 1–11 years in each community. Health data were collected simultaneously from each pair of communities. These consisted of a cross-sectional health survey, daily health diaries, GP consultations, school absenteeism and medication use. Exposure was assessed by proximity to the opencast site and by PM10 (particulate matter) measurement using real-time monitors.

The effect of proximity to the opencast site on health outcomes and PM10 levels were examined. In addition, the association between daily PM10 levels and measures of ill health were examined for both opencast and control communities. Mean PM10 levels were slightly higher for the opencast communities

compared with the controls, but for much of the time, the patterns were similar despite a wide range of values. This reflects the strong regional contribution to PM10 levels rather than contributions from local point sources. The additional PM10 load around opencast sites had a higher shale content. Respiratory illness was similar in the opencast and control communities, and asthmatic children in the opencast communities did not have more frequent or more severe asthma attacks. Respiratory symptoms reported by parents were not significantly different between the two communities, but children in the opencast communities had more GP consultations. Small but significant positive associations between levels of PM10 and daily diary health events were observed in both communities, in line with previously published data. (Source: DETR 1999.)

Case study two: emissions from a factory and asthma

To examine the respiratory health of a population living near a factory producing plastic-coated wallpaper, where there had been concerns about the health effects of air-borne emissions, a geographical information system (GIS) was used to define a set of sectors at 1-km intervals centred on the factory. Asthma prevalence rates standardised for age, sex, socio-economic factors and general practice registration were calculated for each sector. The numerator, i.e. cases of asthma, was derived from a general practitioner computerised repeat prescribing system, and the denominator was obtained from health authority patient registers. Middle-aged and elderly adults living 500–1000 m in a northeastern direction from the factory had a significantly higher prevalence of asthma. (Source: Dunn *et al.* 1995.)

Case study three: active landfill site and congenital malformations

In a study to examine the health effects of living near a landfill site, the health of the exposed population, defined as residents living in the five electoral wards within 3 km of the landfill, was compared with that of a comparison population from 22 other wards matched by quintiles of the Townsend deprivation score. Routinely available health outcome measures were used, including mortality, hospital admission rates, measures of reproductive health, spontaneous abortion and congenital malformations. An increased rate of congenital malformations was found in the area surrounding the landfill. (Source: Fielder *et al.* 2000.)

Case study four: former landfill site and cancer

In a study on the health effects of a former landfill site in the West Midlands, three exposed populations were identified after discussions with a local environmental group. The population for each of these groups was constructed using enumeration districts, and indirectly age–sex standardised cancer incidence ratios were calculated using data from the West Midlands Cancer Registry. The population of the West Midlands region was used as the reference population. This was stratified by Townsend deprivation score quintile to control for socio-economic confounding factors. In none of the three study sites was there a statistically significant excess of cancers. (Source: Saunders *et al.* 1997.)

4.12 Managing acute chemical incidents

An acute chemical incident is defined as an unforeseen event leading to

• exposure of people to a non-radioactive substance resulting in illness and

• a potential threat to health from toxic substances or two or more individuals suffering from a similar illness, which might be due to exposure to toxic substances.

Potentially harmful chemicals may be released into the environment as a result of leakage, spillage, explosion, fire or inappropriate disposal. Deliberate release may be part of a criminal or terrorist activity. Exposure by swallowing, inhalation or contact with skin and mucous membranes may be direct or indirect, via contaminated air, food, water or soil. Chemicals can be dispersed from the site of an accident as gas, vapour or particulate cloud, by water and on clothing, equipment, livestock or vehicles (including on human casualties, emergency service personnel and equipment). Exposure to a harmful chemical may result either in acute injury or poisoning, or in longer-term health effects. Various agencies are involved in the management of an acute chemical incident (Table 4.12.1). In the UK the

Table 4.12.1 Agencies involved in the response to an acute chemical incident

The police	Co-ordinate response of emergency services
	Save lives, protect and preserve the scene
	Advice to the public on sheltering, evacuation
	Secure inner cordon during terrorist incidents
	Chair the strategic co-ordinating group (Gold command)
	Investigation of the incident
	Casualty information
	Media enquiries
The fire service	Fight and prevent fires
	Urban search and rescue
	Save lives
	Manage hazardous materials
	Safety of staff
	Minimise effect of incident on environment
	Decontamination of casualties and exposed persons
	Clean up spillage, arrange with contractor to remove substance, etc.
The ambulance service	Co-ordinate all health service activities on site
	Immediate care and treatment of casualties
	Transport to hospital
	Assist with casualty decontamination (with fire service)
PCTs supported by local health protection team	Protection of health
	Provision of healthcare (resuscitation, decontamination, treatment with antidotes, supportive care, intensive care)
	Planning for chemical incidents
	Assessing health risk
	Sampling
	Health advice to the public
	Monitoring and follow up of affected persons
NHS hospitals	Support the Ambulance Service
	Plan for the treatment and care of people who have been affected by the incident
Local authority departments	Support the emergency services
	Open emergency rest centres if necessary
	Co-ordinate response of other organisations including voluntary agencies
	Restore environment
	Lead the long-term recovery process
Health and Safety Executive	At sites at which chemicals are manufactured or used
	Inspect workplaces
	Investigate accidents and cases of ill-health
	Enforce good standards and legislation
Environment Agency	Advises on environmental impact and disposal of contaminated water and other materials
Local water company	Advises on disposal of contaminated water via sewers and impact on water sources
Food Standards Agency	Advises on chemical contamination of the food chain

Continued

Table 4.12.1 *Continued*

Meteorological Office (CHEMET)	Forecast behaviour of chemical plume according to prevailing weather conditions
National Poisons Information Service (NPIS)	UK-wide clinical toxicology service for healthcare professionals. Advice on diagnosis, treatment and management of patients who have been poisoned. Six UK centres. Online TOXBASE database at http://www.spib.axl.co.uk
Centre for Health and Environment Radiation Protection and Toxicology of the Health Protection Agency	24-hour advice and support to PCTs and health professionals on managing chemical incidents, toxicology, personal protective equipment, decontamination and evacuation, health effects, industrial processes, antidotes and medical treatment, chemical incident surveillance, emergency planning, training, research.

Table 4.12.2 Checklist for local public health officer in acute chemical incidents

Action	Notes
Details of incident: • What type of incident • Where and when • What medium is affected • Source of contamination • What chemical(s) are involved	Initial report may come from Centre for Health and Environment Radiation Protection and Toxicology of the Health Protection Agency, Emergency Services, public, media
Adverse health effects or complaints: • How many people exposed • How many affected • What symptoms • How serious • Decontamination • Antidotes, first aid • Weather conditions	Information from ambulance service, GPs, Accident Department, Water Company, NHS Direct
Initial response: • What agencies are involved • What are the command and control arrangements • Should other agencies be called • Is the site secure • Has sheltering or evacuation been advised • What has been said to media	Consider implementing PCT chemical incident plan, convening response team and setting up incident room
Assessing risk to health: • Review health effects and exposure pathways • Define affected population • Establish register of exposed/symptomatic persons	Obtain toxicological advice Map plume Consider sampling cases, other exposed persons, animals, environment Collect dataset on those affected by the incident or exposed to the chemical(s)
Communications: • Partner agencies (local and national) • Professionals • Media • Public	Set up telephone helpline, use NHS Direct

Table 4.12.2 *Continued*

Post-acute-phase response:	Those affected may require examination, testing, advice,
• Site clean-up	treatment or follow-up, normally carried out by local clinicians
• Environmental effects	Counselling may be considered to avoid stress-related illness
• Epidemiological study	As a minimum there should be a descriptive study, but there may
• Long-term surveillance	be an opportunity for an analytical study to determine the
	strength of any association between the chemical exposure
	and its health effects
Post-incident:	Incident documented, report prepared and circulated
• Written report	
• Audit of response	

CCDC on behalf of the PCT has particular responsibilities for the health aspects of chemical incidents (Table 4.12.2).

Surveillance of chemical incidents

The Health Protection Agency collects standardised information on chemical incidents from a range of agencies. The ten commonest reported chemicals involved in incidents in the UK in 2003 are listed in Table 4.12.3. The number of persons with symptoms in each incident varied from 1–2 to over 50. The most frequently reported types of incidents are spills and leaks followed by air-borne releases and fire and explosion. The most frequently reported location is in residential areas.

Table 4.12.3 Ten commonest chemicals involved in incidents, UK, 2003

Unknown	206
Asbestos	91
Carbon monoxide	83
Petroleum	68
Smoke	43
Mercury	42
Ammonia	39
Chlorine	36
Benzene, toluene & xylenes	35
Sulphuric acid	24

Source: HPA.

4.13 Managing acute radiation incidents

Major radiation incidents, such as accidents involving nuclear reactors, military operations and nuclear-powered satellites crashing to earth, are uncommon. However, because of the widespread use of radioactive materials in medicine, science and industry, small-scale incidents following transportation accidents, leaks and the loss or theft of sources do occur.

In a radiation incident, radioactive material may be released into the atmosphere as a gas or particles. This forms a wind-borne plume, which is dispersed and diluted. Some material will fall to the ground, particularly if there is rain. People may be exposed by direct radiation from the plume, by inhalation, by contamination of the environment leading to direct radiation, or by consumption of contaminated food or drink.

In the UK, health services do not normally take the lead in responding to releases of radioactive materials, but they do have a role in dealing with their health effects and allaying public anxiety (Table 4.13.1). They must have a written plan to cover this and a named person to take overall responsibility. This person is often the CCDC.

Countermeasures

Intervention after a radiation accident is based on countermeasures that aim to do more good

Table 4.13.1 Radiation incidents: responsibilities in the UK

Department of Trade and Industry	Civil nuclear installations.
	Site operators must consult with local agencies and draw up emergency plans including plans for an off-site facility.
	Radiation (Emergency Preparedness and Public Information) Regulations 2001 (REPPIR) require site operators, local authorities and fire services to provide information for the public living near nuclear installations on the action to be taken should an emergency arise.
Department of Transport	Accidents that occur during transportation of civil radioactive material.
	Operators are regulated by the Radioactive Material (Road Transport) Regulations 2002. They must prepare a plan. Operators subscribe to RADSAFE scheme.
Ministry of Defence	Incidents at defence nuclear installations.
Department of Environment, Food and Rural affairs (DEFRA)	Incidents at nuclear installations overseas.
	DEFRA operates the UK's Radioactive Incident Monitoring Network (RIMNET) consisting of some 92 continuous radiation monitoring stations. These automatically raise an alarm if abnormal increases in the levels of radiation are detected at any of the sites.
National Radiological Protection Board (NRPB), now part of Health Protection Agency	Advice to government, other agencies and the public on all aspects of protection from radiological hazards.
	NRPB Nuclear Emergency Plan, Chilton Emergency Centre.
	Co-ordinates National Arrangements for Incidents Involving Radioactivity (NAIR). NAIR covers radiation incidents in public places. NAIR is activated by the Police. First-stage assistance comes from hospital radiation staff and second-stage assistance comes from radiation staff from nuclear power stations or other similar establishments.
Health and Safety Executive	Industrial sites with large amounts of nuclear material.
Health services including PCTs, ambulance service and hospitals	Prepare emergency plans. Reception, treatment and decontamination of casualties at designated hospitals, monitoring people and their personal belongings following exposure, by local medical physics departments, distribution of potassium iodate tablets, information to the public and the media on health aspects of the accident, collating advice from ex-pert sources, telephone advice line, long-term follow-up of exposed persons for clinical or epidemiological purposes.
Food Standards Agency	Advice on what food and drink can be consumed.
Environment agency/water company	Advice on whether radioactive material can be flushed into the drains.
Home office	Nuclear-powered satellite accidents.
	Terrorism.

Box 4.13.1 Checklist for CCDC in acute radiation incidents

- Enquire about
  - nature and scale of the incident,
  - whether anyone has been exposed to radiation as a result of the accident,
  - whether they can be traced,
  - the likely clinical effect of exposure to the source of radiation,
  - the extent and nature of any environmental contamination and
  - the wider population that might have been exposed.
- Carry out an initial risk assessment.
- Consult with local, regional or national sources of expert advice (keep up-to-date contact details in written plan).
- Agree countermeasures, public information, follow-up

Box 4.13.2 Ionising radiation

Ionising radiation is released when an unstable element or radionuclide decays. It is either electromagnetic radiation (X-rays and gamma-rays) or fast-moving particles (alpha particles, beta particles). Ionising radiation releases energy as it passes through biological tissues, resulting in damage. The amount of radioactivity is measured in Bequerels (Bq), the energy deposited by radiation is measured in Grays (Gy) and the effective dose of the radiation or the harm that it causes in measured in Sieverts or millisieverts (mSv). The average annual exposure in the UK is 2.5 mSv. Of this 87% comes from natural background radiation (cosmic rays, granite), 12% comes from medical X-rays, 0.1% from nuclear discharges and 0.4% from fallout. The maximum permitted radiation from artificial sources is 1 mSv. A person will be exposed to ionising radiation by being in close proximity to a radioactive source in their surroundings. Prolonged exposure will follow contamination of skin, clothing and wounds and ingestion. Cells that divide frequently are most sensitive to the effects of ionising radiation. Following exposure to a threshold level of radiation, radiation sickness (1 Gy) and radiation burns (20 Gy) may occur. Any dose of radiation increases the risk of cancers and hereditary diseases. An average individual exposed to 5 mSv as a result of eating contaminated food in the first year after a radiation accident has an additional lifetime risk of about 1 in 4000 of developing fatal cancer. The lifetime risk of dying in a fire is about 1 per 1000 and the lifetime risk of dying in a road traffic accident is 10 per 1000. The average person in the UK received 0.1m Sv from the Chernobyl accident in 1986. In the event of a nuclear accident, sheltering or evacuation would be recommended to prevent a whole-body dose of 30 mSv (the ERL). This is well below the dose that could lead to physical symptoms.

---

than harm. Countermeasures include sheltering, evacuation, iodine prophylaxis and banning contaminated foodstuffs. In an accident involving radioactive iodine-131, 60–70% of uptake can be blocked if potassium iodate tablets are given within 3 hours and 50% at approximately 5 hours. In the UK potassium iodate tablets are part of the UK National Reserve Stock for Major Incidents. However local accident and emergency departments are advised to maintain small stocks for small-scale local incidents. Criteria for countermeasures are based on Emergency Reference Levels (ERL). ERLs are expressed in terms of the radiation dose to an individual that could be averted if the countermeasure is implemented. For each counter-measure a lower and an upper ERL is recommended. The lower ERL is the smallest reduction in dose likely to offset the disadvantages of the countermeasure. If the estimated averted dose exceeds the lower ERL, then implementation of the countermeasure should be considered, but is not essential. The upper ERL is the reduction in dose for which the

countermeasure would be justified in nearly all situations.

4.14 Deliberate release of biological, chemical or radiological agents

Deliberate release (DR) of biological, chemical or radiological agents may be overt or covert. An overt release may be preceded by a warning, may be an immediately apparent substance released into a public place or may present as a number of individuals contaminated by an unknown substance. Those exposed may or may not be acutely ill and a sample of the agent may be available for analysis. The health service may be alerted by the police. Should those exposed develop symptoms within the first few minutes or hours the most likely cause is a chemical agent, followed by a biological toxin or hysteria. Slightly longer incubation periods increase the chances of an infectious or radiological hazard being responsible. Many incidents will turn out to be a hoax or a misinterpretation of a normal event, e.g. the use of powdered silica in packaging triggering a 'white powder' incident. The principles of dealing with such incidents build on those used in managing accidental release of such agents.

A covert incident, e.g. a substance introduced into the food or water supply, may only become apparent when ill patients present to health services. This may be some time after exposure, depending on the nature of the hazard. These cases may not occur in an obvious geographic area or in people with obvious common exposure. Potential indicators of a covert release are given in Box 4.14.1. It is likely that the health services will be the first agency to discover a covert release and will have to inform other agencies of their suspicions. The principles of investigating such incidents build on those used in controlling outbreaks or other longer term incidents (see Chapter 4.3).

As always, advance preparation is the key to success in organising a response and consists of

• multiagency contingency plans.
• ensuring access to equipment, e.g. personal protective clothing, decontamination facilities and therapeutic counter measures.
• training of staff and multiagency exercises.

Organisational response to acute/overt incidents

Co-ordination, command and control of acute DR incidents follow the same principles as that for emergency planning for any incident (e.g. an explosion, plane crash or flooding) and therefore comprise three levels:
• Bronze (operational), usually located at the scene and operating at 'activity' level (e.g. individual patient care).
• Silver (tactical), usually located near the scene and operating at function or range of activities level.
• Gold (strategic), which is usually off-site at a headquarters office and is responsible for multiagency strategic co-ordination.

In the case of suspected DR incidents, an overall lead agency is required to co-ordinate the response. In the UK, this is the police. The multiagency strategic (gold) group will be

---

Box 4.14.1 When to consider possibility of a deliberate release

• Number of ill people with similar disease or syndrome presenting around the same time.
• Number of cases of unexplained disease, syndrome or death.
• Single case of disease caused by uncommon agent.
• Illness occurring in an unusual setting or key sector within a community.
• Failure of a common disease to respond to usual therapy.
• Disease with unusual geographic or seasonal variation.
• Multiple atypical presentations of disease agents.
• Similar typing of agents isolated from temporally or spatially distinct sources.
• Unusual, atypical, genetically engineered or antiquated strain of agents.
• Simultaneous outbreaks of similar illness in non-contiguous areas.
• No local cause for unexpected acute event with syndrome of confusion, nausea, vomiting, respiratory, eye and skin irritation, collapse, difficulty seeing, frightened and possible delayed effects. May be smell or plume without explained cause.
• Deaths or illness among animals that precedes or accompanies illness or death in humans.
• Suspected or known DR in other countries.

supported by a Joint Health Advisory Cell (JHAC) which

• takes advice on the health aspects of the incident from a wide range of sources.

• provides advice to the Police Incident Commander (PIC) on the health consequences of the incident, including the consequences of any evacuation or containment policies.

• agrees the advice to be given to the public on health aspects of the incident with the PIC.

• liaises with the Department of Health and other national and local health agencies.

• formulates advice to health professionals in hospitals, ambulance services and primary care.

• formulates advice on strategic management of the health service response (but does not actually do the strategic management).

The JHAC is chaired by the local Director of Public Health (or someone agreed with him/her) and has multiagency membership similar to that for an accidental incident or outbreak, plus national experts made available via national arrangements.

JHAC arrangements are currently under review in England.

Technical aspects of response

In chemical and biological incidents, the actions in order of priority are containment, decontamination, resuscitation, primary treatment, definitive care and follow up. A schematic illustration of how this might be organised at the scene is given in Figure 4.14.1. In general, only simple, life-saving treatment can be carried out in the 'warm zone' before decontamination. This comprises simple airway opening manoeuvres, bag-valve-mask ventilation and pressure on 'bleeding wounds'.

Advice should be taken on decontamination, but in general follow these guidelines:

• Remove exposed person from scene of contamination.

• Remove all clothing (80% reduction in contamination).

• General decontamination: the decontaminant of choice for most chemicals is water and detergent using the 'rinse-wipe-rinse' method (water or saline only for eyes and mucus membranes).

• Liquid chemical contamination must be removed as soon as possible.

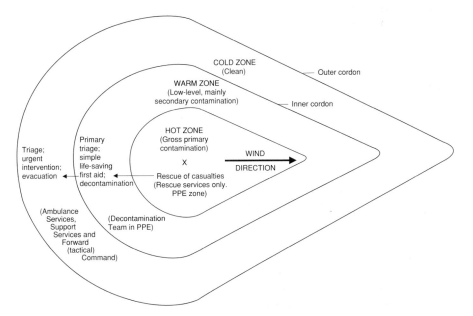

Fig. 4.14.1 Organisation of on-scene response.

Table 4.14.1 Potential chemical terrorism agents

	Symptoms	Speed of action	Antidotes and treatment
Nerve agents (organophosphates and related agents, e.g. Sarin, VX)	Mild: headache, nausea, small pupils, visual difficulties, painful eyes, running nose, excess salivation, mild weakness and agitation. Moderate: dizziness, disorientation, confusion, sneezing, coughing, wheezing, drooling, excess phlegm, vomiting, diarrhoea, marked weakness, difficulty breathing. Severe: respiratory difficulty, convulsions, arrhythmias.	Unconsciousness and convulsions within seconds; death in minutes	Atropine Oximes Diazepam
Mustard	Early: nausea, vomiting, retching, eye irritation, erythema. Hours: nausea, fatigue, headache, painful eyes, lacrimation, blepharospasm, photophobia, runny nose, erythema, sore throat, hoarseness, tachycardia, tachypnoea, oedema. Days: inflammation, blistering, pus, necrosis, coughing.	1.5–2 hours 2–6 hours 13–72 hours	Decontaminate ASAP. No specific antidote. Symptomatic and supportive care only. May need ITU facilities.
Chlorine	Inhalation: irritation of eyes, nose and throat, followed by coughing, wheezing, dyspnoea, sputum, bronchospasm, chest pain. Metabolic complications from mild alkalosis to severe acidosis and hypoxaemia. Cardiorespiratory arrest due to hypoxia may occur. Dermal: skin irritation with burns at high concentration.	Irritation occurs rapidly. Chemical pneumonitis and pulmonary oedema can take 12–24 hours.	Removal from contaminated area. No specific antidote. Symptomatic and supportive care only. May need ITU facilities.
Hydrogen cyanide	Low dose: dyspnoea, headache, dizziness, anxiety, tachycardia, nausea, drowsiness, possibly metallic taste. High dose: hyperventilation, unconsciousness, convulsions, fixed dilated pupils, cyanosis, death.	Unconsciousness and convulsions in seconds. Death in minutes.	Removal from contaminated area and resuscitation. Dicobalt edetate or sodium nitrite.

Agent	Clinical features	Onset	Treatment
Phosgene	Initial phase: eye irritation, lacrimation, nausea, vomiting, chest tightness, retrosternal discomfort, bronchoconstriction, hypertension, brady or tachycardia. Severe exposure can lead to haemolysis and rapid death. Latent phase: may appear well, symptoms precipitated by exercise. Oedema phase: pulmonary oedema, dyspnoea, bronchospasm, frothy sputum, hypotension, tachycardia, hypoxia, ARDS, death (severity of initial phase not related to severity of oedema).	Major effects usually take hours, but may be immediate pain at exposed sites.	Decontaminate ASAP. Symptomatic and supportive. No specific antidote. May need ITU facilities.
Ricin	Fever common. Ingestion causes irritation of oropharynx and oesophagus plus gastroenteritis. Bloody diarrhoea, vomiting, abdominal pain, conjunctivitis, miosis, mydriasis, pulmonary oedema, pneumonia, ARDS, seizures, CNS depression, multiorgan failure, death. Abnormal LFTs, haematuria, proteinuria, high creatinine.	Delayed	Symptomatic and supportive. No specific antidote.
Lewisite (arsenical compound)	Early: very irritating, pain on contact. Damage to eyes, skin, airways (similar to mustard)	Minutes	Decontaminate ASAP. British-Anti-Lewisite.
Saxitoxin	Paralytic shellfish poisoning (see Chapter 3.90). May be confused with nerve agents.	10–120 minutes	Induce vomiting. May need ITU. Avoid Atropine!
Tricothecene mycotoxins ('Yellow rain')	Burning skin, redness, tenderness, blistering, necrosis. Dyspnoea, wheezing, coughing, weakness, prostration, dizziness, ataxia. Tachycardia, hypothermia, hypotension.	Minutes	Decontamination of skin. No specific antidote.

• Water and hypochlorite best for biological contamination (if small numbers).

• Biological contamination of large numbers can usually wait for mass decontamination facilities to be set up.

• Contaminated clothing, equipment and effluent, where possible, to be stored in safe area, awaiting disposal (or evidence collection).

• For radiation, external decontamination is similar to that for non-radioactive chemicals, but extra care is taken with clothes, etc.

• Decontamination team must wear Personal Protective Equipment (PPE).

• Ensure that decontaminated persons are kept separate from those awaiting decontamination (and moved away from contamination).

Following decontamination, triage will separate those exposed into priority groups for treatment and evacuation. Advanced life support procedures and other generic interventions can then be deployed.

It may be possible, based on the symptom profile of those who become ill or the results of screening of samples from the environment and patients, to identify the likely cause of symptoms. This will allow specific countermeasures or antidotes to be deployed (see Table 4.14.1 for symptoms and antidotes of main chemical threats).

Suspicious packages or materials

A package may be considered suspicious if

• suspicious or threatening messages are written on it.

• envelope is distorted, bulky, rigid, discoloured, has an oily stain, has an obvious odour or feels like it has powder inside.

• it is an unexpected envelope, particularly from a foreign country.

• there is no postage stamp, no franking or cancelling of stamp.

• the spelling of common names, places or titles is incorrect.

• It is a handwritten envelope from unknown source, particularly if addressed to individual and marked personal or addressee only.

• on opening, suspicious power or material found.

The immediate response:

• Do not open package.

• Call police immediately for advice.

If package opened or suspect material found, then in addition

• shut windows and doors to room and switch off any room air-conditioning.

• ask room occupants to move to unoccupied adjacent room away from hazard.

• seek medical advice for anyone showing symptoms.

• notify building manager to switch off air-conditioning, close fire doors and close all windows in rest of building.

• do not touch or attempt to clean up any suspect material.

The police should then perform a risk assessment, to decide whether threat is credible. Figure 4.14.2 gives details of action to be taken in response to their assessment. A number of agencies will need to be involved if a credible threat is declared and specialist advice should be taken.

Investigation of incidents of unusual illness

A cluster of an unusual or unknown illness, a single occurrence of an unexpected illness for that community or illness that fails to behave as expected should be investigated according to standard epidemiological and public health practices (see Chapter 4.3). However, there may be some features that should raise the suspicion of a DR (see Box 4.14.1). Infectious agents that are considered to have bioterrorist potential are given in Table 4.14.2; of note is that in DR scenarios, the presentation may be more sudden, more severe and involve larger numbers than in natural outbreaks, particularly if aerosol dispersion has been used. Fortunately most such agents do not spread onwards from person to person, although smallpox and pneumonic plague are important exceptions. Symptoms suggestive of a covert release of a radioactive substance are given in Box 4.14.2.

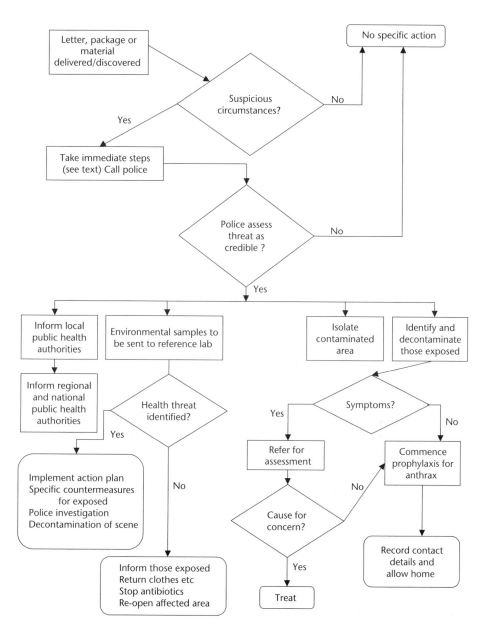

Fig. 4.14.2 Response to suspicious package or material.

In addition to notifying local, regional and national public health authorities, a suspected DR must also be reported to the police, who will have their own investigative needs. As always, meticulous record keeping is essential.

In addition to standard outbreak/incident investigation steps (case definitions, case finding, data collection and recording, laboratory investigations, descriptive epidemiology, hypothesis generation and testing), particular

Table 4.14.2 Potential bioterrorism organisms and toxins

Agent (disease)	Potential source	Ability to cause disease	Incubation period	Ability to spread from person to person	Chemoprophylaxis	Further details
Bacillus anthracis (anthrax)	Aerosol (spores)	Moderate	1–6 days	None	1. Ciprofloxacin 2. Doxycycline 3. Amoxycillin	Chapter 3.2
Brucella sp (brucellosis)	1. Aerosol 2. Food	High	Days to months	None	1. Ciprofloxacin 2. Doxycycline	Chapter 3.5
Burkholderia mallei (glanders)	Aerosol	High	Days to weeks	Low	1. Doxycycline 2. Ciprofloxacin	May survive in environment Potentially fatal Horses may be affected
Burkholderia pseudomallei (melioidosis)	Aerosol	High	1–7 days	Negligible	1. Ciprofloxacin 2. Doxycycline	Stable agent of variable severity
Chlamydia psittaci (psittacosis)	Aerosol	Moderate	4–15 days	Negligible	Doxycycline	Chapter 3.9
Clostridium botulinum toxin (botulism)	1. Food/water 2. Aerosol	High	Hours to days	None	1. None 2. Antitoxin available.	Chapter 3.4
Coccidioides immitis (coccidioidomycosis)	Aerosol	High	1–2 weeks	None	Fluconazole	Stable agent of low lethality
Coxiella burnetii (Q fever)	1. Aerosol 2. Food supply	High	10 days to 5 weeks	Negligible	1. Doxycycline 2. Erythromycin	Chapter 3.60
Ebola/Lassa/CCHF (viral haemorrhagic fevers)	Aerosol	High	3–15 days	Moderate (body fluids)	None available	Chapter 3.84
Francisella tularensis (tularaemia)	Aerosol	High	2–10 days	None	1. Ciprofloxacin 2. Doxycycline	Chapter 3.80
Hantavirus	Aerosol	High	4–42 days	None	None available	Chapter 3.27
Histoplasma. Capsulatum (histoplasmosis)	Aerosol	High	1–2 weeks	None	Fluconazole	Can persist in soil, but low lethality
Influenza virus	Aerosol	High	2–4 days	High (respiratory)	1. Oseltamir 2. Zanamivir	Chapter 3.38

Agent	Transmission	Severity	Incubation period	Person-to-person spread	Treatment/prophylaxis	Notes
Junin virus	Aerosol	Moderate	7–16 days	Low	None (ribavirin if fever)	Chapter 3.90
Machupo virus	Aerosol	Moderate	7–14 days	Low	None (ribavirin if fever)	Chapter 3.90
Rickettsia prowazekii (typhus)	1. Aerosol 2. Infected vectors	High	6–16 days	None	Doxycycline	Chapter 3.82
Rickettsia rickettsia (rocky mountain spotted fever)	1. Aerosol 2. Infected vectors	High	3–10 days	None	Doxycycline	Not very stable but high lethality
Rickettsia tsutsugamushi (scrub typhus)	1. Aerosol 2. Infected vectors	High	4–15 days	None	Doxycycline	Not very stable and low lethality
Rift valley fever virus	Aerosol	Moderate	2–12 days	None	None (ribavirin if fever)	Chapter 3.90 Would also cause disease in sheep and cattle
Salmonella sp (gastroenteritis)	1. Food 2. Water	Low	2–3 days	Moderate (faeco–oral)	Ciprofloxacin	Chapter 3.67
Salmonella typhi (typhoid)	1 Food/water 2. Aerosol	Moderate	7–21 days	Low (faeco–oral)	1. Ciprofloxacin 2. Ceftriaxone	Chapter 3.81
Shigella sp (dysentery)	1. Food 2. Water	High	2–3 days	High (faeco–oral)	Ciprofloxacin	Chapter 3.70
Smallpox virus	Aerosol	High	10–17 days	High (aerosol)	1. None available. 2. Vaccine for contacts.	Chapter 3.71
Staphylococcal enterotoxin B	1. Sabotage 2. Aerosol		1–6 hours	None	None	Stable toxin of low lethality
Venezuelan equine encephalitis virus	Aerosol	High	1–6 days	None	None	Chapter 3.90
Vibrio cholerae (cholera)	1. Food/water 2. Aerosol	Low	1–5 days	low (faeco–oral)	1. Ciprofloxacin 2. Doxycycline	Chapter 3.11
VTEC (haemorrhagic gastroenteritis)	1. Food 2. Water	High	2–3 days	High (faeco–oral)	None	Chapter 3.24
Yellow fever virus	Aerosol	Moderate	3–6 days	None	None	Chapter 3.88
Yersinia pestis (plague)	1. Aerosol 2. Vectors	High	2–3 days	High (pneumonic)	1. Ciprofloxacin 2. Doxycycline	Chapter 3.57

Box 4.14.2 Features of exposure to high doses of external radiation

Whole body exposure
- prodrome of nausea, vomiting, fatigue and possibly fever and diarrhoea.
- latent period of varying lengths (depending on dose).
- illness characterised by infection, bleeding and gastrointestinal symptoms (damage to cells of blood and GI tract).

Local exposure
- erythema, oedema, desquamation, blistering, pain, necrosis, gangrene or epilation (depends on dose).
- local skin injuries evolve over time (weeks to months)
- skin lesions may be very painful and difficult to treat.
- no knowledge of exposure to chemical or heat causes of burns, or to bites or allergen.

---

issues for management include
- defining those 'exposed but not ill' and collecting data on them.
- guidance on investigation and best treatment of rare illnesses or variant organisms.
- risk to contacts, including healthcare staff.
- information for the public.
- communications arrangements.
- environmental contamination.

4.15 Port health

The cholera epidemics that affected Europe between 1830 and 1847 led to international public health co-operation and the first International Sanitary Conference in Paris in 1851. In 1951 WHO member states adopted the International Sanitary Regulations, which were renamed the International Health Regulations (IHR) in 1969. The IHR are a legally binding set of procedures to prevent the spread of disease comprising measures at airports and seaports and reporting of infections to WHO. Under current IHR, only cholera, plague and yellow fever are notifiable. The IHR are undergoing revision to reflect the return of old epidemics such as cholera in South America and the emergence of new infectious agents such as Ebola haemorrhagic fever, SARS, avian influenza and the deliberate use of CBRN agents that may

affect health. The revised IHR will require countries to notify WHO of events constituting an international public health emergency and to provide information so that WHO can respond with appropriate assistance. National IHR Focal Points will be set up and the basic public health capacities a country must have in order to detect, report and respond to an international public health incident will be defined.

In the UK, the Public Health Act 1872 provided for the establishment of Port Sanitary Authorities now called Port Health Authorities (PHA). PHAs are often part of Local Authority environmental health departments and have powers under regulations to control the public health aspects of port activity involving ships, aircraft and international trains (Table 4.15.1). PHAs appoint port health officers and port medical officers.

The port medical officer may also act as Port Medical Inspector (PMI) providing advice to the Immigration and Nationality Service. An immigration officer may refer any person seeking entry to the UK to the PMI for medical examination and may refuse entry if the person is not cleared. In practice only persons intending to remain in the UK for 6 months or more or those who are unwell are required to have medical clearance. Medical clearance may take place in the country of origin. Persons with infectious diseases likely to endanger the health of other persons in the UK, those who are unable for medical reasons to support themselves

Table 4.15.1 Functions of Port Health Authorities

Preventing the importation of disease	Visit and inspect vessels and aircraft.
	Masters of vessels are required to report any illness.
	Advice on illness amongst passengers and crew (viral haemorrhagic fever, yellow fever, plague, cholera, diphtheria, TB), managing outbreaks of infection due to in-flight catering or contaminated water, contamination of the interior of an aircraft with faeces or vomit.
	Contingency plans for assessment and information gathering from a large number of individuals including staff, space (including toilets), questionnaires, faecal sampling, communications and information leaflets.
Rodent control	Ships must be inspected every 96 months for rats.
	PHA can issue de-ratting and de-ratting exemption certificates.
	Airlines required to disinfect aircraft (by use of an aerosol spray) when travelling from countries in which there is a risk of a disease being spread by insects.
Imported food	Border Inspection Post for the inspection and clearance of Products of Animal Origin into the EU.
	Identify and inspect foodstuffs of non-animal origin on a risk-assessment basis to ensure that they comply with the Imported Food Regulations. If necessary carry out sampling.
Fish and shellfish	With Food Standards Agency monitor quality of local shellfish waters and the safety of local shellfish.
Food premises inspections	Monitors standards in shore-based premises as well as on visiting ships and aircraft and in-flight catering.
	Quality of ship and aircraft water supplies.
Animal health	Assist with enforcement of rabies controls.

or their dependants in the UK, or those who require major medical treatment may be refused entry. Those seeking entry at some ports may receive a chest X-ray. Unless entry is refused, details of the immigrant and the results of any examination are passed to the CCDC in the proposed area of residence. Subsequent action taken by the CCDC varies. In some areas new entrants are invited to attend for a further medical assessment. The effectiveness of such arrangements is currently under review.

4.16 Media relations

The media should be considered as an ally in protecting the health of the public. They are one of the most powerful influences upon the public. Relationships with the media should be developed proactively; good routine relationships with the media will make dealing with them during emergency situations much easier.

Communicable disease issues arouse interest and anxiety in the public. This may seem irrational to a professional; however, the public have a right to be informed and the press is often the best route. In some circumstances the public and press may become hostile – avoiding the press, appearing evasive, misleading the public or lying are likely to make the situation worse. Virtually all issues can be presented in a way that the public can understand. Professionals should not hide behind technical obfuscations. Do not expect to have any control over material that you provide, press releases can be selectively quoted and interviews can be edited. However journalists are usually interested in accuracy.

Training

Anyone who is likely to deal with the media should undergo media training. This will help in understanding what the media needs. Journalists often have a similar agenda to public health workers, they wish to inform and educate the public. If they encounter a group of professionals who understand their needs, and are trying to help, then journalists are less likely to be antagonistic.

Identify people within the organisation who are particularly good with the media – they may not be the most senior people.

Routine relationships

Develop regular contact with your local print and broadcast media. Be available to answer their questions, and treat your local reporters as friends. If they trust you and rely on you as an authoritative source it will make things much easier if a story is breaking.

Local papers may be willing to publish a regular column; this is a powerful way of getting health advice across. Use opportunities to publish in local papers, women's magazines, parents' magazines etc. This will probably have a greater influence than publishing in the peer reviewed medical press. Have basic information packs available for journalists. These should describe the clinical features and importance of an infection and the salient epidemiological features and recent trends.

Outbreaks

During outbreak or emergency situations it is important to maintain good relations with the press. Journalists have a job to do, they can become intrusive, but they will understand that you have a job to do. Let the journalists know that they will be kept informed, that there will be regular briefings, daily even twice daily. Ensure that the briefings do happen. Appoint a media spokesperson and ensure that all media briefings are done through that person. The outbreak control team should co-ordinate the flow of information.

Messages

Decide beforehand what your key messages are; if possible discuss these with the journalist and discuss the questions that will be asked. Decide if there are any areas that you do not wish to be drawn into. Be honest and accurate, keep technical details to a minimum. Get the key message across first, then provide the reasoning behind it. Stress the facts and explain the context. Do not try to hide the truth or lie. If you are uncertain of the facts or some detail say so and offer to get the information. Don't be drawn into areas you feel you cannot or should not discuss, be firm and polite and say that you cannot discuss that issue. Try to avoid discussions of money and cost saving, stress public health action and your concern for safeguarding the public health. Avoid being drawn into speculation, or other criticisms of other groups. Behave as if you were always 'on the record'. Make sure that you know if a broadcast is live or recorded.

Press releases

Keep the press release short (8–10 paragraphs); make sure you have considered the message and the audience for the release, consult a press officer. Get the most important message into the first paragraph and support it with a quote from a senior official. In the introduction describe, Who, What, Where, When, Why, How. In the middle expand the story with supporting detail, conclude by summarising and identifying the next steps.

Problems

The press might want access to cases or locations such as outbreak rooms for atmospheric pictures or interviews. These requests should be considered very carefully. Considerations of confidentiality and the smooth running of an investigation must come first. However on occasion such photo opportunities might, by raising public awareness of an issue, be beneficial. If things go wrong remember that they can do in the best of relations. Developing good relations with the media takes time and effort. If errors of fact appear in an article or you feel you have been misrepresented contact the journalist and discuss them; if necessary talk to the editor.

4.17 Clinical governance and audit

Clinical governance provides a framework in which organisations involved in public health protection are accountable for continuously improving the quality of their services and safeguarding public health by creating an environment in which high standards of service are assured and excellence in health protection (HP) practice will flourish.

The main components for clinical governance are
• clear lines of responsibility and accountability for the overall quality of the service provided,
• a comprehensive programme of quality improvement activities,
• clear policies aimed at managing risk and
• procedures to identify and remedy poor performance.

The work of CDC/HP departments does not fit neatly into these compartments, but a suitable breakdown could be as follows.

Responsibility

Clinical governance emphasises that the organisational responsibility for quality lies at board level. As an example, in England this responsibility lies with the Primary Care Trust (PCT) probably via the Director of Public Health as an executive member of the PCT Board. PCTs now share responsibility for

delivery of the district CDC/HP service with the Health Protection Agency (HPA) and both Boards have responsibility for encouraging an environment in which quality can flourish.

The Board of the organisation needs to set clear objectives for the service. It must also take a particular interest in the organisations 'strategic capacity' to deliver a quality service and assess and control the risk to that capacity. This includes
• workforce capacity (see Box 4.17.1) and competence,
• leadership,
• culture or organisational behaviour,
• accountability for key elements of service,
• team working,
• adequate finance,
• information management and technology,
• partnerships,
• facilities and equipment and
• policies and procedures.

The PCT is also responsible for ensuring that other health services involved in CDC/HP (e.g. laboratories, chest clinics, STI clinics) have adequate clinical governance arrangements.

In practice, the executive lead for surveillance, prevention and control of communicable diseases (and other related functions) locally lies with the local health protection unit (HPU), whose Director should therefore take the lead in assuring the quality of the district CDC/HP function. The HPU Director is also responsible for ensuring that support staff provide a quality service by encouraging training, openness, teamwork, the seeking of advice where appropriate and performance review.

Quality improvement

CDC/HP teams should complete a baseline self-assessment of their strengths and weaknesses. This could cover the following areas:
• Service structure, personnel and skills.
• Arrangements for on-call and for covering leave.
• Access to operational support and infrastructure within PCT and HPA, e.g. administrative, IT, statistical expertise, communications, public relations.

Box 4.17.1 Suggested staffing levels for district CDC departments

Medical:
- Minimum of 1.0 whole time equivalent (wte) consultants per 400,000 population.
- Minimum 0.5 wte allocated time and available throughout office hours.
- Extra consultant sessions in districts with more complex workload and for any non-CDC duties.

Nursing:
- Minimum of 1.0 per 400,000 population.
- Extra nurse sessions in districts with large number of community settings (e.g. care homes).

Information Scientist:
- 0.2–0.5 per 400,000 population.
- Minimum of 1 session per week.

Secretarial Clerical/Data entry:
- Minimum of 1.5 wte per 400,000 population.
- Must be telephone cover during working hours.

Source: Report to NHS Executive, England, 1997.

- Access to specialist advice, library services and relevant Internet sites (e.g. Medline, Cochrane).
- Arrangements for multiagency working, particularly with Environmental Health Departments and hospital Control of Infection teams. Should include relevant operational support from other health organisations (e.g. PCTs and NHS Trusts) for activities such as surveillance, contact tracing and incident control.
- Clarity of roles and responsibilities of different organisations and individuals.
- How well the unit functions as a team.
- Adequacy of surveillance: data access (timeliness, quality), analysis and dissemination.
- Completeness and updating of policies and plans.
- Use of evidence-based practice and mechanisms for disseminating good practice.
- Support to prevention and control in community settings.
- Mechanisms to maintain patient confidentiality.
- Multiagency fora and committees (e.g. district control of infection, immunisation) for agreeing policies and procedures.
- Patient, service user, carer and public involvement.
- Audit and evaluation (see later).

Departments may also wish to invite an external peer reviewer to comment on how their services compare with standard/best practice elsewhere.

The HPU Director should formulate a risk register in the light of the baseline assessment, with a prioritised action plan with clearly assigned responsibilities and timescales. This should then be discussed with the appropriate clinical governance lead for the organisation. Progress on the action plan needs to be regularly reviewed.

One important element of quality improvement will be continuing professional development (CPD) for CDC/HP staff. Each staff member should have a personal development plan, which should be discussed with their line manager. This could include training and updating in

- epidemiology and control of communicable diseases.
- epidemiological methods and statistics for surveillance, outbreaks and research.
- information technology.
- infection control and environmental health.
- management methods such as leadership, organisation, supervisory skills, team working, time management, presentation and media skills.
- new governmental, organisational or professional priorities.
- non-communicable risks to health (if relevant).

Departmental CPD should include training and updating in on-call issues for all staff on the out of hours rota. Those whose routine work does not include a large component of CDC/HP would benefit from attendance at a specialist course at least every 3 years. In UK, the role of the General Medical Council in revalidation will mean that doctors will need to be able to regularly demonstrate that they are keeping themselves up to date and remain fit to practise in their chosen field.

Policies for managing risk

Such policies should include the following:
- Incident response plans for:
  community outbreaks,
  hospital outbreaks,
  water-borne diseases,
  instances requiring patient tracing, notification and helplines,
  chemical incidents,
  radiation incidents,
  major emergencies and
  deliberate release.

These plans need regular revision. If used in an incident, a written report should be produced. If not recently used, consideration should be given to a simulation exercise.
- Policies and procedures for dealing with common or serious diseases.
- A regularly updated on-call pack, which includes relevant policies and contact details for staff and other organisations.
- Good documentation of incidents and requests for advice.
- A system for reporting and learning lessons from complaints, problems encountered in delivering service, or poor outcomes. The system should include a mechanism for ensuring that action is taken in response to lessons learned.

Rectifying poor performance

In CDC/HP this primarily revolves around clinical audit and CPD (there is obvious overlap with quality improvement processes).

- Clinical audit involves
  setting standards,
  comparing actual performance to standards and
  rectifying identified deficiencies.
- Audit should involve an element of peer review. One useful mechanism is to involve staff in neighbouring teams, perhaps as part of a Regional Audit Group. Where national standards do not exist, this group can devise regional ones on which to base audit.
- Suitable topics for audit might be:
  adequacy of contingency plans,
  adequacy of district surveillance systems for spotting outbreaks and analysing trends,
  response of on-call staff (including partner organisations),
  review of management of an actual outbreak,
  review of response to (randomly selected) cases of meningococcal disease,
  immunisation uptake rates and methods used to improve them and
  appropriateness of HIV prevention strategy.
- A report should be written on all significant outbreaks and incidents detailing the lessons learnt. More minor episodes (e.g. sporadic case of typhoid) can be discussed informally, e.g. at weekly departmental surveillance and information meetings.
- Discussion and monitoring of formal and informal complaints from the public or health professionals.
- It is important in all cases to ensure that someone is responsible for ensuring that identified deficiencies in the service are rectified. Methods of rectifying poor performance are given in Section 2 above.

It is clear that the quality of CDC/HP work and the ability to carry out clinical governance and audit are both dependent upon the level of resources available to the CDC/HP department and the overall culture of the organisation. Nonetheless, the individual practitioner can use his/her leadership, management and professional skills to maximise the resources available and to prioritise their use: clinical governance is a tool that can be used to further those objectives.

Section 5
Communicable disease control in Europe

5.1 Introduction

Infectious diseases do not respect national boundaries, and international travel and trade increase the risk that an outbreak involves more than one country. The WHO has been responsible for collecting international data on infectious diseases and administering the International Health Regulations – the mainstay of the international response to communicable disease. New patterns of collaboration are developing to enable countries to respond appropriately to international threats to health. This has particularly been the case in Europe. The EU is a free trade area within which goods, people and their infections can circulate; several collaborations, largely been funded by the European Commission, have developed between national surveillance centres in response to this problem (Table 5.1.1). These have shown some remarkable successes in identifying outbreaks that would probably not have been identified otherwise, in assisting in the response to international outbreaks and in developing the framework for international collaborative action. These collaborations are based around experts in particular infections and around infrastructure developments, such as training. There is a legal basis whereby national surveillance systems collaborate around a common list of diseases under surveillance, common case definitions and common laboratory methods. An Early Warning and Response System connects EU member states to communicate information on countermeasures and risks.

European Centre for Disease Prevention and Control

In Spring 2004 the Council and the European Parliament adopted enabling legislation to create a European Centre for Disease Prevention and Control (ECDC). This new EU agency will provide a structured and systematic approach to the control of communicable diseases and other serious health threats that affect EU citizens. The ECDC will also mobilise and sig-nificantly reinforce the synergies between the existing national centres for disease control. It is due to start work in May 2005 and will be based in Stockholm. The ECDC was formally launched in September 2004 and Zsuzsanna Jakab has been appointed as the first Director of the centre.

The main tasks of the ECDC, as described by the EU, will be as follows:

• *Epidemiological surveillance and networking of laboratories*: The centre will develop epidemiological surveillance at European level. In this work, the centre could either use its own staff, staff from the dedicated surveillance networks (see Table 5.1.1), or, in some instances, it could subcontract tasks to a national centre of excellence. The centre could also identify and maintain networks of reference laboratories, and enhance the quality assurance schemes of microbiological laboratories.

• *Early warning and response*: To be effective, the early warning and response system (EWRS) requires 'around the clock' availability of specialists in communicable diseases. Whilst the responsibility for action will remain with Member States and the Commission, technical operation of the EWRS would be undertaken by the centre and its networks.

• *Scientific opinions*: Public health decisions have to be based on independent scientific evidence. Scientific issues arising in the area of communicable diseases vary widely, ranging from questions of clinical medicine and epidemiology through to standardisation of laboratory procedures. Creating one permanent scientific committee to cover all these issues would not, therefore, be appropriate. The centre would, instead, bring together scientific expertise in specific fields through its various EU-wide networks and via ad hoc scientific panels.

• *Technical assistance and communication*: The centre's rapid reaction capacity could cover more than the EU itself, to similar structures in such areas as the EEA/EFTA, and candidate countries. When requested, it would send an EU-team to investigate an outbreak of an unknown human disease in a European country. The centre should also have the ability to support, if necessary, those Commission services

Table 5.1.1 EU collaborations in communicable disease surveillance

Description	Internet URL
Enhanced Laboratory Surveillance of Measles aims to develop, harmonise and co-ordinate the wider use of standard and oral-fluid based diagnostic methods within Europe in order to enhance the surveillance of measles.	www.elsm.net
Enter-Net is the international surveillance network for the enteric infections, e.g. Salmonella and VTEC O157, and involves all 25 countries of the EU, plus Switzerland and Norway.	http://www.hpa.org.uk/hpa/inter/enter-net_menu.htm
DIPNET, the European Diphtheria Surveillance Network and the European Laboratory Working Group on Diphtheria (ELWGD), is a definitive expansion of the ELWGD and encompasses the key epidemiologists and microbiologists from most EU member states and accession countries.	http://www.hpa.org.uk/hpa/inter/elwgd_menu.htm
European Sero-Epidemiology Network 2 (ESEN2) aims to co-ordinate and harmonise throughout Europe the serological surveillance of immunity to a variety of vaccine preventable infections.	http://www.hpa.org.uk/hpa/inter/esen2_menu.htm
European Union Invasive Bacterial Infections Surveillance (EU-IBIS) network aims to improve epidemiological information and laboratory capacity to characterise isolates of invasive *Haemophilus influenzae* and *Neisseria meningitidis* within the EU.	http://www.euibis.org/
European Working Group for Legionella Infections (EWGLI) aims to improve the detection and control of Legionnaires disease. EWGLI now has 36 collaborating countries.	http://www.hpa.org.uk/hpa/inter/ewgli.htm
Eurosurveillance is dedicated to the surveillance, prevention and control of infectious and communicable disease. Eurosurveillance produces a weekly and a monthly bulletin.	http://www.eurosurveillance.org/index-02.asp
The HARMONY project – Harmonisation of antibiotic resistant methods of typing organisms and ways of using these and other tools to increase the effectiveness of Nosocomial infection control.	http://www.harmony-microbe.net/
Salmgene aims to strengthening international Salmonella surveillance through strain typing and differentiation (Salm-gene).	http://www.salmgene.net/
EARSS (European Antimicrobial Resistance Surveillance System) is an international network of national surveillance systems, collecting comparable and validated antimicrobial resistance data for public health purposes.	http://www.earss.rivm.nl/
EISS (European Influenza Surveillance Scheme) aims to contribute to a reduction in morbidity and mortality due to influenza in Europe.	http://www.eiss.org/
EuroHIV (European Centre for the Epidemiological Monitoring of AIDS) co-ordinates HIV/AIDS surveillance in the 52 countries of WHO's European Region.	http://www.eurohiv.org
EuroTB aims for surveillance of tuberculosis in Europe.	http://www.eurotb.org
EUVAC.NET, the European surveillance network for vaccine preventable diseases, involves surveillance institutions in the EU countries plus Iceland, Malta, Norway and Switzerland.	http://www.euvac.net
StrepEuro aims to improve our understanding of the burden, risk-factors, microbiological characteristics of invasive group A streptococcal disease.	http://www.hpa.org.uk/hpa/inter/strep-EURO.htm

that give humanitarian aid or other types of assistance in response to disease outbreaks in third-world countries.

5.2 Austria

Contacts

Bundesministerium für Arbeit, Gesundheit und Soziales (Federal Ministry for Labour, Health, Social Affaires), http://www.bmags.gv.at.

Statutory notification systems

The details regarding statutory notification systems are given in Table 5.2.1.

Flow chart of statutory notification

See Figure 5.2.1.

Outbreak detection and investigation

Physicians' notifications and laboratory reports are collected at district and regional level. In the case of an outbreak the Ministry of Health has to be informed. District and regional health administrations have the legal responsibility for detection, investigation and public health action in co-operation with regional food and veterinary administration.

Prevention/prophylaxis

• Vaccine programme: DTPa-IPV, MMR, Hib, HBV.
• Vaccination coverage: >90 % for MMR1, 65% for MMR2 vaccinations, with strong regional variation.
• Antibiotics and malaria prophylaxis available only on prescription.

Table 5.2.1 Statutory notification systems (Austria)

Legal framework	Ministry of Health is responsible for introducing changes in the statutory notification system.
Levels of responsibility	
Local responsiblility for reporting	Physicians and laboratories.
Local responsiblility for action	Notifier is responsible for case management. Public health officers are responsible for contact tracing and contact management.
National surveillance	Federal Ministry for Health and Women.
Notifiable diseases	39 diseases are notifiable. No financial incentives for notifying physicians.
Case definitions	In use for TB, AIDS, CJD, acute poliomyelitis and measles.
Levels of reporting	Local level for reporting: 122 Local Health Departments with an average population of 66,000. Regional level: 9 regions with an average population of 1,006,600.
Estimated time to inform national level	Up to 30 days.
Public health action	The responsibility for case management is held by the notifier. Control measures including contact tracing and outbreak investigation is generally the responsibility of the Public Health Service, primarily at local level with support from regional and national level.
Data dissemination	A list of notifiable diseases is published by the Ministry monthly/yearly. In addition the national AIDS-Statistics (Östereichische AIDS-Statistik) are published monthly.

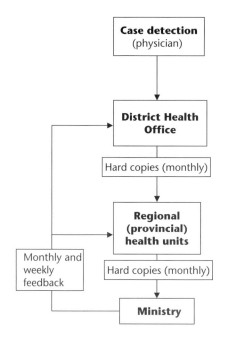

Fig. 5.2.1 Flow chart of statutory notification (Austria).

5.3 Belgium

Belgium is a federal state, which comprises communities and regions. On the basis of language and culture, Belgium can be divided into three communities: the Flemish community, the French community and the German community. The communities have the responsibility towards control of infectious diseases. Each has its own ministry (Ministry of *respective* Community, Administration of Public Health). In Brussels, where the Flemish community and the French community both share the responsibility, a Community Commission manages the control of infectious diseases. The country is also divided into three regions, which also have responsibility towards public health in their tasks of environmental and zoonotic disease control. Again, each has its own ministry.

Contacts

Institut Scientifique de Sante Publique – Wetenschappelijk Instituut Volksgezondheid (Scientific Institute of Public Health), http://www.iph.fgov.be.

Statutory notification systems

The details regarding statutory notification systems are given in Table 5.3.1.

Flow chart of statutory notification

See Figure 5.3.1.

Outbreak detection and investigation

A variety of sources of information are used to detect possible outbreaks (physicians' notifications/reporting, laboratory reporting, telephone calls from the public). The Health Inspectors of the Communities have the legal responsibility for detection, investigation and public health action within their community in co-operation with other local/regional authorities (environmental health, veterinarians, etc.). Other national authorities may also then be involved.

Prevention/prophylaxis

• Vaccine programme: DTPa-IPV, Hib, HBV, MMR, Men C
• Vaccination coverage (Flemish community, data 1999): 96% for polio, 95% for DTP, ~80% for other vaccinations (report at: http://www.wvc.vlaanderen.be/vaccinatie, or http://www.wvc.vlaanderen.be/epibul/index_archief.htm - bulletin 2000/4).
• Antibiotics and malaria prophylaxis available only on prescription.

Table 5.3.1 Statutory notification systems (Belgium)

Legal framework	Ministry of Health for each community is responsible for introducing changes in the statutory notification system.
Levels of responsibility	At *Federal level* the Ministry for Public Health is responsible for, e.g • inspection of drugs and food products and • control of imported diseases. Governments at *Community level* are responsible for, e.g • prevention and • social and environmental-hygienic aspects of health. The administration of these Community governments has a 'health inspector' per province in charge of surveillance and control of infectious diseases. The tasks are • registration of notified cases of infectious diseases, • co-ordination and follow up of control measures, • investigation and follow up of outbreaks and • vaccination policy and its implementation.
Notifiable diseases	About 40 diseases are notifiable in the three communities and case definitions are in use for each of them. No financial incentives are given for notifying physicians or laboratories in Belgium.
Case definitions	Since 2003, the European case definitions are in use in all the three communities (decision 2002/253/EC).
Levels of reporting	*Local level for reporting*: Usually at the level of the province with an average population size of 900,000 (250,000–1,600,000).
Time to inform national level	Regional level: 24–48 hours, depending on the specific disease. National level is involved only in certain cases (see below).
Public health action	The responsibility for case management is held by the treating physician. Control measures including contact tracing and outbreak investigation is generally the responsibility of the Community Health Inspection. In certain cases (e.g. food-related outbreaks, bioterrorism, health problem of international dimension), the federal (national) authority is involved.
Data dissemination	In Flanders, data are compiled and a monthly summary sheet is sent to the notifying physicians and laboratories and a number of other institutions. In addition, a quarterly epidemiological bulletin, the *Epidemiologisch Bulletin van de Vlaamse Gemeenschap,* is published (http://www.wvc.vlaanderen.be/epibul/). It contains tables with notification data. In addition an annual report is disseminated. At the Scientific Institute of Public Health, the data from sentinel and reference laboratories are accessible via internet (http://www.iph.fgov.be/epidemio/epien/index8.htm).

Flemish Communities

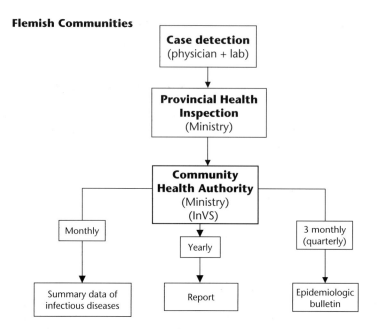

French community (including data from the German community)

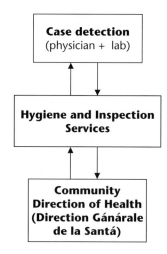

Fig. 5.3.1 Flow chart of statutory notification (Belgium).

5.4 Cyprus

Contacts

• Ministry of Health – http://www.moh.gov. cy.
• Network for Surveillance of Communicable Diseases – cycomnet@cytanet.com.cy.

Statutory notification systems

The details regarding statutory notification systems are given in Table 5.4.1.

Flow chart of statutory notification

See Figure 5.4.1.

Prevention/prophylaxis

Vaccination coverage (Survey 2003): fully immunised for DTP + OPV = 97.5%; DTP + OPV + MMR = 85.6%

Table 5.4.1 Statutory notification systems (Cyprus)

Legal framework	According to the Quarantine (Public Health) Law and Regulations and its amendments, the Medical and Public Health Services of the Ministry of Health of Cyprus is the competent authority. The Director of Medical and Public Health Services is the person responsible for the implementation of all necessary measures related to the prevention and control of communicable diseases.
Levels of responsibility	
Local responsibility for reporting	All registered medical practitioners
Local responsibility for action	District medical officers/district health inspectors
Headquarters Medical and Public Health Services, Ministry of Health	Network unit for surveillance and control of communicable diseases
Notifiable diseases	43 communicable diseases are notifiable: 11 to be notified within 24 hours
Case definitions	Case definitions recommended by the EU (which categorise cases as probable, possible or confirmed) are used for all diseases.
Levels of reporting	Reporting at the local level (District Medical Officer) that forwards the information to the Medical and Public Health Services. For those diseases notified within 24 hours simultaneous reporting locally and directly to the Medical and Public Health Services. Districts: 5, population size range(40,100–289,100) Population: 730400 inhabitants (Government controlled area 2003)
Estimated time to inform national level	24-hour notification system to the central level for 11diseases. For the rest in general less than a week.
Public health action	The notifier holds the responsibility for case management. Control measures including contact tracing and outbreak investigation is generally the responsibility of the District Medical Officer and his team, supported by the Medical and Public Health Services, at the central level.
Data dissemination	The system will provide feedback through a six monthly newsletter and will inform countries in the EU of communicable disease developments in Cyprus.

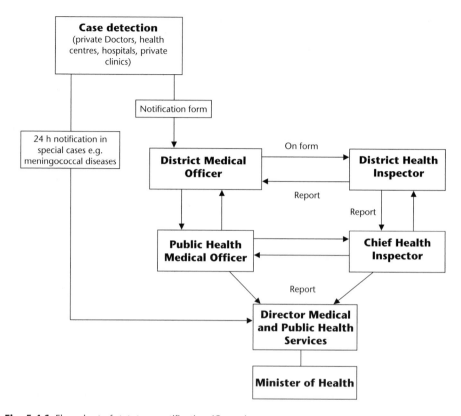

Fig. 5.4.1 Flow chart of statutory notification (Cyprus).

5.5 Czech Republic

Contacts

• Ministry of Health of the Czech Republic (MZd), http://www.mzcr.cz/.
• National Institute of Public Health (NIPH), http://www.szu.cz/
• Center for Epidemiology and Microbiology of NIPH, http://www.szu.cz/cem/hpcem.htm.

Statutory notification systems

The details regarding statutory notification systems are given in Table 5.5.1.

Flow chart of statutory notification

See Figure 5.5.1.

Outbreak detection and investigation

Various sources are used to detect possible outbreaks (physicians' notifications, laboratory reporting, telephone calls from the public). Notifications from physicians and laboratory reports are sent to the DRIPH. When appropriate, the DRIPH sends a notification form to the Center for Epidemiology and Microbiology of NIPH (administrative action). When necessary, they provide consultations. Directors of all health care facilities are required by law to notify unusually high occurrence or severity. The Regional Institutes of Public Health

Table 5.5.1 Statutory notification systems (Czech Republic)

Legal framework	The Ministry of Health is responsible for changes in the statutory notification system (Act. No.: 258/2000).
Levels of responsibility	Under the MOH, all public health services (central governmental and regions) are centralised. The Public Health Service is responsible for the collection and processing of notifiable disease data. The National Institute of Public Health in Prague carries the main responsibility for this activity and coordinates the reporting system (EPIDAT) of notifiable diseases at the national level. Regional Institutes of Public Health and Detached Regional Institutes of Public Health (DRIPH) form links between the top and basic levels of Public Health Service. Data on the occurrence of notifiable diseases are reported by the DRIPH service to the Regional Public Health Service, which in turn is forwarded to the National Institute of Public Health.
Local responsibility for reporting	Physicians, laboratories and DRIPH service.
Local responsibility for action	DRIPH service.
National surveillance	National Institute of Public Health (SZU).
Notifiable diseases	Classical infectious diseases ($n = 36$), TB, STD, ARI and influenza (reporting to EISS). No financial incentive is given to physicians to notify.
Case definitions	In use for all notifiable diseases.
Levels of reporting	10,246,178 (2004) inhabitants.
Estimated time to inform national level	In general less than a week.
Public health action	The responsibility for case management is held by the notifier. Control measures including contact tracing and outbreak investigation is generally the responsibility of the Public Health Service, primarily at regional level with detached workplace with support from national level in some cases.
Data dissemination	An epidemiological bulletin, the *Zprávy CEM*, is published at national level every 4 weeks (http://www.szu.cz/cem/hpcem.htm; select "Zpravy CEM"). Feedback of data, updated monthly, is given via Internet (http://www.szu.cz/cem/hpcem.htm; select EPIDAT). Also a 'Weekly Communicable Diseases Monitor' is released regularly. The 'Monitor' is provided to all participating institutes of Public Health Service and to the MoH (available in printed or computerised format). A monthly and yearly analysis is regularly produced and provided to human and veterinary health authorities.

co-ordinate investigations and inform decision makers. The national outbreak management team recommends the most appropriate interventions.

- Vaccination coverage: 97% for all vaccinations.
- Antibiotics and malaria prophylaxis available only on prescription.

Prevention/prophylaxis

- Vaccine programme: BCG, DTPa-IPV, Hib, MMR, HBV.

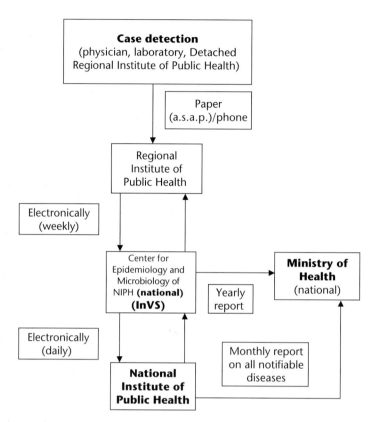

Fig. 5.5.1 Flow chart of statutory notification (Czech Republic).

5.6 Denmark

Contacts

• Sundhedsstyrelsen (SST) – National Board of Health – http://www.sst.dk.
• Department of Epidemiology, Statens Serum Institute (SSI) – http://www.ssi.dk.

Statutory notification systems

The details regarding statutory notification systems are given in Table 5.6.1.

Flow chart of statutory notification

See Figure 5.6.1.

Outbreak detection and investigation

Physicians are required by law to report any abnormal event or outbreak of any disease immediately by phone to the local health department. They also have to notify to the national level (SSI) by mail using a written form. Local and national reference laboratories also detect and report outbreaks. The local health authorities have the responsibility for outbreak control at regional/local level. The SSI has the national responsibility as a reference

Table 5.6.1 Statutory notification systems (Denmark)

Legal framework	The National Board of Health and the Ministry of Health have the responsibility for modifications.
Levels of responsibility	
Local responsibility for reporting	All physicians are obliged by law to notify all cases who fulfil the criteria for notifiable diseases.
Local responsibility for ACTION	Medical Officers of Health at departmental level.
National surveillance	SSI
Notifiable diseases	33 diseases are notifiable on person identifiable basis; 4 diseases are notifiable on an anonymous basis. No financial incentives are given to physicians to notify. Laboratories report 5 diseases to SSI as well as the number of positive and negative HIV-test results. All blood banks report screening results of blood donors for virological markers.
Case definitions	In use for all notifiable diseases.
Levels of reporting	Local level for reporting: 15 departments with an average population size of 350,000 (45,000–625,000). National population: 5.3 million inhabitants.
Estimated time to inform national level	Vary for different diseases. Considerable time delays occur; range from 2 days to several weeks for national level between diagnosis and receipt at national level.
Public health action	The responsibility for case management is held by the notifier. Control measures including contact tracing and outbreak investigation is the responsibility of the local health department, with support from national level (SSI).
Data dissemination	An epidemiological bulletin, the *Epi-Nyt (Epi-news),* is published weekly at national level (http://www.ssi.dk). Data for notifiable diseases are published quarterly/yearly. On local level feedback is given in yearly reports.

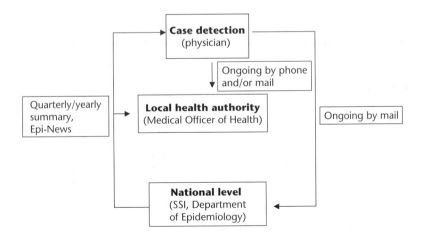

Fig. 5.6.1 Flow chart of statutory notification (Denmark).

centre for surveillance and will be involved in outbreak investigation/control on request. SSI has a microbiologist on duty 24 hours/day.

Prevention/prophylaxis

• Vaccination programme: DTPa-IPV, HIB, MMR.
• Vaccination coverage: ~85% for MMR vaccinations.
• Antibiotics and malaria prophylaxis available only on prescription.

5.7 Estonia

Contacts

• Ministry of Social Affairs (MoSA) – Sotsiaalministeerium (SM) – http://www.sm.ee/.

• Health Protection Inspectorate (HPI) – Tervisekaitseinspektsioon (TKI) – http://www.tervisekaitse.ee/.
• State Statistical Board (Statistikaamet), http://www.stat.ee/.

Statutory notification systems

The details regarding statutory notification systems are given in Table 5.7.1.

Flow chart of statutory notification

See Figure 5.7.1.

Outbreak detection and investigation

A variety of information sources are used to detect possible outbreaks. The information

Table 5.7.1 Statutory notification systems (Estonia)

Legal framework	'Communicable Diseases Prevention and Control Act' The MoSA is responsible for changes in the statutory notification system and legislation.
Levels of responsibility	
Local responsibility for reporting	Physicians and laboratories.
Local responsibility for action	County HPI (Tervisekaitsetalituse osakond) in co-operation with physicians and hospitals.
National surveillance	HPI in co-operation with 15 County Health Protection Offices.
Notifiable diseases	Four groups, which differ by disease-related events and differing amount of data to be notified within different time intervals. No financial incentives are given for notifying physicians and laboratories.
Case definitions	These are developed for most diseases.
Levels of reporting	The country is divided into 15 counties, each with a County Health Protection Office. Average population size covered by an office is 90,400 (10,300–520,000). Total Estonian population is 1,356,045.
Estimated time of outbreak report to inform national level	24 hours
Public health action	The responsibility for case management is held by the physicians (including contact tracing). The main responsibilities of HPI and local epidemiologists are surveillance of CD, management of specific surveillance programmes (polio, measles elimination, tularaemia, diphtheria, TBE), outbreak management, early warning and response and collaboration with EU CD networks.
Data dissemination	An epidemiological bulletin by HPI *EstEpi Report* is published monthly and is available at http://www.tervisekaitse.ee/.

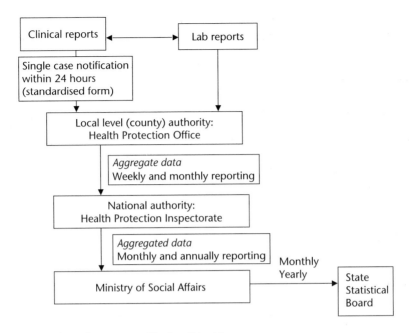

Fig. 5.7.1 Flow chart of statutory notification (Estonia).

is forwarded to Local County Health Protection Office (LCHPO) (Tervisekaitsetalituse osakond), responsible for investigation and public health action at local level. The LCHPO reports to the HPI and is responsible for outbreak detection and management at national level.

Prevention/prophylaxis

• Recommended vaccinations (94–99% infants immunised in 2003): HBV, BCG, DTP, MMR, OPV, DT.
• Antibiotics and malaria prophylaxis available only on prescription.

5.8 Finland

Contacts

• Kansanterveyslaitos (KTL) – National Public Health Institute – http://www.ktl.fi

• Elintarvikevirasto – National Food Agency – http://www.elintarvikevirasto.fi/
• Eläinlääkintä-ja elintarvikelaitos (EELA) – National Veterinary and Food Research Institute – http://www.eela.fi
• National Infectious Disease Register (NIDR) – www.ktl.fi/ttr

Statutory notification systems

The details regarding statutory notification systems are given in Table 5.8.1.

Flow chart of statutory notification

See Figure 5.8.1.

Outbreak detection and investigation

In outbreak situations local health authorities are primarily responsible for situation analysis

Table 5.8.1 Statutory notification systems (Finland)

Legal framework	The law and act of communicable diseases (1986, last amendment 2003) regulates surveillance and control of infectious diseases. Ministry of Health is responsible for introducing changes in the statutory notification system.
Levels of responsibility	
Local responsibility for reporting and action	Physicians are responsible for detection and notification of cases and for necessary action to stop spread. They are assisted by infectious disease specialists and microbiologists. Laboratories report directly to NIDR about diseases and other microbes specified to be registered. In addition, laboratories send microbes to a national strain collection. Municipal health authorities are in primary charge of control measures.
National surveillance	KTL
Notifiable diseases	79 diseases are notifiable. They are classified into three categories. Two complementary components form the data collection. For some diseases both the physician and the laboratory must report the case, for others only laboratory reports are collected (more than half of all infections). During routine reporting, laboratories remind clinics about the duty of the treating physician to notify any notifiable infectious diseases. The information is entered into the NIDR and duplicate notifications are merged. Data from individual cases are linked by the unique personal identifying number. There are no financial incentives for notifying physicians.
Case definitions	Are in use for all notifiable diseases
Levels of reporting	452 local health units (average population size of 11,000) and 21 regions (average population size of 240,000).
Estimated time to inform national level	Laboratory notifications are sent directly to the national level at KTL with an average of 5 working days from sampling date. Physician notifications are sent through the regional level to the national level, in approximately 2 weeks.
Public health action	Responsibility for case management is held by the notifier. Control measures including contact tracing and outbreak investigation are generally the responsibility of the Public Health Service, primarily at local level with support from national level.
Data dissemination	All registry data are compiled and arranged at KTL and accessible through encrypted www-communication to health authorities in charge at district and municipal levels. A weekly updated www-version is available for the public and includes comments and epidemiological observations. The data format allows compilations of tables, trend analysis, etc., by the user. Actual figures and summary comments are also routinely reported in the monthly bulletin, the *Kansanterveys-lehti*. In addition, annual reports are published.

and action. In cases where several municipalities are involved, the hospital district specialist and/or the provincial veterinary and food authorities act as co-ordinator and consultant. KTL is involved in wider outbreaks and provides co-ordination and expert help. It has built up its capacity for rapid response.

Prevention/prophylaxis

- Vaccine programme: For 0–24 months BCG, DTaP-IPV-Hib, MMR.
- Vaccination coverage: ~93% for all vaccinations by the age of 24 months.
- Antibiotics and malaria prophylaxis available only on prescription.

Flow of data and information in the National Infectious Disease Register (NIDR)

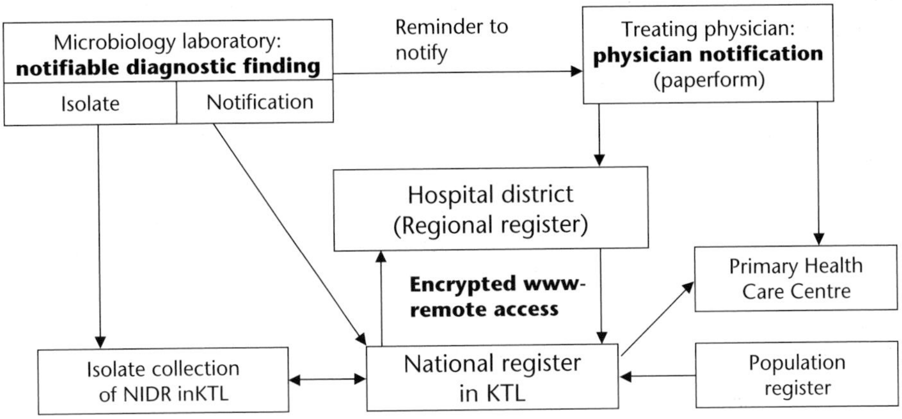

Fig. 5.8.1 Flow chart of statutory notification (Finland).

5.9 France

Contacts

• Direction Générale de la Santé (DGS) – Directorate of Health belonging to the Ministry of Health – http://www.sante.gouv.fr.

• Institut de Veille Sanitaire (InVS) – National Public Health Center – http://www.invs.sante.fr.

Mandatory notification system

The details regarding mandatory notification systems are given in Table 5.9.1.

Table 5.9.1 Mandatory notification system (France)

Legal framework	Ministry of Health is responsible for introducing changes in the mandatory notification system.
Levels of responsibility	
Local responsibility for notification	All physicians, biologists and hospitals are obliged by law to notify all cases that fulfil the criteria for mandatory notifiable diseases.
Local responsibility for action	Local Health Departments (DDASS) are responsible for public Health action.
National surveillance	Ministry of Health is responsible for introducing modifications in the notification system. InVS and DGS are involved in managing surveillance at national level.
Notifiable diseases	For 26 diseases, notification is mandatory. Individual cases are anonymously notified to the DDASS with the use of standardised forms. No financial incentive is given to notifiers. According to the disease, a case detection may lead to two levels of action. All the diseases, except for HIV/AIDS, acute hepatitis B and tetanus, have to be reported in emergency and then notified for immediate action.
Case definitions	In use for all mandatory notifiable diseases.
Levels of reporting	Local level for reporting: 100 DDASS, with an average population size of 570,000 (75,000–2,500,000). National population: 61 million inhabitants.

Continued on p. 348

Table 5.9.1 *Continued*

Estimated time to inform national level	Between 1 and 5 days, for local and national level and according to the diseases.
Public health action	The responsibility for case management is held by the notifier. Control measures including outbreak investigation is generally the responsibility of the Public Health Services, primarily on local level with support from regional and national level. InVS performs trend analysis and outbreak detection based on the surveillance data. A computerised alert system is used (http://www.invs.sante.fr).
Communication	A weekly epidemiological bulletin, the *Bulletin Épidemiologique Hebdomadaire*, is published at national level (http://www.invs.sante.fr) by the Direction Générale de la Santé. In addition annual reports are provided (http://www.invs.sante.fr).

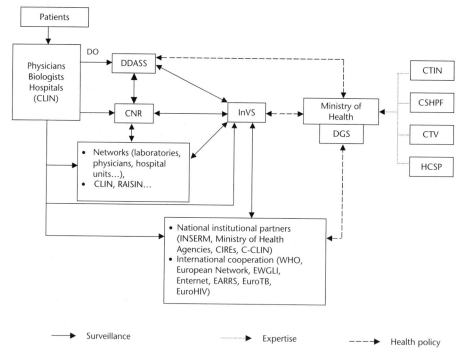

CIRE = Inter-Regional Epidemiology Unit; CLIN = Nosocomial Infections Control Committee; C-CLIN = Coordination Center for Nosocomial Infections Control; CNR = National Reference Center; CSHPF = French Council for Public Health; CTIN = Technical Committee for Nosocomial Infections; CTV = Technical Committee Vaccinations; DDASS = Local Health Departments; DGS = Directorate of Health; DO = Mandatory Notification; EARRS = European Antimicrobial Resistance Surveillance System; EnterNet = International Surveillance Network for Enteric infections due to *Salmonella* et VTEC O157; EuroTB = European Surveillance Programme for Tuberculosis; EuroHIV = European Surveillance Programme for HIV/AIDS; EWGLI = European working group on Legionella infection; HCSP = High Committee of Public Health; InVS = Institut de veille sanitaire; WHO = World Health Organisation; RAISIN = Alert, Investigation and Surveillance Network for Nosocomial Infections.

Fig. 5.9.1 Flow chart of notification system for infectious diseases (France).

Flow chart of French notification system for infectious diseases

See Figure 5.9.1.

Non-statutory surveillance systems (NSSS)

There are a number of national NSSS. In addition the European networks for HIV/Aids surveillance, Euro-TB and Eurosurveillance are located in France. Information concerning these can be obtained from InVS (http://www.invs.sante.fr).

Outbreak investigation

Any health professional should inform the local health authority (DDASS) of any abnormal health event or outbreak of any disease. The local health authority is responsible for investigation and control. The DDASS can respond by asking the help of regional (CIREs) or national level (InVS) in order to investigate. Control of the outbreak is the responsibility of the DDASS and the Ministry of Health. Depending on the disease involved in the outbreak (e.g. food-borne outbreaks) the

Ministries of Agriculture, Finance, Consumers or others can be involved.

Reference: D.Che, J.C. Desenclos. L'alerte dans la surveillance actuelle des maladies infectieuses. *Med Mal Inf* 2002; **32**, 704–716.

5.10 Germany

Contacts

• Bundesministerium für Gesundheit und Soziale Sicherung (BMGS) – Federal Ministry for Health – http://www.bmgs.bund.de.
• Robert Koch Institute (RKI) – Federal Institute of Communicable and Non-Communicable Diseases – http://www.rki.de.

Statutory notification systems

The details regarding statutory notification systems are given in Table 5.10.1.

Flow chart of statutory notification

See Figure 5.10.1.

Table 5.10.1 Statutory notification systems (Germany)

Legal framework	The Ministry of Health is responsible for introducing changes in the statutory notification system. New legislation was enforced in 2001.
Levels of responsibility	
Local responsibility for reporting	Physicians and medical microbiology laboratories are obliged to report notifiable diseases.
Local responsibility for action	Local health departments (Gesundheitsämter) in co-operation with physicians and hospitals.
National surveillance	RKI in co-operation with the 16 states as in the federal system of Germany, the responsibility for health is at state level.
Notifiable diseases	47 diseases/infections are notified including identifiers of the patient. Six other diseases/infections are notified without personal identifiers. No financial incentives are given for notifying physicians.
Case definitions	For all diseases case definitions are in use.
Levels of reporting	The country is divided into 439 districts, each with a local health department. The average population size is 186,000 (20,000–3,500,000). These districts belong to regions that form 16 states with an average population size of 5,100,000 inhabitants (700,000–18,000,000).

Continued on p. 350

Table 5.10.1 *Continued*

Estimated time to inform national level	Up to 7 days for regional level and 14 days for national level.
Public health action	The responsibility for case management is held by the notifier. Control measures including contact tracing and outbreak investigation are generally the responsibility of the Public Health Service, primarily on local level with support from state and national level.
Data dissemination	A weekly epidemiological bulletin, the *Epidemiologisches Bulletin* (http://www.rki.de/INFEKT/EPIBULL/EPI.HTM) and an annual report is published at national level (http://www.rki.de/INFEKT/IFSG/JAHRBUCH-2003.PDF). The data can also be accessed and used via an internet application (http://www3.rki.de/SurvStat). In addition, regular feedback is given by institutions on regional and state level.

Outbreak detection and investigation

A variety of information sources are used to detect possible outbreaks. The information is forwarded to local health departments (Gesundheitsamt), which are responsible for investigation and for public health action at the local level. The Gesundheitsamt reports to the State Health Department, which is responsible for outbreak detection and management at the regional level. The State Health Department reports to the RKI, which has the national responsibility for outbreak control.

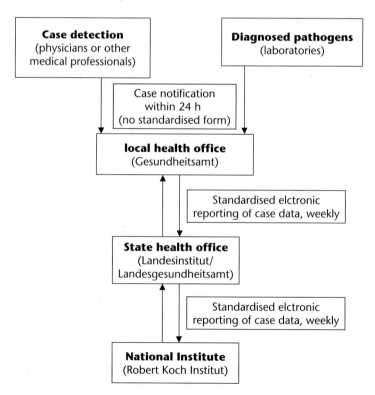

Fig. 5.10.1 Flow chart of statutory notification (Germany).

Prevention/prophylaxis

• Recommended vaccinations: DTPa, MMR, Hib, IPV, HBV, Varicella.
• Vaccination coverage: ~85%.
• Antibiotics and malaria prophylaxis available only on prescription.

5.11 Greece

Contacts

• Ministry of Health and Welfare, http://www.minagric.gr/greek/index.shtml.
• National Centre for Surveillance and Intervention, http://www.keel.org.gr.

Statutory notification systems

The details regarding statutory notification systems are given in Table 5.11.1.

Flow chart of statutory notification

See Figure 5.11.1.

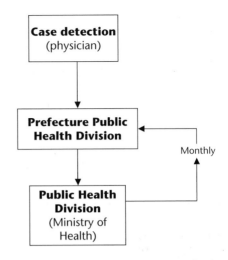

Fig. 5.11.1 Flow chart of statutory notification (Greece).

Outbreak detection and investigation

Physicians notify cases to the prefecture public health division, which is responsible for case investigation. Monthly aggregate data is sent to the Ministry of Health. Here a monthly report is generated and disseminated as feedback. The National Centre for Surveillance and Intervention was established in 1997. It aims to

Table 5.11.1 Statutory notification systems (Greece)

Legal framework	Ministry of Health is responsible for introducing changes in the statutory notification system.
Notifiable diseases	29 diseases are notifiable. No financial incentive is given to physicians to notify.
Case definitions	In use for acute polio and AIDS.
Levels of reporting	54 local health units with an average population size of 200,000 and 13 regions with an average population size of 800,000.
Estimated time to inform national level	1 week.
Public health action	The responsibility for case management is held by the notifier. Control measures including contact tracing and outbreak investigation are generally the responsibility of the Public Health Service, primarily on local level with support from national level
Data dissemination	A monthly report is published.

computerise the notification system and transmission of data. Here data is analysed to detect and investigate outbreaks.

Prevention/prophylaxis

• Vaccine programme: DTP, MMR, Men C in case of outbreak, HBV.
• Antibiotics and malaria prophylaxis available only on prescription.

5.12 Hungary

Contacts

Országos Epidemiológiai Központ (Hungarian National Centre for Epidemiology, NCE), http://www.antsz.hu/oek.

Statutory notification systems

The details regarding statutory notification systems are given in Table 5.12.1.

Table 5.11.2 Statutory notification systems (Hungary)

Legal framework	The reporting system of communicable diseases is regulated by Decree No 63/1997 (XII.21) of the Minister of Welfare (based on the authorisation by Act 47 of 1997).
Levels of responsibility	
Local responsibility for reporting	Communicable diseases, even the suspicion of the disease, are reported by health service providers to the local level of the National Public Health and Medical Officers' Service. The report is sent by mail on paper forms. The reported data are forwarded electronically to the county institutes and from the county institutes to the National Centre for Epidemiology.
Local responsibility for action	Healthcare providers
National surveillance	The National Centre for Epidemiology provides the scientific background (including research and training) for the surveillance of communicable diseases.
Notifiable diseases	For 69 diseases mandatory notification with personal identifying data and for 13 diseases mandatory notification without identifying data is required.
Case definitions	A national surveillance manual (1998) provides clinical definitions, laboratory criteria for diagnosis and case definitions. The implementation of EU case definitions and the amending of the surveillance manual are in progress.
Levels of reporting	The basis of the institutional network is the National Public Health and Medical Officers' Service (NPHMOS). The system of the NPHMOS relies on an institutional network, covering the entire country; 136 municipal institutes are the principal enforcement authorities.
Estimated time to inform national level	24 hours to 1 week.
Public health action	The case management is held by notifying doctors, hospitals and health care providers. Control measures including contact tracing and outbreak investigations are generally the responsibility of municipal and regional institutes, with support of the National Centre for Epidemiology.
Data dissemination	The National Centre for Epidemiology provides a weekly printed epidemiological bulletin (EPINFO), a weekly electronic bulletin, regularly printed special editions of the epidemiological bulletin, and guidelines.

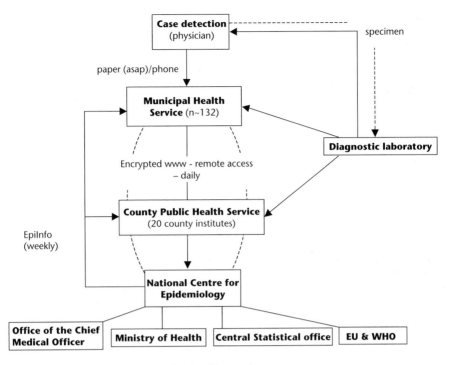

Fig. 5.12.1 Flow chart of statutory notification (Hungary).

Flow chart of statutory notification

See Figure 5.12.1.

Flow chart of statutory notification

See Figure 5.13.1.

5.13 Ireland

Contacts

• An Roinn Sláinte agus Leanaí – Department of Health and Children – http://www.doh.ie.
• National Disease Surveillance Centre (NDSC), http://www.ndsc.ie.

Statutory notification systems

The details regarding statutory notification systems are given in Table 5.13.1.

Outbreak detection and investigation

The NDSC has the responsibilities regarding national outbreak control, liasing with laboratories and the Food Safety Authority.

Prevention/prophylaxis

• Vaccine programme: DTP, MMR, Hib, Men C.
• Vaccination coverage: uptake at 12 months of 78–79% for all vaccinations in 2002.
• Antibiotics and malaria prophylaxis available only on prescription.

Table 5.13.1 Statutory notification systems (Ireland)

Legal framework	On 1st July 2000, the Infectious Diseases (Amendment) Regulations, 2000 (S.I. No 151 of 2000) came into force, which were revised in 2003 (S.I. No. 707 of 2003). The Ministry of Health is responsible for introducing changes in the statutory notification system.
Levels of responsibility	
Local responsibility for reporting	As soon as a medical practitioner becomes aware of or suspects that a person on whom he/she is in professional attendance is suffering from or is the carrier of an infectious disease, or a clinical director of a diagnostic laboratory as soon as an infectious disease is identified in that laboratory, he is required to transmit a written or electronic notification to a Medical Officer of Health.
Local responsibility for action	Coordinated through the regional health boards.
National surveillance	The NDSC is responsible for the collation and analysis of weekly notifications of infectious diseases.
Notifiable diseases	68 diseases are notifiable. €2.00 is given to physicians as financial incentive to notify.
Case definitions	In use for all notifiable diseases.
Levels of reporting	8 Regional Health Boards with an average population size of 250,000.
Estimated time to inform national level	10 days for regional level and 17 days for national level.
Public health action	The responsibility for case management is held by the notifier. Control measures including contact tracing and outbreak investigation is generally the responsibility of the Public Health Service, primarily at local level with support from national level.
Data dissemination	NDSC provides, on a weekly basis, figures available on notifiable infectious diseases at national level by health board region (http://www.ndsc.ie/IDStatistics/WeeklyIDReport/). In addition the *EPI-INSIGHT*, a monthly report on infectious disease in Ireland (http://www.ndsc.ie/Publications/EPI-Insight/) and an annual report is published.

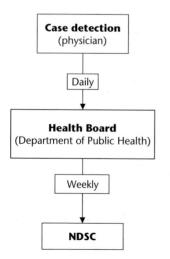

Fig. 5.13.1 Flow chart of statutory notification (Ireland).

5.14 Italy

Contacts

- Ministry of Health, http://www.sanita.it.
- Instituto Superiore di Sanità (ISS) – National Institute of Health – http://www.iss.it.

Statutory notification systems

The details regarding statutory notification systems are given in Table 5.14.1.

Flow chart of statutory notification

See Figure 5.14.1.

Table 5.14.1 Statutory notification systems (Italy)

Legal framework	Ministry of Health is responsible for introducing changes in the statutory notification system, which is defined by law.
Levels of responsibility	
Local responsibility for reporting	All physicians are obliged by law to notify all cases that fulfil the criteria for notifiable diseases.
Local responsibility for action	The local health units (USL) are responsible for public health action.
National surveillance	The ISS is responsible for managing surveillance at national level.
Notifiable diseases	48 diseases are notifiable. These are divided into 5 classes, which differ by flow of information and by the degree of ascertainment requested. For each class a specific form exists. No financial incentive is given to physicians to notify.
Case definitions	In use for most notifiable diseases.
Levels of reporting	228 USLs with an average population size of 250,000 and 20 regions with an average population size of 2,850,000.
Estimated time to inform national level	7 days for local level, 40 days for regional level and 90 days for national level.
Public health action	The responsibility for case management is held by the notifier. Control measures including contact tracing and outbreak investigation is generally the responsibility of the Public Health Service, primarily at local level with support from national level.
Data dissemination	An epidemiological bulletin, the *Bollettino epidemiologico*, is published by the Ministry of Health at national level every 6 months on paper.

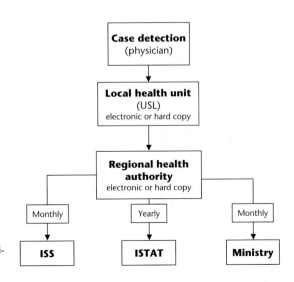

Fig. 5.14.1 Flow chart of statutory notification (Italy).

Outbreak detection and investigation

Unusual events are reported informally to the ID Unit at regional and national level by telephone calls. Outbreak investigations are mainly performed by local health departments. ISS performs field investigations only upon request of the Ministry of Health or the regional authority.

Prevention/prophylaxis

- Vaccine programme: DTP, IPV/OPV, MMR.
- Vaccination coverage: ~60% for MMR and >95% for DTP vaccinations.
- Antibiotics and malaria prophylaxis available only on prescription.

5.15 Latvia

Contacts

State Public Health Agency (PHA), http://www.sva.lv.

Case notification

The details regarding case notification are given in Table 5.15.1.

Flowchart of case notification data

See Figure 5.15.1.

Table 5.15.1 Case notification (Latvia)

Legal framework	Law on Epidemiological Safety (1997); Procedure of Notification of Infectious Diseases (Regulations of the Cabinet of Ministers, 1999); Procedure of epidemiological surveillance of infectious diseases (Order of the Ministry of Welfare, 2001).
Levels of responsibility	
Local responsibility for reporting and action	Physicians in public and private healthcare sectors.
Surveillance institutions	State Public Health Agency including local branches, State Centre of Sexually Transmitted and Dermal Diseases, AIDS Prevention Centre and the State Centre of Tuberculosis and Lung Diseases.
Notifiable diseases	By law physicians are obliged to report two groups of 99 notifiable diseases: • Individually (every single case) notified and registered infectious diseases and conditions; • Summary notified and registered cases (influenza and other acute respiratory infections, enterobiasis).
Case definitions	Guidelines with case definitions are available for several diseases. Elaboration of case definitions is in the process.
Levels of reporting	The territory of Latvia is divided into 27 districts. The population in districts varies from 26,020 (eastern part) to 892,418 inhabitants (central part). PHA branches (10) or subbranches (17) from each district collect the regional information to be processed by the central PHA office.

Table 5.15.1 *Continued*

Notification time	72 hours for TB, STD, skin diseases, HIV and AIDS; weekly for influenza, ARI and pneumonia during influenza epidemic season from 100 sentinel sites; monthly for enteritis, influenza and other ARI.
Public health action	Physicians are responsible for case management. Epidemiologists of PHA branches organise preventive and control measures and perform case investigations (outbreaks).
Dissemination of information	The *Epidemiological Bulletin* is disseminated regularly (weekly/monthly) by e-mail and mail to ministries, institutions and media and is available at http://www.sva.lv.

Outbreak investigation and health emergencies

A variety of information sources are used to detect possible outbreaks. Information received by PHA branches from different sources is forwarded to PHA and Centre of Emergency and Disaster Medicine. The PHA is responsible for the outbreak control.

Prevention

- Recommended childhood vaccinations: DTPa, MMR, Hib, IPV, HBV, BCG.
- Recommended vaccination for adults: DT.
- Vaccination coverage in children: 89–99.5% for MMR vaccinations.
- Antibiotics and malaria prophylaxis available only on prescription.

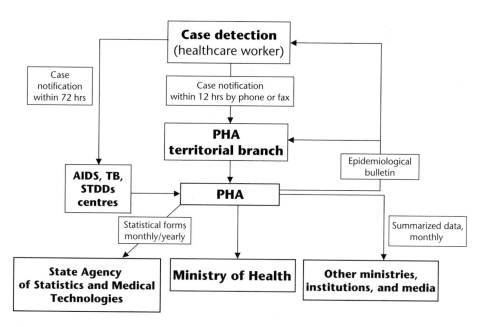

Fig. 5.15.1 Flow chart of case notification (Latvia).

Table 5.16.1 Statutory notification systems (Lithuania)

Notifiable diseases	84 communicable diseases are notifiable.
Levels of reporting	36 district public health institutions and 11 regional public health centres report for a population of 3,592,600 (2003) inhabitants.
Estimated time to inform national level	Primary healthcare institutions report every suspected case to regional public health centres within 12 hours.
Public health action	Physicians and laboratories report by phone or fax their district public health centre. These then report to the regional public health centre. District and regional public health centres investigate outbreaks. For food-borne outbreaks, food and veterinary services are also involved. The CCDPC supports systematic outbreak investigations and informs Media, the State Public Health services and the MoH.
Data dissemination	Monthly and annual communicable diseases report forms are completed by every regional public health centre and sent to the CCDPC.

5.16 Lithuania

Contact

Centre for Communicable Diseases Prevention and Control (CCDPC), http://www.vvspt.lt/.

Statutory notification systems

The details regarding statutory notification systems are given in Table 5.16.1.

Flow chart of statutory notification

See Figure 5.16.1.

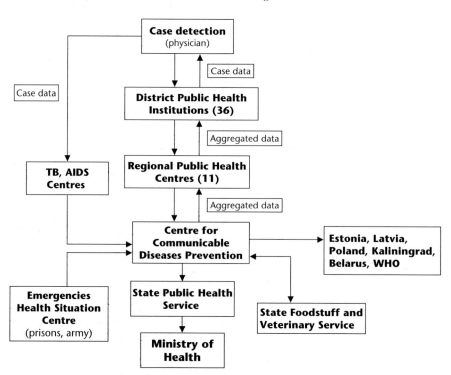

Fig. 5.16.1 Flow chart of statutory notification (Lithuania).

Prevention/prophylaxis

CCDPC organises the National Immunopro-phylaxis Programme and provides health institutions with vaccines and syringes.

The most significant communicable disease problems are food – and water-borne disease outbreaks. There is a high number of tick-borne disease cases (tick-borne encephalitis). There is a high prevalence of rabies in wild animals and thus there is a threat of rabies to humans.

5.17 Luxembourg

Contact

Direction de la Santé, http://www.sante.lu.

Statutory notification systems

The details regarding statutory notification systems are given in Table 5.17.1.

Flow chart of statutory notification

See Figure 5.17.1.

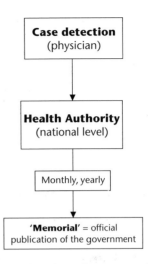

Fig. 5.17.1 Flow chart of statutory notification (Luxembourg).

Prevention/prophylaxis

- Vaccine programme: MMR, HBV, DTPa-IPV.
- Vaccination coverage: 98% for all vaccinations.
- Antibiotics and malaria prophylaxis available only on prescription.

Table 5.17.1 Statutory notification systems (Luxembourg)

Legal framework	Notification of communicable diseases is defined by law. This was last changed in 2004. The Ministry of Health (MoH) is responsible for introducing changes in the statutory notification system.
Notifiable diseases	The diseases that are notifiable are grouped in 8 classes. The list was revised in September 2004. €2.00 is given to physicians as financial incentive to notify.
Case definitions	The revised list includes no case definitions.
Levels of reporting	One level of reporting with 420,000 inhabitants.
Estimated time to inform national level	2 days.
Public health action	The notifier is responsible for case management. Control measures including contact tracing and outbreak investigation is the responsibility of the Public Health Service, a technical administration of the MoH.
Data dissemination	The *Memorial* is published by the MoH at national level every month with a yearly summary report.

Table 5.18.1 Statutory notification systems (Malta)

Legal framework	Prevention of Disease Ordinance; Public Health Act.
Notifiable diseases	67 specified communicable diseases are notifiable by law for all doctors in both public and private sectors. A supplementary system of reporting key infections also operates from the laboratories of the main state hospital and private medical diagnostic laboratories. The laboratories on the island detect infections at a primary level. For further investigations and confirmatory tests, clinical samples are occasionally carried out at reference laboratories overseas.
Case definitions	Definitions based on European case definitions are in use.
Levels of reporting	One level of reporting with 376,513 (1997) inhabitants.
Estimated time to inform national level	2 days.
Public health action	Reports of outbreaks are collected at the Department of Public Health. Outbreak control teams are set up centrally by the DSU to investigate and follow up outbreaks so that timely control measures can be taken.
Data dissemination	Reports on notified and confirmed cases are issued on a weekly and monthly basis (http://www.health.gov.mt/dph/dsuhome.htm

5.18 Malta

Contacts

• Ministry of Health, the Elderly and Community Care, http://www.health.gov.mt.
• Department of Public Health, Disease Surveillance Unit (DSU), http://www.health.gov.mt/dph/dsuhome.htm.

Statutory notification systems

The details regarding statutory notification systems are given in Table 5.18.1.

Flow chart of statutory notification

See Figure 5.18.1.

Prevention/prophylaxis

• Vaccine programme (coverage): MMR (90%), Hib (93%), HBV (70%), DTP (94%), OPV (94%).
• Antibiotics and malaria prophylaxis are available only on prescription.

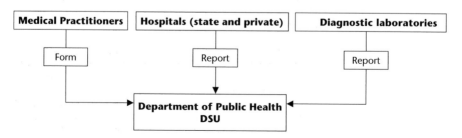

Fig. 5.18.1 Flow chart of statutory notification (Malta).

5.19 The Netherlands

Contacts

• Ministry of Health, Welfare and Sports (VWS), http://www.minvws.nl.
• National Institute for Public Health and the Environment (RIVM), http://www.rivm.nl.
• National Coordinating Centre for Communicable Disease Outbreak Management (LCI), http://www.infektieziekten.info.
• The Dutch Health Care Inspectorate (IGZ), http://www.igz.nl.

Statutory notification systems

The details regarding statutory notification systems are given in Table 5.19.1.

Flow chart of statutory notification

See Figure 5.19.1.

Non-statutory surveillance systems (NSSS)

There are a number of NSSS. Information concerning these can be obtained from RIVM.

Outbreak detection and investigation

Various sources are used to detect possible outbreaks (physicians' notifications, laboratory reporting, telephone calls from the public). Notifications from physicians and laboratory reports are sent to the Municipal Health Departments (GGD). When appropriate, the

Table 5.19.1 Statutory notification systems (The Netherlands)

Legal framework	Ministry of Health is responsible for changes in statutory notification; new legislation implemented 1999.
Levels of responsibility	
Local responsibility for reporting	Physicians, Laboratories, Municipal Health Services (GGD).
Local responsibility for action	Municipal Health Services (GGD).
National surveillance	RIVM.
Notifiable diseases	35 diseases are notifiable in three groups: Group A (Polio and SARS) cases to be notified immediately by the physician to the GGD if there is a suspected case; Group B (23 diseases) cases to be notified by the physician after diagnosis within 24 hours; for Group C (10 diseases) positive laboratory test results to be notified within 48 hours. No financial incentive is given to physicians to notify.
Case definitions	In use for all notifiable diseases.
Levels of reporting	Local level for reporting: Municipal Health Services (GGD) with an average population size of 369.070 (160.943–1.003.452). National population: 16.2 million inhabitants.
Estimated time to inform national level	In general less than a week.
Public health action	The responsibility for case management is held by the notifier. Control measures including contact tracing and outbreak investigation is generally the responsibility of the Public Health Service, primarily at local level with support from national level.
Data dissemination	An epidemiological bulletin, the *Infectieziekten Bulletin*, is published at national level every 4 weeks (http://www.rivm.nl/infectieziektenbulletin/). Feedback of data, which are updated daily, is given via Internet (http://www.rivm.nl/isis/).

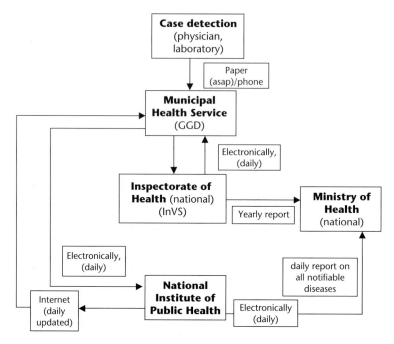

Fig. 5.19.1 Flow chart of statutory notification (The Netherlands).

GGD sends a notification form to the Health Inspectorate (administrative action). When necessary, the National Co-ordinating Centre for Communicable Disease Outbreak Management (LCI) is informed (consultation and assistance). Directors of all healthcare facilities are required by law to notify unusually high occurrence or severity. The LCI co-ordinates investigations, summons the outbreak management team and informs those individuals responsible for decision-making (under the responsibility of the Ministry of Health). The national outbreak management team recommends the most appropriate interventions.

Prevention/prophylaxis

• Vaccine programme: DTPa-IPV, MMR, Men C, Hib, HBV for risk groups (children whose parents are from endemic areas).
• Vaccination coverage: 95% for all vaccinations.
• Antibiotics and malaria prophylaxis available only on prescription.

5.20 Norway

Contacts

• Ministry of Health (Helsedepartmentet), http://odin.dep.no/hd/.
• Norwegian Institute of Public Health, http://www.fhi.no.
• Directorate for Health and Social Affairs, http://www.shdir.no.

Statutory notification systems

The details regarding statutory notification systems are given in Table 5.20.1.

Flow chart of statutory notification

See Figure 5.20.1.

Table 5.20.1 Statutory notification systems (Norway)

Legal framework	Notification is based on the Communicable Diseases Control Act from 1995 and Health Register Act from 2002. The Ministry of Health is responsible for introducing changes in the statutory notification system.
Levels of responsibility	
Local responsibility for reporting	Physicians and medical microbiology laboratories are obliged to report notifiable disease.
Local responsibility for action	The Public Health Officer (head physician in the municipality) is responsible for infectious disease control.
National surveillance	Norwegian Institute of Public Health is responsible for managing the surveillance system.
Notifiable diseases	51 diseases are reported with full patient identification. HIV, gonorrhoea and syphilis are reported anonymously using non-unique identifier linking reports from clinicians and laboratories. There are no financial incentives for notifying physicians.
Case definitions	In use for all notifiable diseases.
Levels of reporting	432 local health units with an average population size of 10,000.
Estimated time to inform national level	3 days.
Public health action	The responsibility for case management (including contact tracing) is held by the notifier. Control measures including outbreak investigation are generally the responsibility of the Public Health Service, primarily at local level with support from national level.
Data dissemination	An epidemiological bulletin, the *MSIS-Rapport,* is published by the National Institute of Public Health at national level every week (http://www.fhi.no). Infectious disease statutory notification data are accessible on the Internet via http://www.fhi.no.

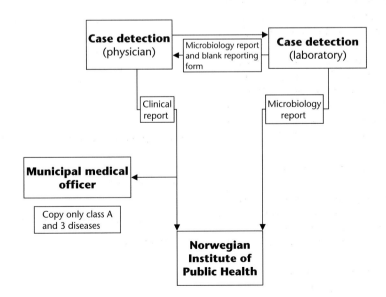

Fig. 5.20.1 Flow chart of statutory notification (Norway).

Outbreak detection and investigation

The main sources for information on outbreaks are an early warning system whereby doctors must report immediately to local, regional and central health authorities (Norwegian Institute of Public Health) on suspected or confirmed outbreaks. In addition, through the national notification system for infectious diseases (combined clinical and laboratory) outbreaks may be detected. The municipal medical officers have the legal responsibility for detection, investigation and public health actions within their municipality, in co-operation with other local authorities (e.g. food safety authorities). If more than one municipality is involved or if the outbreak is unusually severe, outbreak investigations and public health actions are done in close co-operation with the NIPH. On request, field epidemiologists from the NIPH will assist local health authorities.

Prevention/prophylaxis

• Vaccine programme: DTPa-IPV, HiB, MMR, BCG.
• Vaccination coverage: 90–95% for all vaccinations.
• Antibiotics and malaria prophylaxis available only on prescription.

5.21 Poland

Contacts

• The Ministry of Health, http://www.mz.gov.pl/.
• Chief Sanitary Inspectorate, www.gis.mz.gov.pl.
• National Institute of Hygiene (NIH), http://www.pzh.gov.pl/aindex.html.

Statutory notification systems

The details regarding statutory notification systems are given in Table 5.21.1.

Flow chart of statutory notification

See Figure 5.21.1.

Outbreak detection and investigation

A variety of information sources are used to detect possible outbreaks. The information is forwarded to district public health departments (PSSE), which are responsible for investigation and for public health action at the local level. PSSE report to the Province Public Health Department (WSSE), which is responsible for

Table 5.21.1 Statutory notification systems (Poland)

Legal framework	The Parliament and the Ministry of Health are responsible for introducing changes in the statutory notification system. New legislation is being developed.
Levels of responsibility	
Local responsibility for reporting	Physicians and laboratories.
Local responsibility for action	Sanitary-Epidemiological Stations (SES) and Border SES in co-operation with physicians and hospitals. May be dedicated service for TB and STIs.
Regional responsibility for action	Regional SES for selected diseases and larger health threats. May be dedicated service for TB and STIs.
National surveillance	Chief Sanitary Inspectorate in co-operation with consulting bodies that have responsibility for public health at the national level (National Institutes of Hygiene, Pulmonary Diseases Dermatology and Venerology).

Table 5.21.1 *Continued*

Notifiable diseases	78 diseases and syndromes reportable. For some specific case based epidemiological information is collected. Flu-like illness cases are reported in aggregate form. No financial incentives are given for notifying physicians.
Case definitions	Case definitions available for all reportable diseases, based where appropriate on the EU definitions.
Levels of reporting	The country comprises 16 provinces (population range 1–5 million, average 2.4 million) each with a public health department – Voivodeship Sanitary-Epidemiological Stations (WSSE). Provinces are divided into districts, where Poviat (PSSE) and Border (GSSE) Sanitary-Epidemiological Stations are located. There are 373 districts (population 22,000–1.7 million, average 104,000) served by 318 PSSE and 15 GSSE.
Estimated time to inform national level	Up to 14 days.
Public health action	The notifier has the responsibility for case management. Control measures including contact tracing and outbreak investigation are generally the responsibility of the district level Public Health Service, with support from provincial and national level.
Data dissemination	An epidemiological bulletin is published by the National Institute of Hygiene at national level every other week. It includes tables of notified diseases and can be accessed via Internet (http://www.pzh.gov.pl/epimeld/index_a.html). Annual reports are also published by the National Institute of Hygiene and the Institute of Pulmonary Diseases (TB).

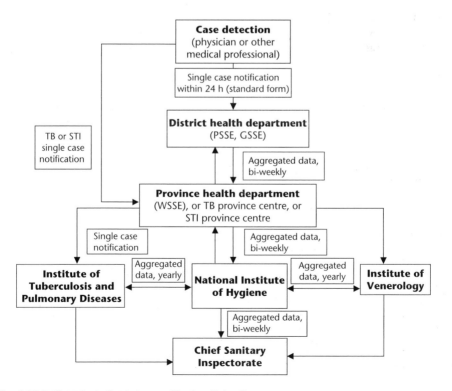

Fig. 5.21.1 Flow chart of statutory notification (Poland).

outbreak detection and management at the regional level. The WSSE reports to the National Institute of Hygiene and Chief Sanitary Inspectorate, which has the national responsibility for outbreak control.

Prevention/prophylaxis

• Vaccine programme: mandatory – hepatitis B, DTP, DTPa, Td, TB, IPV/OPV, MMR; recommended in special cases, financed by the government – Hib (for children in orphanages), additional TB, HBV (for special populations), diphtheria, typhoid fever, rabies, tetanus (in selected situations).
• Vaccination coverage: >95% for MMR.

5.22 Portugal

Contacts

• Direccao General de Saùde (Directorate General for Health – Ministry of Health), http://www.dgsaude.pt.
• Instituto Nacional de Saúde Dr Ricardo Jorge (National Institute of Health), http://www.insarj.pt.

Statutory notification systems

The details regarding statutory notification systems are given in Table 5.22.1.

Table 5.22.1 Statutory notification systems (Portugal)

Legal framework	Ministry of Health is responsible for introducing changes in the statutory notification system.
Levels of responsibility	
Local responsible for reporting	Every physician identifying a case (within 48 hours).
Local responsible for action	Treatment of individual cases by identifying physician; public health action and epidemiological control by local Public Health Department.
National surveillance	National Director of Health from the Directorate General of Health. The National Institute of Health is by law responsible for Communicable Disease surveillance although it is not directly involved in the management of notifications.
Notifiable diseases	46 diseases are notifiable. There are no financial incentives for notifying physicians.
Case definitions	Available for all notifiable diseases since 1999.
Levels of reporting	630 local health units with an average population size of 16,000 and 20 regions (18 districts and 2 autonomic regions) with an average population size of 500,000 (128,000–2,050,000).
Estimated time to inform national level	2 days for local level and national level.
Public health action	The responsibility for case management is held by the notifier. Control measures including contact tracing and outbreak investigation is generally the responsibility of the Public Health Service, primarily at local level with support from national level.
Data dissemination	The *Saúde em números* (Epidemiological Bulletin) is published by the Directorate General for Health at national level four times a year. Yearly statistics on mandatory notifiable diseases are published on the internet (http://www.dgsaude.pt). Special bulletins are released when needed.

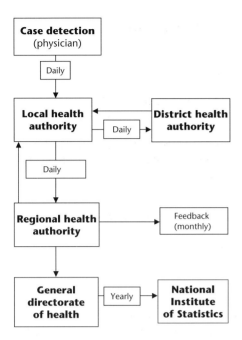

Fig. 5.22.1 Flow chart of statutory notification (Portugal).

Flow chart of statutory notification

See Figure 5.22.1.

Outbreak detection and investigation

Notifications are checked daily in the Division of Epidemiology of the Ministry of Health. If necessary, the information is checked through contact with the notifier or the respective local health department. An epidemiological investigation can be initiated through the decision of the Agency responsible for Communicable Disease surveillance. This should then be carried out by the local health department.

Prevention/prophylaxis

• Vaccine programme: BCG, HBV, OPV, Hib, DTP, Td, MMR .
• Vaccination coverage: near 95% for all vaccinations.
• Antibiotics and malaria prophylaxis are available only on prescription.

5.23 Slovakia

Contacts

• Ministry of Health of the Slovak Republic, http://www.health.gov.sk.
• The Public Health Authority of the Slovak Republic, http://www.uvzsr.sk/.
• Regional Public Health Authority in Banská Bystrica, http://www.szubb.sk/.

Statutory notification systems

The details regarding statutory notification systems are given in Table 5.23.1.

Table 5.23.1 Statutory notification systems (Slovakia)

Legal framework	MoH is the direct superior to the Public Health Authority of the Slovak Republic and is responsible for changes in the statutory notification system.
Levels of responsibility	
Local responsibility for reporting	Physicians, laboratories, regional public health authorities.
Local responsibility for action	Regional public health authorities.
National surveillance	The Public Health Authority of the Slovak Republic. Central Register of communicable diseases is at the Regional Public Health Authority in Banská Bystrica.

Continued on p. 368

Table 5.23.1 *Continued*

Notifiable diseases	44 diseases are mandatory reporting (according to the Decision 2002/253/EC and 2003/534/EC).
Case definitions	In use for all 44 mandatory reporting diseases.
Levels of reporting	5,423,567 (2004) inhabitants.
Estimated time to inform national level	In general less than a week.
Public health action	The responsibility for case management is held by the notifier. Control measures including contact tracing and outbreak investigation is generally the responsibility of the Regional Public Health Authorities with support from Public Health Authority of the Slovak Republic.
Data dissemination	Numbers of infectious diseases in the Slovak Republic are published monthly via Internet (www.health.gov.sk). An epidemiological bulletin is published at national level annually.

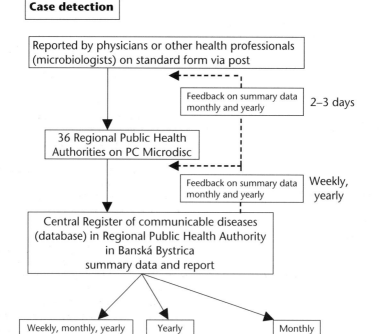

Fig. 5.23.1 Flow chart of statutory notification (Slovakia).

Flow chart of statutory notification

See Figure 5.23.1.

Prevention/prophylaxis

• Vaccine programme: Compulsory vaccination for DTPa-IPV, HiB, HBV, TB and MMR.
• Recommended vaccination for risk group: Tick-borne encephalitis, influenza, pneumococcal infection, meningococcal infection and HAV.
• Vaccination coverage: 98–99% for all compulsory vaccinations.
• Antibiotics and malaria prophylaxis available only on prescription.

5.24 Slovenia

Contacts

Centre for Communicable Diseases of the Institute of Public Health of the Republic of Slovenia, http://www.sigov.si/ivz/.

Statutory notification systems

The details regarding statutory notification systems are given in Table 5.24.1.

Table 5.24.1 Statutory notification systems (Slovenia)

Legal framework	Ministry of Health is responsible for changes in statutory notification; last legislation implemented 1995, draft of new legislation 2004.
Levels of responsibility	
Local responsibility for reporting	Physicians and laboratories.
Responsibility for control	Regional Institutes for Public Health (nine RIPH).
Responsibility for national surveillance	National Institute for Public Health (NIPH).
Notifiable diseases	75 notifiable diseases (1995). Diseases are grouped according to urgency of public health action. Group 1 disease must be reported by physicians within 6 hours of diagnosis to the RIPH and NIPH. Reconciliation of notifications and laboratory reports is undertaken at regional level.
Case definitions	In use for some notifiable diseases (EU case definitions).
Levels of reporting	Local level for reporting – RIPH, with an average population size of 221,746 (73,994–603,374). National population: 1,995,718 inhabitants.
Estimated time to inform national level	In general within 1 week. Group 1 disease and outbreaks within 6–24 hours.
Public health action	The responsibility for case management is held by the notifier. Control measures such as contact tracing, clusters and outbreak investigation is under the responsibility of the RIPH with support from NIPH.
Data dissemination	Most of the results on national surveillance are published in an annual communicable disease surveillance report. *CDC NEWS* issued monthly; http://www.sigov.si/ivz/.

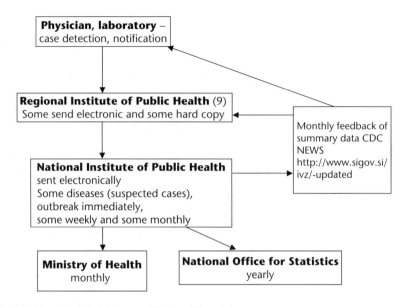

Fig. 5.24.1 Flow chart of statutory notification (Slovenia).

Surveillance

Whilst most reporting is passive, active surveillance is established for vaccine-preventable diseases, sexually transmitted infections, HIV/AIDS, invasive bacterial infections (meningococcal, *Haemophilus*, pneumococcal disease) and tick-borne meningoencephalitis.

Flow chart of statutory notification

See Figure 5.24.1.

Outbreak detection and investigation

Outbreaks are detected at the regional level, either through (direct) notification by physicians and institutions like schools, telephone calls from the public or media, by analysing the lab reports (microbiological laboratories are integrated in the regional public health institutes) or by analysing the notifications. Reporting on outbreaks is obligatory and must be immediate and on suspicion using the quickest way possible (telephone, fax). Outbreaks are reported to the RIPH, which directly informs the NIPH, which then informs MoH. Outside office hours, outbreaks are reported to the 112 emergency services or directly by phone to the epidemiologist on duty. Both at regional and national level, a formal system of contacting the relevant persons outside office hours is in place. A national protocol is presently prepared for responding to outbreaks. When necessary, Centre for Communicable Diseases, NIPH, is asked for consultation and assistance. The outbreak management team recommends the most appropriate interventions.

Prevention/prophylaxis

• Vaccination (DTPa-IPV, Hib, HBV, MMR, BCG, Td) is obligatory and provided free of charge by public and private nominated doctors.
• Vaccination coverage: 90–95% for all vaccinations.

5.25 Spain

Contacts

• Ministerio de Sanidad y Consumo Dirección General de Salud Publica (Ministry of Health and Consumers Affairs), http://www.msc.es.
• Instituto de Salud "Carlos III" (National Institute of Health), http://www.isciii.es.

Statutory notification systems

The details regarding statutory notification systems are given in Table 5.25.1.

Flow chart of statutory notification

The primary notifications are forwarded using a variety of systems: mail, fax, telephone, e-mail, etc. (Figure 5.25.1). Presently all the regions transmit data via e-mail. A network is being developed for the National Epidemiological Surveillance Network, which will permit the flow of data from the local level.

Non-statutory surveillance systems

The laboratory reporting system (SIM), based on the notification of microbiological identifications at the laboratories of hospitals.

Outbreak detection and investigation

The notification of outbreaks is mandatory and standardised. All the outbreaks must be reported immediately at regional level. At national level it is obligatory to report immediately only those outbreaks that, by law, are

Table 5.25.1 Statutory notification systems (Spain)

Legal framework	Ministry of Health is responsible for introducing changes in the statutory notification system. The autonomous regions are influential; national decisions are usually taken by consensus.
Levels of responsibility	All physicians are obliged by law to notify cases that fulfil the criteria for notifiable diseases.
Local responsibility for reporting and action	The regional health departments in each autonomous region are responsible for public health reporting and action.
National surveillance	Ministry of Health is responsible for introducing modifications in the notification system. The Centro Nacional de Epidemiología is involved in managing surveillance at national level.
Notifiable diseases	33 diseases are notifiable. There are no financial incentives for notifying physicians.
Case definitions	In use for all notifiable diseases.
Levels of reporting	52 Provincial Health Units with an average population size of 756,000 and 19 regions with an average population size of 2,100,000.
Estimated time to inform national level	Maximum: 21 days for national level. It depends on the protocol for each disease.
Public health action	The responsibility for case management is held by the notifier. Control measures including contact tracing and outbreak investigation are generally the responsability of the Public Health Service, primarily at local level with support from national level.
Data dissemination	An epidemiological bulletin, the *Boletín Epidemiológico Semanal*, is published by the National Institute of Health at national level (http://www.isciii.es/cne). Other regional and local bulletins are also published.

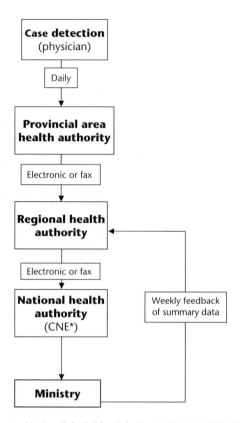

*CNE = Centro Nacional de Epidemiologia, Instituto de Salud "Carlos III"

Fig. 5.25.1 Flow chart of statutory notification (Spain).

defined as being 'supracomunitario' (considered to be of national interest), in order to facilitate their rapid control, whereas the rest of the outbreaks are reported quarterly. Outbreak investigations as well as necessary control measures are carried out by the health authorities of the autonomous regions.

Prevention/prophylaxis

• Vaccine programme: DTPa-IPV, MMR, Hib, HBV.
• Vaccination coverage: >95% for DTP, polio, MMR.

5.26 Sweden

Contacts

• Swedish Institute for Infectious Disease Control (SMI),
http://www.smittskyddsinstitutet.se.
• National Board of Health and Welfare, http://www.sos.se.

Statutory notification systems

The details regarding statutory notification systems are given in Table 5.26.1.

Table 5.26.1 Statutory notification systems (Sweden)

Legal framework	Ministry of Health is responsible for introducing changes in the Communicable Disease Act.
Levels of responsibility	
Local responsibility for reporting	All physicians and laboratories are obliged by law to notify all cases that fulfil the criteria for notifiable diseases.
Local responsibility for action	The County Medical Officers for Communicable Disease Control are responsible for public health action.
National surveillance	The National Board of Health and Welfare is responsible for introducing modifications in the notification system. The SMI is responsible for managing surveillance at national level.
Notifiable diseases	54 diseases and 55 pathogens are notifiable. There are no financial incentives for notifying physicians. Physicians notify individual cases with a unique identification number. A code is used for STDs. Notification is done in parallel to the County Medical Officer and to the SMI. A computerised notification system (SmiNet), both on county and national level, is in use since 1997.
Case definitions	In use for all notifiable diseases.
Levels of reporting	21 counties with an average population size of 422,000 (median 274,000; 57,000–1,803,000). National population 8,900,000.
Estimated time to inform national level	Notification should in general be done within 24 hours.
Public health action	The notifier holds the responsibility for case management. Control measures including contact tracing and outbreak investigation are generally the responsibility of the County Medical Officer, with support from the national level.
Data dissemination	Information is feed back via the SMI homepage, the Yearly Report of Department of Epidemiology and the weekly bulletin *EPI-aktuellt* (in Swedish). Longer reports are published in the bimonthly periodical *Smittskydd* (also in Swedish). Local data and compiled national data are accessible to the County Medical Officer through the *SmiNet*. Compiled national statistics are published in the yearly report of the SMI. Monthly and yearly national data are accessible to the public on http://gis.smittskyddsinstitutet.se/mapapp/build/intro_eng.html.

Flow chart of statutory notification

See Figure 5.26.1.

Non-statutory surveillance systems

STDs are notified numerically by all regional labs on voluntary basis.

Outbreak detection and investigation

Physicians' notifications, laboratory reporting and telephone calls from the public are used for outbreak detection at local and national level. The County Medical Officer is responsible for investigation and control, and can ask the help of regional epidemiological units or the national level (SMI). Depending on the kind of the outbreak the National Veterinary Institute (http://www.sva.se), Swedish Board of Agriculture (http://www.sjv.se) and the National Food Administration (http://www.slv.se) are involved as well.

Prevention/prophylaxis

• Vaccine programme: See http://www. smittskyddsinstitutet.se/SMItemplates/ Article_3699.aspx.

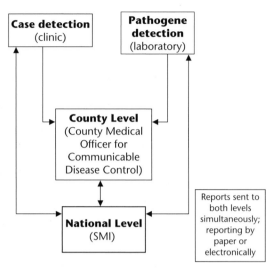

SMI = Smittskyddsinstitutet = Swedish Institute for Infectious Disease Control

Fig. 5.26.1 Flow chart of statutory notification (Sweden).

• Vaccination coverage: >95% for MMR vaccinations.
• Antibiotics and malaria prophylaxis available only on prescription.

5.27 Switzerland

Contacts

Bundesamt für Gesundheit (BAG) – Swiss Federal Office of Public Health – http://www.bag.admin.ch.

Statutory notification systems

The details regarding statutory notification systems are given in Table 5.27.1.

Flow chart of statutory notification

See Figure 5.27.1.

Outbreak detection and investigation

There is no national system for outbreak control in Switzerland. Outbreak management is the responsibility of the 26 cantons. The role of the Swiss Federal Office of Public Health is mainly a co-ordinating one. Action can only be taken by the Federal Office in exceptional situations. Physicians and laboratories are required by law to report unusual high frequencies of infectious diseases to the cantonal physician, who then have to inform the Federal Office, which issues guidelines for outbreak investigations and supports local actions on demand.

Prevention/prophylaxis

• Vaccine programme: DTPa-IPV, MMR, Hib.
• Vaccination coverage: 50–99% varying for vaccination and cantons.
• Antibiotics and malaria prophylaxis available only on prescription.

Table 5.27.1 Statutory notification systems (Switzerland)

Legal framework	Ministry of Health is responsible for introducing changes in the statutory notification system.
Levels of responsibility	
Local responsibility for reporting	The majority of diseases are to be reported primarily by the laboratories to both the cantonal physician and the BAG. Statutory notification by physicians is restricted to diseases that may require prompt public health action in case of suspicion (e.g. meningococcal disease) or for those where the diagnosis is on clinical rather than laboratory grounds (e.g. AIDS).
Local responsibility for action	Physician treating the patient and cantonal physician.
National surveillance	The responsibility for the control of infectious diseases lies with the 26 cantons. The Federal Office of Public Health has a co-ordinating and supervisory function and issues national recommendations for surveillance and control.
Notifiable diseases	35 diseases are notifiable. There are no financial incentives for notifying physicians.
Case definitions	Not in use.
Levels of reporting	26 cantons with a population size varying from 15,000–1,250,000.
Estimated time to inform national level	24 hours to 7 days (depending on the disease).
Public health action	Control measures including contact tracing and outbreak investigation is the responsibility of the Public Health Service, primarily on local level with support from national level.
Data dissemination	An epidemiological bulletin, the *Bulletin de l'Office fédéral de la santé publique / Bulletin des Bundesamtes für Gesundheit,* is published by the Federal Office at national level every week (http://www.bag.admin.ch/ dienste/publika/bulletin/d/index.htm) and infectious disease statutory notification data are published on the Internet (http://www.bag.admin.ch/infreporting).

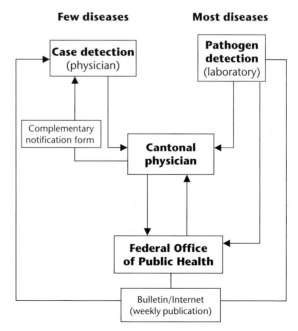

Fig. 5.27.1 Flow chart of statutory notification (Switzerland).

5.28 United Kingdom

Contacts

• Department of Health, England, http://www.dh.gov.uk/Home/fs/en.
• Health Department, Scottish Executive, http://www.show.scot.nhs.uk/sehd.
• Health and Social Care Department, Welsh Assembly Government, http://www.wales.gov.uk/subihealth/index.htm.
• Department of Health, Social Services and Public Safety, Northern Ireland Executive, http://www.dhsspsni.gov.uk/.

Statutory notification systems

The details regarding statutory notification systems are given in Table 5.28.1.

Flow chart of statutory notification

See Figure 5.28.1.

Prevention/prophylaxis

• Vaccine programme: See Box 4.7.1.
• Vaccination coverage: For MMR at 24 months of age approximately 80% in England and Wales and 88% in Northern Ireland and

Table 5.28.1 Statutory notification systems (United Kingdom)

Legal framework	The relevant department of health is responsible for introducing changes in the statutory notification system.
Levels of responsibility	
Local responsibility for reporting	General practitioners and hospital physicians report to proper officer (statutory).
	Laboratory reporting (non-statutory but encouraged) is to the local health protection units and the HPA regional surveillance units (RSU) via an electronic reporting system (CoSurv), which then reports to the national centre.
Local responsibility for action	*England*
	• 302 Primary Care Trusts
	• 600+ acute trusts, ambulance trusts, mental health trusts, care trusts and foundation trusts
	• 388 District and unitary local government authorities
	• Local Units of Health Protection Agency (CCDC)
	Northern Ireland
	• 4 local Health and Social Services Boards
	• 18 hospital trusts
	• 26 local government authorities
	Scotland
	• 15 area health boards
	• 28 hospital trusts
	• 32 local government authorities
	Wales
	• 22 local health boards
	• 22 local authorities
Regional responsibility for action	*England*
	• 28 Strategic health authorities
	• Government offices (9) and regional assemblies
	Wales
	• 3 regional offices

Table 5.28.1 *Continued*

National surveillance	*England:* Health Protection Agency Centre for Infections, http://www.hpa.org.uk/infections/about/about.htm.
	Northern Ireland: Communicable Disease Surveillance Centre, Northern Ireland, http://www.cdscni.org.uk/.
	Wales: The Infection and Communicable Disease Service (ICDS), which includes the Communicable Disease Surveillance Centre and a network of eight microbiology laboratories, is part of the National Public Health Service of Wales. Six CCDCs (http://www2.nphs.wales.nhs.uk/icds/).
	Scotland: The Scottish Centre for Infection and Environmental Health (SCIEH), http://www.show.scot.nhs.uk/scieh/about.html. From November 2004 SCIEH became part of Health Protection Scotland.
Notifiable diseases	In England and Wales 30 diseases are notifiable (see Table 4.2.1). The lists of notifiable diseases are slightly different for Scotland and Northern Ireland; *ca.* 4 Euro is given to physicians as financial incentive to notify.
Case definitions	For statutory notifications, case definitions are in use only for food poisoning. Increasingly case definitions are available for enhanced surveillance schemes and specialist systems such as the Wales GP scheme.
Levels of reporting	Data is reported at a variety of levels including national, regional, local authority, PCT.
Estimated time to inform national level	Variable: Statutory notifications reach national level within 7 days, laboratory reports reach local level within 1–2 days and regional level within 7 days.
Public health action	The notifier has the responsibility for case management. Control measures, including contact tracing and outbreak investigation, are generally the responsibility of the CCDC of the local HPA unit.
	Regional and national support is available from the HPA in England, ICDS in Wales, SCIEH in Scotland and CDSCNI in Northern Ireland.
Data dissemination	*England and Wales:* An epidemiological bulletin, *the CDR Weekly*, is published by the HPA every week. It is available on-line at the HPA website at http://www.hpa.org.uk/cdr/index.html. Summary epidemiological data is also available at the HPA website.
	Northern Ireland: Monthly and annual reports are available via the CDSC Northern Ireland website, http://www.cdscni.org.uk/.
	Scotland: SCIEH produces a weekly report available on-line, http://www.show.scot.nhs.uk/scieh/wrhome.html.
	Wales: CDSC surveillance reports can be accessed via the National Public Health Service of Wales website, http://www2.nphs.wales.nhs.uk/icds/page.cfm?pid=193.

Scotland. For infant schedule at 12 months of age 90% in England and Wales and 95% in Northern Ireland and Scotland.

• Antibiotics available only on prescription. Chloroquine and proguanil can be purchased without a prescription.

Scotland

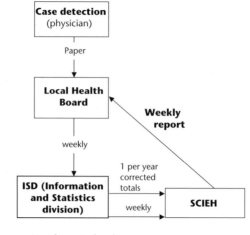

Northern Ireland

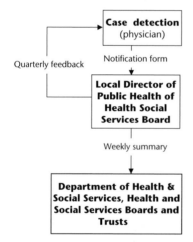

England and Wales

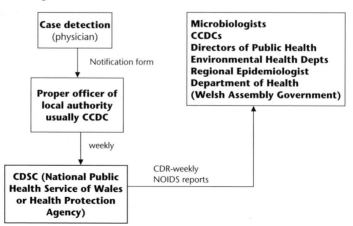

Fig. 5.28.1 Flow chart of statutory notification (United Kingdom).

Appendices

Appendix 1: Useful addresses and telephone numbers

World Health Organization
Headquarters
Avenue Appia 20, 1211 Geneva 27, Switzerland
Tel: 0041 22791 2111

Regional Office for Europe (EURO)
8, Scherfigsvej, DK-2100 Copenhagen 0,
Denmark
Tel: 0045 3917 1717

European Union
European Commission Directorate-General
Health and Consumer Protection
Rue de la Loi 200 / Wetstraat 200, B-1049
Bruxelles/Brussel, Belgium
Tel: 0035 243011

European Centre for Disease Prevention and Control
Solna Stadhus,
SE-171 86 Solna,
Sweden
Tel: (+46-8) 7342050

Health Protection Agency
HPA Central Office,
7th Floor, Holborn Gate,
330 High Holborn,
London,
WC1V 7BA
Tel: 0207 061 3270

• Centre for Infection
61 Colindale Avenue, London, NW9 5EQ
Communicable Disease Surveillance Centre
(CDSC)
Tel: 0208 200 6868
Specialist and Reference Microbiology
Tel: 0208 200 4400

• Centre for Radiation, Chemical and
Environmental Hazards
Chilton, Didcot, Oxon OX11 0RQ
Chemical Hazards and Poisons:

Tel: 01235 822895
Radiological Protection:
Tel: 01235 831600

• Centre for Emergency Preparedness and
Response
HPA Porton Down, Salisbury, Wiltshire SP4
0JG
Tel: 01980 612100

• Local and Regional Services Division
6th Floor, New Court, 48 Carey Street, London,
WC2A 2JE
Divisional Office
Tel: 0207 492 0400
East of England
Tel: 01223 372 824
East Midlands
Tel: 0115 962 7948
London
Tel: 020 7492 0470
North East
Tel: 0191 261 2577
North West
Tel: 0151 482 5688
South East
Tel: 020 7492 0555
South West
Tel: 01453 829740
West Midlands
Tel: 0121 634 8700
Yorkshire and Humber
Tel: 0113 284 0600

Health Protection Scotland (includes SCIEH)
Clifton House, Clifton Place, Glasgow,
G3 7LN
Tel: 0141 300 1100

CDSC Wales
Abton House, Wedal Road, Roath, Cardiff,
CF14 3QX
Tel: 029 20521997

Communicable Disease Surveillance Centre (Northern Ireland)
McBrien Building, Belfast City Hospital,
Lisburn Rd, Belfast BT9 7AB
Tel: 02890 263765

Departments of Health
1 England
• Richmond House, 79 Whitehall, London SW1A 2NL
Switchboard: 0207 210 4850
Duty medical officer (out of hours): 0207 210 5025
Press Office: 0207 210 5221

• Skipton House, 80 London Road, London SE1 6LH
Communicable Disease, Emergency Planning
Tel: 0207 972 3000

2 Scotland: Scottish Executive Health Department
St Andrew's House, Regent Road, Edinburgh EH1 3DG
Tel: 0131 556 8400

3 Wales: National Assembly for Wales
Cathays Park, Cardiff CF10 3NQ
Tel: 02920 825111

4 Northern Ireland: Department of Health, Social Services and Public Safety
Castle Buildings, Stormont, Belfast, BT 4 3SJ
Tel: 028 90520500

Food Standards Agency
1 UK Headquarters: Aviation House, 125 Kingsway, London, WC2B 6NH
Switchboard: 0207 276 8000
Emergencies only: 0207 270 8960

2 Scotland: St Magnus House, 6th Floor, 25 Guild Street, Aberdeen, AB11 6NJ
Switchboard: 01224 285100

3 Wales: 11th Floor, Southgate House, Wood Street, Cardiff, CF10 1EW
Switchboard: 02920 678999

4 Northern Ireland: 10c Clarendon Road, Belfast, BT1 3BG
Switchboard: 02890 417700

HPA Malaria Reference Laboratory
London School of Hygiene and Tropical Medicine, Keppel Street, London, WC1E 7HT

Advisory Service (Health professionals only): 0207 636 3924
Laboratory: 0207 927 2427

Clinical Infectious Disease Units
Hospital for Tropical Diseases, London
Tel: 0207 387 9300/4411
Heartlands Hospital, Birmingham
Tel: 0121 424 3359
Churchill Hospital, Oxford
Tel: 01865 741841
University Hospital (Fazakerley), Liverpool
Tel: 0151 525 5980
North Manchester General
Tel: 0161 795 4567
Southmead Hospital, Bristol
Tel: 0117 950 5050

Poisons Information Service
National Helpline: 0870 600 6266

National Travel Health Network and Centre (NaTHNaC)
Tel: 0207 380 9234

Advice Lines Available to General Public
National AIDS Helpline
Tel: 0800 567123
Hospital for Tropical Diseases Travel Clinic
Tel: 0906 133 7733*
Malaria Reference Laboratory Helpline
Tel: 0906 550 8908*
Medical Advisory Service for Travellers Abroad
Tel: 0113 238 7575
Liverpool School of Tropical Medicine Travel Advice Line
Tel: 0906 701 0095*
National Meningitis Trust
Tel: 0845 6000 800
Meningitis Research Foundation
Tel: 080 880 3344
*Subject to premium rate call charges

Appendix 2: Guidance documents and books

Links to many of these can be found on the UK National Electronic Library for Infection www.neli.org.uk

Blood-borne viruses

UK Health Departments. *AIDS/HIV Infected Health Care Workers: Guidance on the Management of Infected Health Care Workers and Patient Notification.* London: Department of Health, 1998. (Revised guidance out to consultation at time of writing, available at http://www.dh.gov.uk/assetRoot/04/01/85/96/04018596.pdf.)

Department of Health. *HIV Post-Exposure Prophylaxis: Guidance from the UK Chief Medical Officers' Expert Advisory Group on AIDS.* London: Department of Health, 2004. (Available at http://www.dh.gov.uk/assetRoot/04/08/36/40/04083640.pdf.)

European Commission. *Recommendations for Post-Exposure Prophylaxis Against HIV Infection in Health Care Workers in Europe.* Project number SI2.322294, March 2002.

European Commission. *Management of Non-Occupational Post-Exposure Prophylaxis to HIV: Sexual, Injecting Drug User or Other Exposures.* Project number 2000CVG4-022, April 2002.

Department of Health. *Protecting Health Care Workers and Patients from Hepatitis B: HSG (93) 40.* London: Department of Health, 1993. (Addendum issued under cover of EL(96)77.)

NHS Executive (England). *Hepatitis B Infected Health Care Workers. Guidance on Implementation of Health Service Circular 2000/020.* Leeds: NHS Executive, 2000. (Available at http://www.dh.gov.uk/assetRoot/04/05/75/38/04057538.pdf.)

Department of Health. *Hepatitis C Infected Health Care Workers.* London: Department of Health Publications, 2002. (Available at http://www.dh.gov.uk/assetRoot/04/05/95/44/04059544.pdf.)

UK Health Departments. *Guidance for Clinical Health Care Workers: Protection Against Infection with Blood-Borne Viruses. Recommendations of the Expert Advisory Group on AIDS and the Advisory Group on Hepatitis.* London: UK Health Departments, 1998.

Department of Health. *Hepatitis C Strategy for England.* London: DH, 2003. (Available at: http://www.publications.doh.gov.uk/cmo/hcvstrategy/77097dhhepcstrat.pdf.)

Gastrointestinal disease

PHLS Salmonella Subcommittee. The prevention of human transmission of gastrointestinal infections, infestations and bacterial infections. *Commun Dis Rep CDR Rev* 1995, **5**: R158–172. (Revised guidelines should become available on HPA website in 2005).

Department of Health. *Management of Outbreaks of Food-borne Illness.* London: Department of Health, 1994.

Subcommittee of the PHLS Advisory Committee on Gastrointestinal Infections. Guidelines for the control of infections with Verocytotoxin producing *Escherichia coli* (VTEC). *Commun Dis Public Health* 2000, **3**: 14–23.

PHLS Viral Gastroenteritis Working Group. Managements of hospital outbreaks of gastroenteritis due to small round structured viruses. *J Hosp Inf* 2000, **45**: 1–10.

Bouchier IT (Chairman). *Cryptosporidium in water supplies.* Third report of the group of experts to Department of Environment, Transport, and the Region and the Department of Health. London: DETR, 1998.

Hunter PR. Advice on the response from public and environmental health to the detection of cryptosporidial oocysts in treated drinking water. *Commun Dis Public Health* 2000, **3**: 24–27.

Crowcroft NS, Walsh B, Davison KL, Gungabissoon, U. Guidelines for the control of hepatitis A infection. *Commun Dis Public Health* 2001, **4**: 213–227.

Department of Health Expert Working Party. *Food Handlers, Fitness to Work, Guidance for*

Food Businesses, Enforcement Officers and Health Professionals. London: Department of Health, 1995.

Immunisation

Department of Health. *Immunisation Against Infectious Diseases*. London: HMSO, 1996. ISBN 0-11-321-815-X. (Available at www.immunisation . nhs.uk.)

Department of Health. *Immunisation Against Infectious Disease. The 'Green book' chapters on Hib, Pertussis, Polio and Tetanus*. London: DH Publications, 2004. (Available at http://80.168.38.66/files/greenbook.pdf.)

Royal College of Paediatrics and Child Health. *Immunisation of the Immunocompromised Child: Best Practice Statement*. February 2002. (Available at http://www.rcpch.ac.uk/publications/recent_publications/Immunocomp.pdf.)

Imported infection and travel advice

World Health Organization. *International Travel and Health*. Geneva: WHO, 2004. (Available at http://www.who.int/ith/.)

Department of Health. *Health Information for Overseas Travel*. London: The Stationary Office, 2001. ISBN 0-11-322329-3. (Available at https://www.the-stationery-office.co.uk/doh/hinfo/index.htm.)

Bradley DJ, Bannister B. Guidelines for malaria prevention in travellers from the United Kingdom for 2003. *Commun Dis Public Health* 2003, **6**: 180–199.

Advisory Committee on Dangerous Pathogens. *Management and Control of Viral Haemorrhagic Fevers*. London: The Stationary Office, 1996. ISBN: 0-11-321860-5. (Available at http://www.hpa.org.uk/infections/topics_az/VHF/ACDP_VHF_guidance.pdf.)

Bonnet JM, Begg NT. Control of diphtheria: guidance for consultants in communicable disease control. *Commun Dis Public Health* 1999, **2**: 242–249.

Department of Health. *Memorandum on Rabies. Prevention and Control*. London: Department of Health, 2000. (Available at http://www.dh.gov.uk/assetRoot/04/08/06/57/04080657.pdf.)

Health Protection Agency. *SARS and Avian Influenza (H5N1) Algorithm: Recognition, Investigation and Initial Management of Potential Cases*. December 2004. (Available at http://www.hpa.org.uk/infections/topics_az/avianinfluenza/pdfs/Algorithm.pdf.)

Infection control and healthcare-acquired infection

Public Health Medicine Environmental Group. *Guidelines for the Control of Infection in Residential Homes and Nursing Homes*. London: Department of Health, 1996.

National Institute for Clinical Excellence. *Prevention of Healthcare-Associated Infection in Primary and Community Care*. London: NICE, 2003. (Available at http://www.nice.org.uk/page.aspx?o=71774.)

Ward V, Wilson J, Taylor L, Cookson B, Glynn A. *Preventing Hospital-Acquired Infection: Clinical Guidelines*. A supplement to Hospital-Acquired Infection: Surveillance, Policies, and Practice. London: HPA, 1997. ISBN 0 901144 41 X.

Healing TD, Hoffman PN, Young SEJ. The infection hazards of human cadavers. *Commun Dis Rep CDR Rev* 1995, **5**: R61–R68.

Combined working party of the British Society of Antimicrobial Chemotherapy, the Hospital Infection Society and the Infection Control Nurses Association. Revised guidelines for the control of methicillin-resistant Staphylococcus aureus in hospital. *J Hosp Inf* 1998, **39**: 253–290.

Chief Medical Officer for England. *Winning Ways: Working Together to Reduce Healthcare*

Associated Infection in England. London: Department of Health, 2004. (Available at: http://www.dh.gov.uk/assetRoot/04/06/46/89/04064689.pdf.)

Meningitis and meningococcal infection

PHLS Meningococcus Forum. Guidelines for the public health management of meningococcal disease in the UK. *Commun Dis Public Health* 2002, **5**: 187–204.

Cartwright KAV, Begg NT, Rudd P. Use of vaccines and antibiotic prophylaxis in contacts and cases of *Haemophilus influenzae* type b (Hib) disease. *Commun Dis Rep CDR Rev* 1994, **4**: R16–R17.

Tuberculosis

Joint Tuberculosis Committee of the British Thoracic Society. Control and prevention of tuberculosis in the United Kingdom: Code of Practice 2000. *Thorax* 2001, **55**: 887–901.

Interdepartmental Working Group on Tuberculosis. *Recommendations for the Prevention and Control of Tuberculosis at Local Level.* London: Department of Health and Welsh Office, 1996.

Interdepartmental Working Group on Tuberculosis. *The Prevention and Control of Tuberculosis in the United Kingdom. UK Guidance on the Prevention and Control of Transmission of: 1. HIV related Tuberculosis, 2. Drug resistant, including multiple drug-resistant tuberculosis.* London: Department of Health and Welsh Office, 1998.

Joint Tuberculosis Committee of the British Thoracic Society. Chemotherapy and management of tuberculosis in the United Kingdom: recommendations 1998. *Thorax* 1998, **53**: 536–548.

Chief Medical Officer for England. *Stopping Tuberculosis in England: An Action Plan from the Chief Medical Officer.* London: Department of

Health, 2004. (Available at: http://www.dh.gov.uk/assetRoot/04/10/08/60/04100860.pdf.)

Other

Lee JV, Joseph C. Guidelines for investigating single cases of Legionnaires' disease. *Commun Dis Public Health* 2002, **5**: 157–161

Morgan-Capner P, Crowcroft NS. Guidelines on the management of and exposure to rash illness in pregnancy. *Commun Dis Public Health* 2002, **5**: 59–71

Dodhia H, Crowcroft N, Bramley JC, Miller E. UK guidelines for use of erythromycin chemoprophylaxis in persons exposed to pertussis. *J Public Health Med* 2002, **24**: 200–206.

Guidance for the control of parvovirus B19 infection in healthcare settings and the community. *J Public Health Med* 1999, **21**: 439–446.

CDSC. *Guidelines for Managing Outbreaks of Sexually Transmitted Infections at a Local, District or Regional Level. An Outbreak Plan.* July 2002. (Available at: http://www.hpa.org.uk/infections/topics_az/hiv_and_sti/guidelines/sti_outbreakplan.pdf.)

Department of Health. *Better Prevention, Better Services, Better Sexual Health – The National Strategy for Sexual Health and HIV.* London: Department of Health, 2001. (Available at: http://www.dh.gov.uk/assetRoot/04/05/89/45/04058945.pdf.)

Health Protection Agency. *Initial Investigation and Management of Outbreaks and Incidents of Unusual Illness.* (Available at www.hpa.org.uk/infections/topics_az/deliberate_release/unknown/unusual_illness.pdf.)

Murray V (Ed). *Major Chemical Disasters – Medical Aspects of Management.* Oxford: Royal Society of Medicine Services, 1990.

NHS Executive. *Planning for Major Incidents. The NHS Guidance.* London: Department of Health, 1998.

General

Guidance on Infection Control in Schools and Nurseries (poster). London: Department of Health, 1999. (Summary database of the evidence for the exclusion periods and comments on poster available via HPA Website).

Joint Formulary Committee. *British National Formulary*. London: British Medical Association, 2004.

Directory of CsCDC and MOsEH in England and Wales and Northern Ireland. PHLS Communi-cable Disease Surveillance Centre, 8th edition (*or* 'ComDisc' from CDSC).

Department of Health and Welsh Office Public Health Legal Information Unit. *Communicable Disease Control: A Practical Guide to the Law for Health and Local Authorities in England and Wales*. London: Department of Health, 1994.

Chief Medical Officer for England. *Getting Ahead of the Curve: A Strategy for Combating Infectious Diseases (Including Other Aspects of Health Protection)*. London: Department of Health, 2002.

Index

Note: Page numbers in *italics* refer to figures and boxes, those in **bold** refer to tables.